Dosage Calculations made Incredibly Easy!®

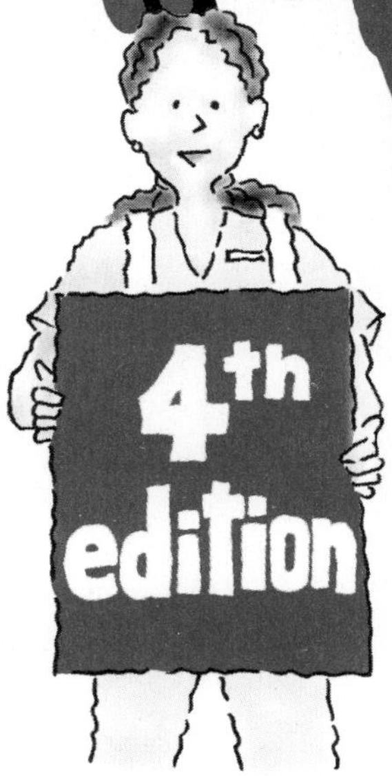

Wolters Kluwer Health | Lippincott Williams & Wilkins
Philadelphia • Baltimore • New York • London
Buenos Aires • Hong Kong • Sydney • Tokyo

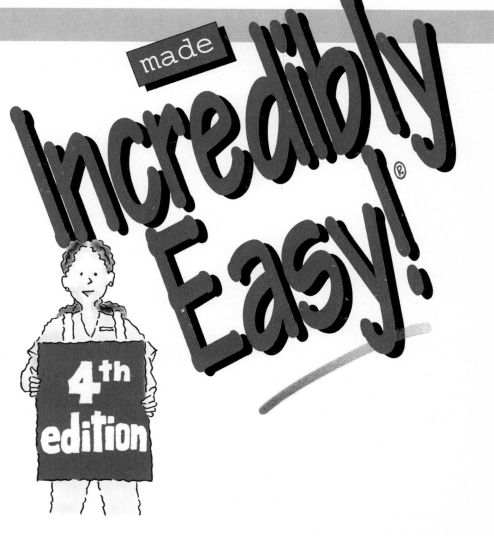

Staff

Executive Publisher
Judith A. Schilling McCann, RN, MSN

Clinical Director
Joan M. Robinson, RN, MSN

Art Director
Elaine Kasmer

Clinical Project Managers
Kathryn Henry, RN, BSN, CCRC;
Jennifer Meyering, RN, BSN, MS, CCRN

Editor
Diane Labus

Clinical Editor
Collette Bishop Hendler, RN, MS

Illustrator
Bot Roda

Design Assistant
Kate Zulak

Associate Manufacturing Manager
Beth J. Welsh

Editorial Assistants
Karen J. Kirk, Jeri O'Shea, Linda K. Ruhf

DCMIE4010109

We thank the following companies for permission to include photographs of their products in this book: Schering-Plough (Noxafil, p. 164), GlaxoSmithKline (Bactroban, p. 190), APP Pharmaceuticals (Diprivan, pp. 211, C5), Pfizer, Inc. (Solu-Medrol, p. 222).

Library of Congress Cataloging-in-Publication Data

CIP data available upon request

ISBN13 978-1-60547-197-6
ISBN10 1-60547-197-6

RRC1108

Contents

Contributors and consultants

Rita Bates, RN, BS, MSN
Assistant Professor
University of Arkansas
Fort Smith

Julie A. Calvery Carman, RN, MS
Instructor
University of Arkansas
Fort Smith

Kim Cooper, RN, MSN
Nursing Department Chair
Ivy Tech Community College
Terre Haute, Ind.

Cheryl DeGraw, RN, MSN, CRNP, CNE
Instructor
Florence-Darlington Technical College
Florence, S.C.

MaryAnn Edelman, RN, MS
Assistant Professor of Nursing
Kingsborough Community College
Brooklyn, N.Y.

Judith Faust, RN, MSN
Associate Professor
Ivy Tech Community College
Lafayette, Ind.

Virginia Lester, RN, MSN
Assistant Professor of Nursing
Angelo State University
San Angelo, Tex.

Dana Reeves, RN, MSN
Assistant Professor
University of Arkansas
Fort Smith

Peggy Thweatt, RN, MSN
Nursing Instructor
Medical Careers Institute School of Nursing
Newport News, Va.

Trinidad Villaruel, RN, MSN
Clinical Nurse Specialist
New York–Presbyterian Hospital
New York

Not another boring foreword

If you're like me, you're too busy caring for your patients to have the time to wade through a foreword that uses pretentious terms and umpteen dull paragraphs to get to the point. So let's cut right to the chase! Here's why this book is so terrific:

1. It will teach you all the important things you need to know about dosage calculations. (And it will leave out all the fluff that wastes your time.)
2. It will help you remember what you've learned.
3. It will make you smile as it enhances your knowledge and skills.

Don't believe me? Try these recurring logos on for size:

Before you give that drug!—Contains urgent advice on how to avoid dangerous drug errors

Advice from the experts—Provides pointers on how to maintain dosage accuracy

For math phobics only—Offers hints, tips, and illustrations to help you get over the "I hate math" hurdles

Dosage drill—Poses real-life practice problems to hone your skills

Memory jogger—Reinforces learning through easy-to-remember anecdotes and mnemonics

See? I told you! And that's not all. Look for me and my friends in the margins throughout this book. We'll be there to explain key concepts, provide important care reminders, and offer reassurance. Oh, and if you don't mind, we'll be spicing up the pages with a bit of humor along the way, to teach and entertain in a way that no other resource can.

I hope you find this book helpful. Best of luck throughout your career!

Joy

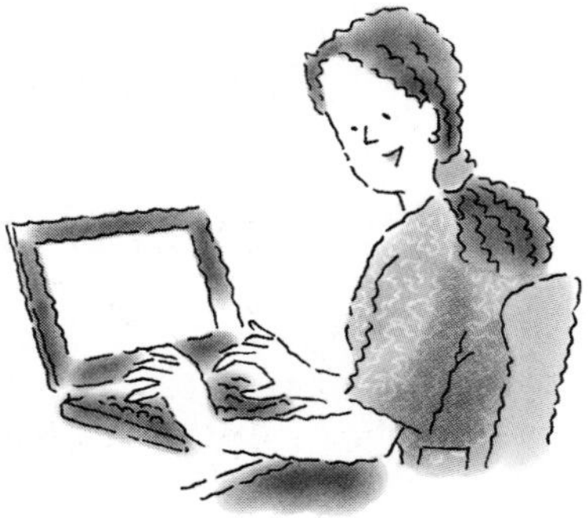

Part I Math basics

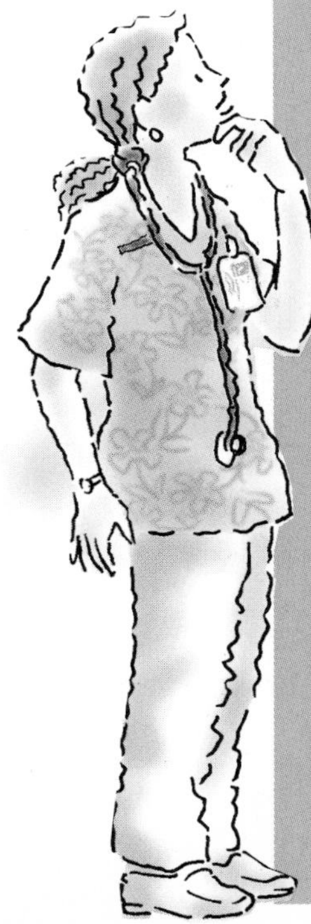

1

Fractions

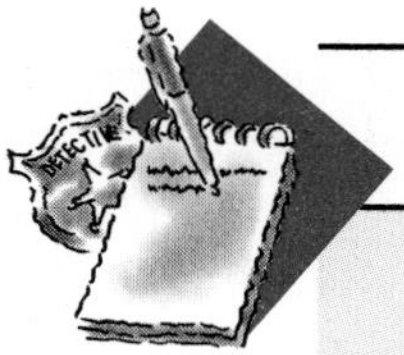

Just the facts

In this chapter, you'll learn:

- what a fraction is
- about different types of fractions you may use
- how to convert fractions, reduce them to their lowest terms, and find the lowest common denominator
- how to add, subtract, multiply, and divide fractions.

A look at fractions

A fraction represents the division of one number by another number. It's a mathematical expression for parts of a whole. (See *Parts of a whole.*)

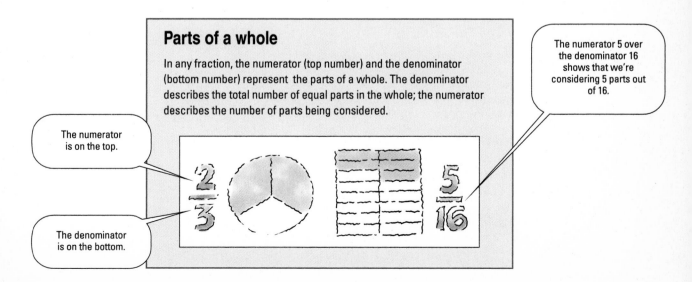

Parts of a whole

In any fraction, the numerator (top number) and the denominator (bottom number) represent the parts of a whole. The denominator describes the total number of equal parts in the whole; the numerator describes the number of parts being considered.

The numerator is on the top.

The denominator is on the bottom.

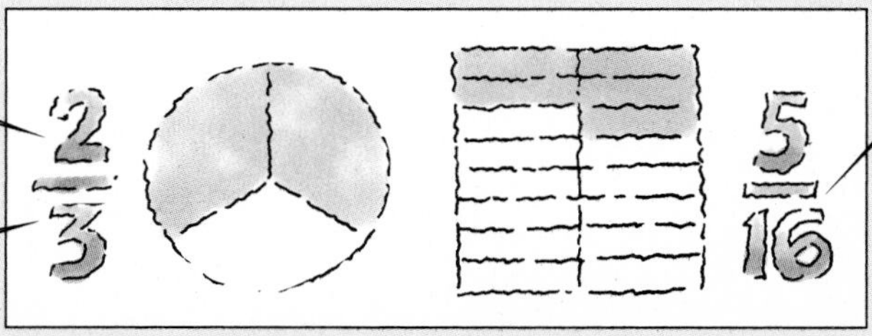

The numerator 5 over the denominator 16 shows that we're considering 5 parts out of 16.

Getting to the bottom of it

The bottom number, or *denominator*, represents the total number of equal parts in the whole. The larger the denominator, the greater the number of equal parts. For example, in the fraction $3/5$, the denominator 5 indicates that the whole has been divided into five equal parts. In the fraction $7/12$, the denominator 12 indicates that the whole has been divided into 12 equal parts. So, as the denominator becomes larger, the size of the parts becomes smaller.

Staying on top of it

The top number, or *numerator*, signifies the number of parts of the whole being considered. For example, in the fraction $3/5$, only 3 of the 5 equal parts are being considered. In the fraction $7/12$, only 7 of the 12 equal parts are being considered.

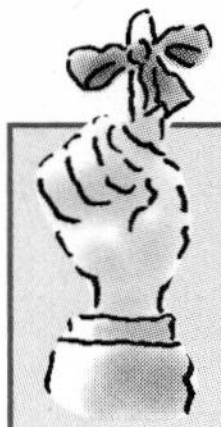

Memory jogger

To remember which number is the numerator and which is the denominator in a fraction, think of:

Nursing

Diagnosis

The **N**umerator is on the top; the **D**enominator, on the bottom.

Types of fractions

There are four types of fractions:

- common
- complex
- proper
- improper.

Common and complex

In a common fraction, such as $2/3$, both the numerator and denominator are whole numbers.

In a complex fraction, the numerator and denominator are fractions. For example:

$$\frac{2/7}{5/16}$$

Proper and improper

In a proper fraction, such as $1/4$, the numerator is smaller than the denominator.

In an improper fraction, such as $8/7$ or $11/4$, the numerator is larger than the denominator. In other words, it's top heavy. An improper fraction represents a number that's greater than 1.

An improper fraction can also be expressed as a mixed number — a whole number and a fraction. Therefore, $8/7$ can be rewritten as $1\,1/7$ and $11/4$ can be rewritten as $2\,3/4$.

Working with fractions

You can manipulate fractions in three ways, including:

- converting mixed numbers to improper fractions and vice versa
- reducing fractions to their lowest terms
- finding a common denominator.

Converting mixed numbers to improper fractions

To convert a mixed number to an improper fraction, follow these steps:

1. Multiply the denominator by the whole number to get the product (or resulting number).
2. Add the product from the first step to the numerator (this gives you a new numerator).
3. Leave the denominator as it is.

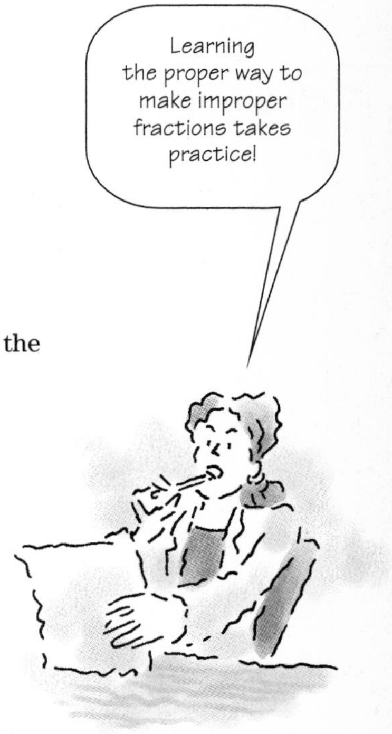

Learning the proper way to make improper fractions takes practice!

Three incredibly easy steps

For example, to convert the mixed number $5\frac{1}{3}$ to an improper fraction:

1. Multiply the denominator 3 by the whole number 5, to get the product of 15.
2. Add 15 to the numerator 1, for a new numerator of 16.
3. Leave the denominator as it is. The improper fraction is $\frac{16}{3}$.

$$5\frac{1}{3} \text{ is } \frac{16}{3}$$

Encore!

Here's another example! To convert the mixed number $8\frac{4}{5}$ to an improper fraction:

1. Multiply the denominator 5 by the whole number 8, to get the product, 40.
2. Add 40 to the numerator 4, for a new numerator of 44.

Memory jogger

Here's a way to remember how to convert mixed numbers to improper fractions. Think **MAST:** "**M**ultiply, **A**dd, and **S**tack on **T**op."

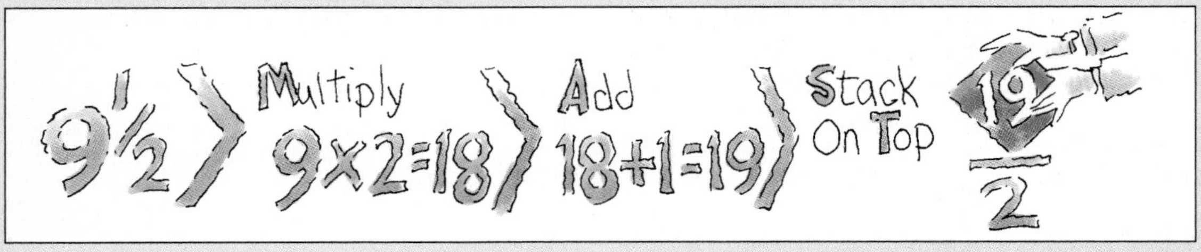

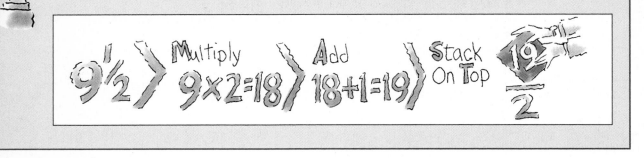

Leave the denominator as it is. The improper fraction is $\frac{44}{5}$.

$$8\tfrac{4}{5} \text{ is } \frac{44}{5}$$

Putting it in reverse

At times, you may want to convert improper fractions back to mixed numbers. To convert the improper fraction $\frac{16}{3}$ back to a mixed number:

Divide the numerator 16 by the denominator 3. When you do this, you get 5 with 1 left over.

The 1 becomes the new numerator, and the denominator stays the same.

The mixed number is $5\tfrac{1}{3}$:

$$\frac{16}{3} \text{ is } 5\tfrac{1}{3}$$

One more time

To convert the improper fraction $\frac{44}{5}$ back into a mixed number:

Divide the numerator 44 by the denominator 5. The answer is 8 with 4 left over.

Place the 4 over the 5.

The mixed number is $8\tfrac{4}{5}$.

$$\frac{44}{5} \text{ is } 8\tfrac{4}{5}$$

Reducing fractions to lowest terms

For simplicity's sake, a fraction should usually be reduced to its lowest terms — that is, to the smallest numbers possible in the numerator and denominator. To simplify a fraction, follow these steps:

1. Determine the largest common divisor of the numerator and the denominator — the largest number by which both can be divided equally.

2. Divide both the numerator and denominator by that number to reduce the fraction to its lowest terms.

Example numero uno

To reduce the fraction $8/10$ to its lowest terms:

1. Determine the largest common divisor of 8 and 10, which is 2.

2. Divide the numerator and denominator by 2 to reduce the fraction to its lowest terms, or $4/5$.

$$\frac{8}{10} \text{ is } \frac{8 \div 2}{10 \div 2} \text{ is } \frac{4}{5}$$

Missed it? Watch again!

To reduce the fraction $7/14$ to its lowest terms:

1. Determine that the number 7 is the largest divisor that 7 and 14 have in common.

2. Divide the numerator and the denominator by 7 to reduce the fraction to its lowest terms, or $1/2$. This fraction can't be reduced further.

$$\frac{7}{14} \text{ is } \frac{7 \div 7}{14 \div 7} \text{ is } \frac{1}{2}$$

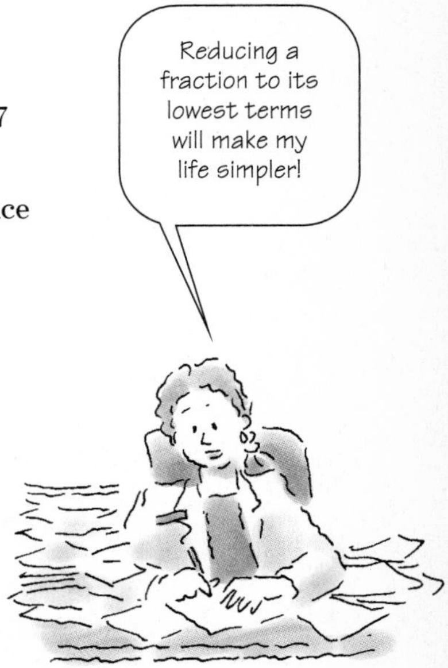
Reducing a fraction to its lowest terms will make my life simpler!

One more time

To reduce the fraction $2/10$ to its lowest terms:

1. Determine that the number 2 is the largest divisor that 2 and 10 have in common.

2. Divide the numerator and the denominator by 2 to reduce the fraction to its lowest terms, or $1/5$.

$$\frac{2}{10} \text{ is } \frac{2 \div 2}{10 \div 2} \text{ is } \frac{1}{5}$$

Finding a common denominator

One way to find a common denominator for a set of fractions is to multiply all the denominators. For example, to find a common denominator for the fractions $2/5$ and $7/10$, multiply the denominators 5 and 10 to get the multiplied common denominator 50:

Multiply the denominators...

$$\frac{2}{5} \quad \frac{7}{10}$$
$$\downarrow \quad \downarrow$$
$$5 \times 10 = 50$$

...to find the multiplied common denominator.

To find the multiplied common denominator of the set of fractions $1/8$, $1/4$, and $1/5$, simply multiply all the denominators together to find the common denominator 160:

$$8 \times 4 \times 5 = 160$$

Lowest common denominator

Unfortunately, multiplying all the denominators of a set of fractions won't always give you the lowest common denominator. The *lowest common denominator* or *least common multiple* — the smallest number that's a multiple of all the denominators in a set of fractions — is an important tool for working with fractions.

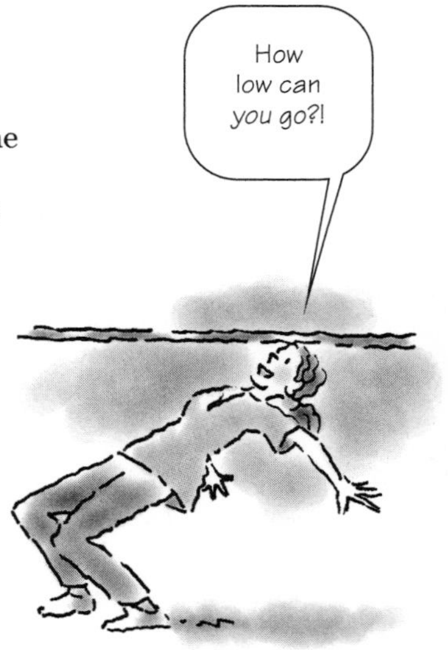

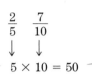

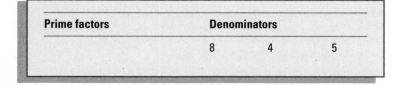

How low can you go?

One way to find the lowest common denominator of a set of fractions is to work with its prime factors. A *prime number* is a number that's evenly divisible only by 1 and itself. Some prime numbers are 2, 3, 5, and 7. *Prime factors* are prime numbers that can be divided into some part of a mathematical expression, in this case, the denominators in a set of fractions.

Prime factoring

Let's say you want to find the lowest common denominator for $1/8$, $1/4$, and $1/5$. Here's a useful technique, called *prime factoring:*

- Make a table with two headings: "Prime factors" and "Denominators."
- Write the denominators 8, 4, and 5 over the top right columns.

Prime factors	**Denominators**		
	8	4	5

• Divide the three denominators by the prime factors for each, starting with the smallest prime factor by which one of the denominators can be divided — in this case, 2. Write 2 in the left-hand column and divide the denominators by it. (Divide the denominator 8 by the prime factor 2 and write the answer, 4, in the column under the 8. Then divide the denominator 4 by the prime factor 2 and write the answer, 2, in the column under the denominator 4.)
• Bring down the numbers in the right-side columns that aren't evenly divisible by the prime factor in the left column. (In this case, the denominator 5 isn't divisible by the prime factor 2, so just bring the 5 down.)

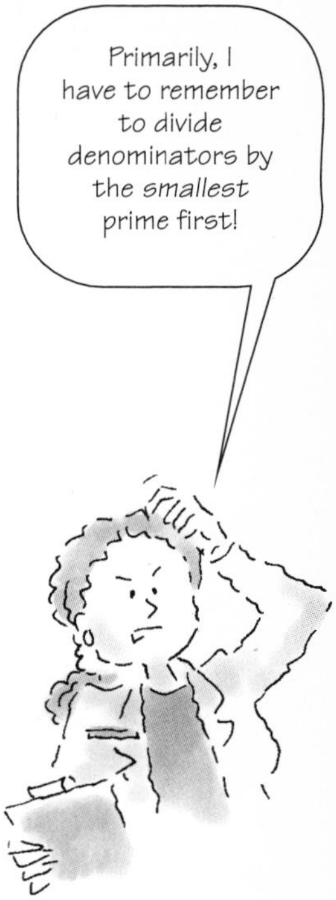
Primarily, I have to remember to divide denominators by the smallest prime first!

Prime factors	Denominators		
÷	8	4	5
2 =	4	2	5

• Repeat this process until the numbers in the bottom row can't be divided further.

Prime factors	Denominators		
	8	4	5
2	4	2	5
2	2	1	5
2	1	1	5

• Then multiply the prime factors in the left column by the numbers in the bottom row. To say it with numbers:

$$2 \times 2 \times 2 \times 1 \times 1 \times 5 = 40$$

• The lowest common denominator for this set of fractions is 40.

Wow! Can you show me again?

OK. Let's use prime factoring to find the lowest common denominator for $\frac{3}{8}$ and $\frac{5}{6}$. Create a table that lists the denominators horizontally; then find the prime factors.

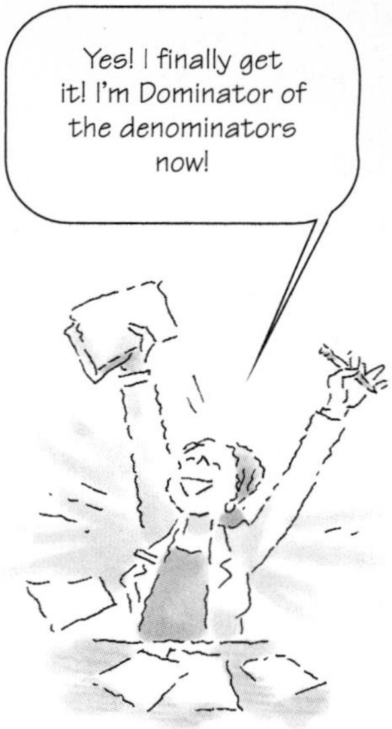

Yes! I finally get it! I'm Dominator of the denominators now!

- Set up a table like this:

Prime factors	Denominators	
	8	6
2	4	3
2	2	3
2	1	3

- Then multiply the prime factors in the left column by the numbers in the bottom row:

$$2 \times 2 \times 2 \times 1 \times 3 = 24$$

Lowest common denominator

Once more, please

Now, use prime factoring to find the lowest common denominator for ⅓, ¼, and ½.

- Set up the table:

Prime factors	Denominators		
	3	4	2
2	3	2	1
2	3	1	1

- Then multiply the prime factors in the left column by the numbers in the bottom row:

$$2 \times 2 \times 3 \times 1 \times 1 = 12$$

Lowest common denominator

Converting fractions

When you know the lowest common denominator of a set of fractions, you can *convert* the fractions so they'll all have the same denominator — the *lowest common denominator.*

One way to convert a set of fractions is to multiply each fraction by 1 in the form of a fraction — that is, a fraction with the same number in the numerator and denominator. You can find this fraction by taking the lowest common denominator and dividing it by the original denominator.

Here's what the formula looks like:

$$\text{original fraction} \times \frac{\text{lowest common denominator} \div \text{original denominator}}{\text{lowest common denominator} \div \text{original denominator}}$$

This is how you convert a fraction using 1 in the form of a fraction.

Conversion excursion

Convert the set of fractions ⅛, ¼, and ⅕ so that each has the lowest common denominator. We already know that the lowest common denominator for this set of fractions is 40.

- Here's the conversion of the first fraction, ⅛, to 5⁄40:

$$\frac{1}{8} = \frac{1}{8} \times \frac{40 \div 8}{40 \div 8} = \frac{1}{8} \times \frac{5}{5} = \frac{1 \times 5}{8 \times 5} = \frac{5}{40}$$

- Convert the next fraction, ¼, to 10⁄40:

$$\frac{1}{4} = \frac{1}{4} \times \frac{40 \div 4}{40 \div 4} = \frac{1}{4} \times \frac{10}{10} = \frac{1 \times 10}{4 \times 10} = \frac{10}{40}$$

- Convert the last fraction in the set, ⅕, to 8⁄40:

$$\frac{1}{5} = \frac{1}{5} \times \frac{40 \div 5}{40 \div 5} = \frac{1}{5} \times \frac{8}{8} = \frac{1 \times 8}{5 \times 8} = \frac{8}{40}$$

Do it again

This is how to convert ⅜ and ⅚ to fractions with the lowest common denominator, which is 24.

- Convert the first fraction, ⅜, to 9⁄24:

$$\frac{3}{8} = \frac{3}{8} \times \frac{24 \div 8}{24 \div 8} = \frac{3}{8} \times \frac{3}{3} = \frac{3 \times 3}{8 \times 3} = \frac{9}{24}$$

- Convert the other fraction, ⅚, to 20⁄24:

$$\frac{5}{6} = \frac{5}{6} \times \frac{24 \div 6}{24 \div 6} = \frac{5}{6} \times \frac{4}{4} = \frac{5 \times 4}{6 \times 4} = \frac{20}{24}$$

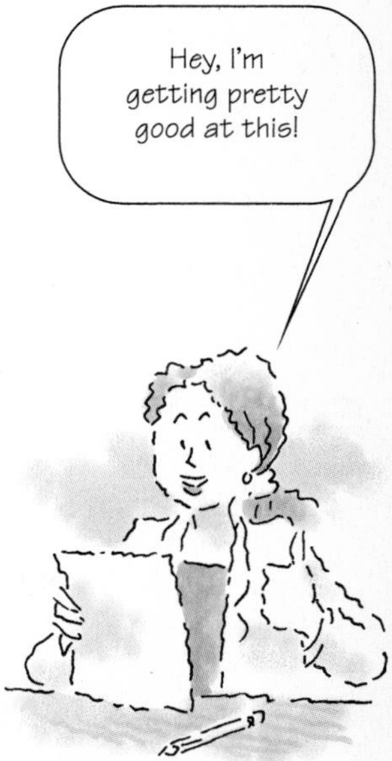
Hey, I'm getting pretty good at this!

Once more

OK. Now convert ⅓, ¼, and ½ to fractions with the lowest common denominator, which is 12.

- Convert ⅓ to 4⁄12:

$$\frac{1}{3} = \frac{1}{3} \times \frac{12 \div 3}{12 \div 3} = \frac{1}{3} \times \frac{4}{4} = \frac{1 \times 4}{3 \times 4} = \frac{4}{12}$$

- Convert ¼ to 3⁄12:

$$\frac{1}{4} = \frac{1}{4} \times \frac{12 \div 4}{12 \div 4} = \frac{1}{4} \times \frac{3}{3} = \frac{1 \times 3}{4 \times 3} = \frac{3}{12}$$

- Convert the last fraction, ½, to 6⁄12:

$$\frac{1}{2} = \frac{1}{2} \times \frac{12 \div 2}{12 \div 2} = \frac{1}{2} \times \frac{6}{6} = \frac{1 \times 6}{2 \times 6} = \frac{6}{12}$$

Divide and conquer

You can also convert a set of fractions by using long division. To convert each fraction, follow these steps:

1. Divide the lowest common denominator by the original denominator.
2. Multiply the *quotient*, or resulting number, by the original numerator to determine the new numerator.
3. Place the new numerator over the lowest common denominator.

Here's how to set up the conversion for each fraction:

$$\text{original denominator}\overset{\text{quotient}}{\overline{)\text{lowest common denominator}}} \times \text{original numerator} = \frac{\text{new numerator}}{\text{lowest common denominator}}$$

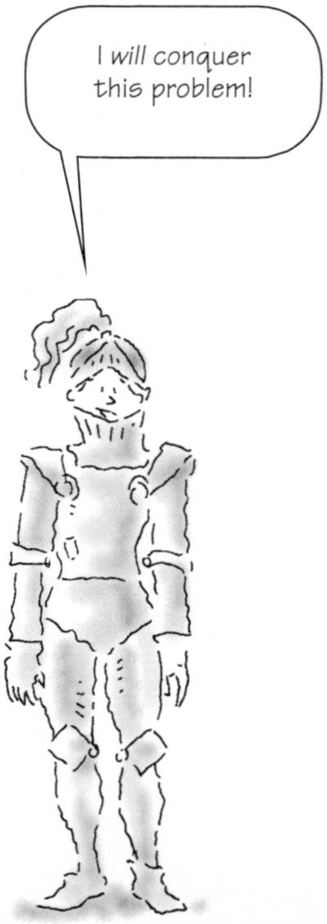
I will conquer
this problem!

Set 'em up

This is how to convert 3⁄8, ¼, and 2⁄5. The lowest common denominator is 40.

- Convert the first fraction in the set, 3⁄8, to 15⁄40:

$$\frac{3}{8} = 8\overset{5}{\overline{)40}} \times 3 = \frac{15}{40}$$

- Convert ¼ to 10⁄40:

$$\frac{1}{4} = 4\overset{10}{\overline{)40}} \times 1 = \frac{10}{40}$$

- Convert 2⁄5 to 16⁄40:

$$\frac{2}{5} = 5\overset{8}{\overline{)40}} \times 2 = \frac{16}{40}$$

Amazing! Let's see that again

This is how to convert 3/8 and 5/6. The lowest common denominator is 24.

- Convert the fraction 3/8 to 9/24:

$$\frac{3}{8} = 8\overset{3}{\overline{)24}} \times 3 = \frac{9}{24}$$

- Convert 5/6 to 20/24:

$$\frac{5}{6} = 6\overset{4}{\overline{)24}} \times 5 = \frac{20}{24}$$

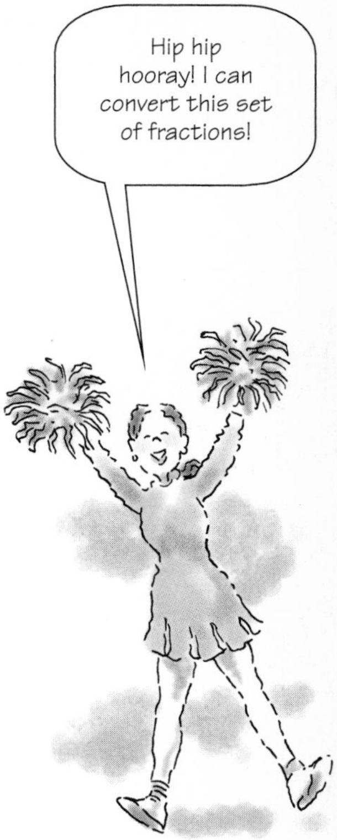

Hip hip hooray! I can convert this set of fractions!

One last time

And this is how to convert 1/3, 1/4, and 1/2. The lowest common denominator is 12.

- Convert 1/3 to 4/12:

$$\frac{1}{3} = 3\overset{4}{\overline{)12}} \times 1 = \frac{4}{12}$$

- Convert 1/4 to 3/12:

$$\frac{1}{4} = 4\overset{3}{\overline{)12}} \times 1 = \frac{3}{12}$$

- Convert 1/2 to 6/12:

$$\frac{1}{2} = 2\overset{6}{\overline{)12}} \times 1 = \frac{6}{12}$$

Comparing fraction size

Why are these calculations important? Because finding the lowest common denominator in a set of fractions allows you to compare the relative size of the fractions. This concept is extremely useful for comparing the strengths of medications. (See *Denominators can be deceptive*, page 14.)

Suppose you want to compare the strengths of sublingual nitroglycerin tablets, which are available in 1/100-grain, 1/150-grain, and 1/200-grain strengths. Follow these steps:

Using the prime factor method, first find the lowest common denominator for these three fractions. The table looks like this:

Prime factors	Denominators		
	100	150	200
2	50	75	100
2	25	75	50
5	5	15	10
5	1	3	2

Then multiply the prime factors in the left column and the numbers in the bottom row. In other words:

$$2 \times 2 \times 5 \times 5 \times 1 \times 3 \times 2 = 600$$

Lowest common denominator

Finding common ground

Next, convert all three fractions — $\frac{1}{100}$, $\frac{1}{150}$, and $\frac{1}{200}$ — to new fractions with the lowest common denominator of 600. To do this, multiply each fraction by 1 in the form of a fraction (create this

For math phobics only

Denominators can be deceptive

If you were hungry, would you rather have 1 slice from a pie that was cut into 4 slices, 8 slices, or 16 slices? You'd choose 4, of course, because the slices would be bigger. You can judge the size of fractions the same way. When the fractions all have the same numerators — in this case, $\frac{1}{4}$, $\frac{1}{8}$, and $\frac{1}{16}$ — the fraction with the lowest denominator is the biggest one. Don't fall into the trap of thinking that the bigger the denominator, the bigger the fraction. Think in terms of a pie, as shown below.

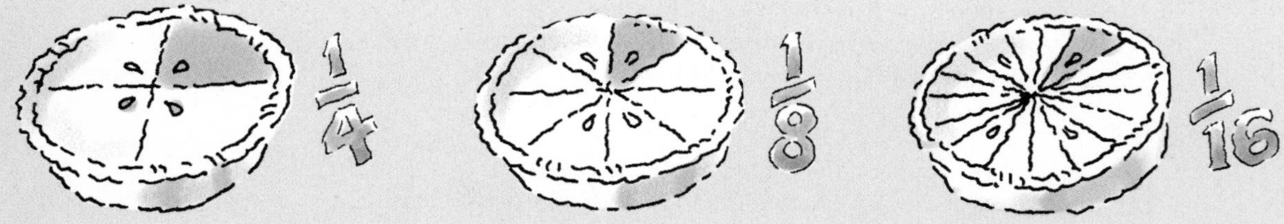

fraction by dividing the lowest common denominator by the original denominator).

Here's the conversion:

- The fraction $\frac{1}{100}$ is converted to $\frac{6}{600}$:

$$\frac{1}{100} = \frac{1}{100} \times \frac{600 \div 100}{600 \div 100} = \frac{1}{100} \times \frac{6}{6} = \frac{1 \times 6}{100 \times 6} = \frac{6}{600}$$

- $\frac{1}{150}$ is converted to $\frac{4}{600}$:

$$\frac{1}{150} = \frac{1}{150} \times \frac{600 \div 150}{600 \div 150} = \frac{1}{150} \times \frac{4}{4} = \frac{1 \times 4}{150 \times 4} = \frac{4}{600}$$

- $\frac{1}{200}$ is converted to $\frac{3}{600}$:

$$\frac{1}{200} = \frac{1}{200} \times \frac{600 \div 200}{600 \div 200} = \frac{1}{200} \times \frac{3}{3} = \frac{1 \times 3}{200 \times 3} = \frac{3}{600}$$

Comparing the three final fractions, you'll see that the $\frac{1}{100}$-grain nitroglycerin tablet offers the largest dose: $\frac{6}{600}$.

Same destination, different route

You can arrive at the same conclusion by dividing the lowest common denominator (600) by the denominator, multiplying the numerator by the number obtained, and placing the result over the lowest common denominator.

- The fraction $\frac{1}{100}$ is converted to $\frac{6}{600}$ this way:

$$\frac{1}{100} = 100\overline{)600}^{\,6} \times 1 = \frac{6}{600}$$

- $\frac{1}{150}$ is converted to $\frac{4}{600}$:

$$\frac{1}{150} = 150\overline{)600}^{\,4} \times 1 = \frac{4}{600}$$

- $\frac{1}{200}$ is converted to $\frac{3}{600}$:

$$\frac{1}{200} = 200\overline{)600}^{\,3} \times 1 = \frac{3}{600}$$

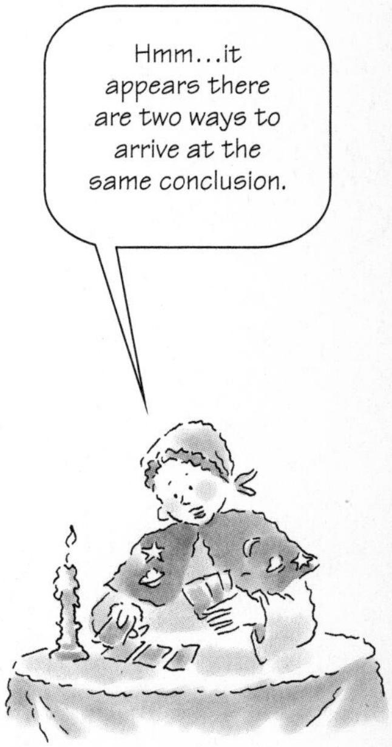
Hmm...it appears there are two ways to arrive at the same conclusion.

Fraction fact

When comparing fractions with common denominators, the fraction with the largest numerator is the largest number. In the set of fractions above, $\frac{6}{600}$ is the largest number.

A common hero

The lowest common denominator also enables you to add and subtract fractions. Reducing fractions to their lowest terms and converting improper fractions to mixed numbers lets you present the answers to addition, subtraction, multiplication, and division problems in a useful way.

Remember: Whenever you perform these functions, always reduce the final answer to its lowest terms and, if it's an improper fraction, convert it to a mixed number.

Adding fractions

To add fractions, first convert them to fractions with common denominators. (See *Comparing apples to apples.*)

It all adds up

Here's an example of adding fractions. Follow the steps below to add the fractions $1/7$ and $1/3$.

1. Find the lowest common denominator. Because the denominators in $1/7$ and $1/3$ are both prime numbers, multiply 7 by 3 to find the lowest common denominator, 21.

2. Then convert the fractions by multiplying each by 1 (in the form of a fraction) to yield fractions with the lowest common denominator.

3. Start by converting $1/7$ to $3/21$:

$$\frac{1}{7} = \frac{1}{7} \times \frac{21 \div 7}{21 \div 7} = \frac{1}{7} \times \frac{3}{3} = \frac{1 \times 3}{7 \times 3} = \frac{3}{21}$$

4. Then convert $1/3$ to $7/21$:

$$\frac{1}{3} = \frac{1}{3} \times \frac{21 \div 3}{21 \div 3} = \frac{1}{3} \times \frac{7}{7} = \frac{1 \times 7}{3 \times 7} = \frac{7}{21}$$

5. Now, add the new fractions. To add fractions with a common denominator, add the numerators and place the result over the common denominator. The resulting fraction is your answer. (Reduce it to its lowest terms, if possible.)

$$\frac{3}{21} + \frac{7}{21} = \frac{3 + 7}{21} = \frac{10}{21}$$

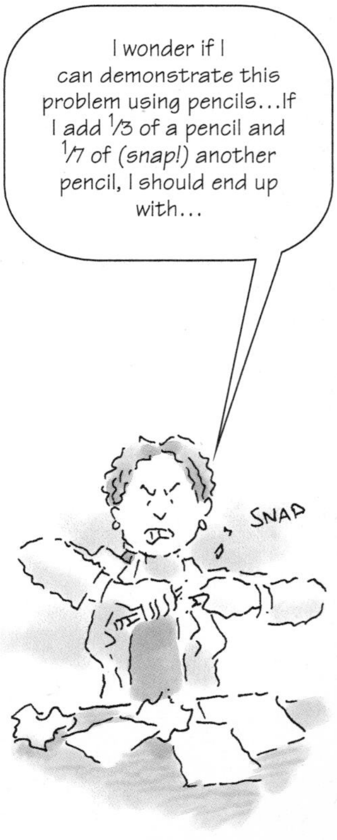

I wonder if I can demonstrate this problem using pencils...If I add 1/3 of a pencil and 1/7 of (snap!) another pencil, I should end up with...
SNAP

Additional addition

To add $1/2$ and $1/5$, follow these steps:

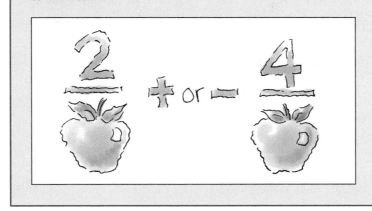

Comparing apples to apples

When adding or subtracting fractions, don't forget to convert them to fractions with common denominators. That way, you'll be comparing apples to apples.

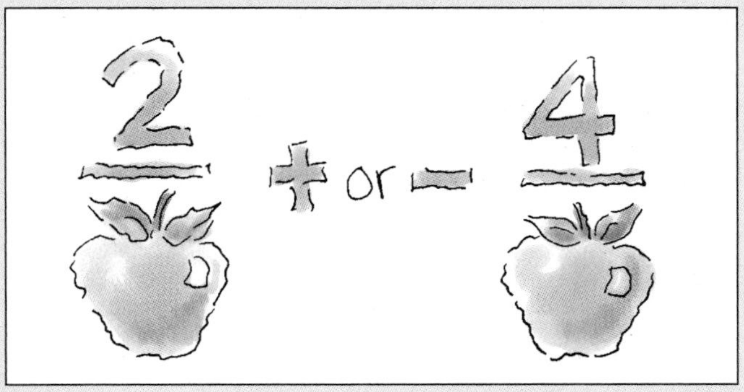

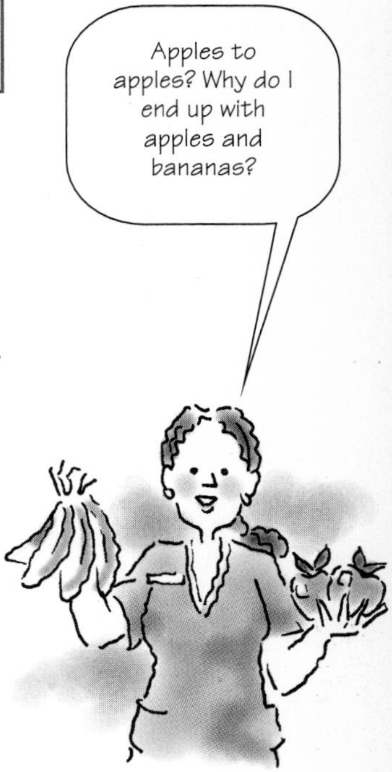
Apples to apples? Why do I end up with apples and bananas?

Find the lowest common denominator. In this case, because the denominators 2 and 5 are both prime numbers, multiply 2 by 5 to find the lowest common denominator, 10.

Convert the fractions by multiplying each by 1 (in the form of a fraction) to yield fractions with the lowest common denominator.

Convert the fraction $\frac{1}{2}$ to $\frac{5}{10}$:

$$\frac{1}{2} = \frac{1}{2} \times \frac{10 \div 2}{10 \div 2} = \frac{1}{2} \times \frac{5}{5} = \frac{1 \times 5}{2 \times 5} = \frac{5}{10}$$

Then convert $\frac{1}{5}$ to $\frac{2}{10}$:

$$\frac{1}{5} = \frac{1}{5} \times \frac{10 \div 5}{10 \div 5} = \frac{1}{5} \times \frac{2}{2} = \frac{1 \times 2}{5 \times 2} = \frac{2}{10}$$

Now, add the converted fractions. To do this, add the numerators and place the result over the common denominator:

$$\frac{5}{10} + \frac{2}{10} = \frac{5 + 2}{10} = \frac{7}{10}$$

Another additional addition

To add 3⁄5 and 2⁄3, follow these steps:

Find the lowest common denominator — in this case, 15.

Convert the fractions by multiplying each by 1 (in the form of a fraction) to yield fractions with the lowest common denominator.

Convert 3⁄5 to 9⁄15:

$$\frac{3}{5} = \frac{3}{5} \times \frac{15 \div 5}{15 \div 5} = \frac{3}{5} \times \frac{3}{3} = \frac{3 \times 3}{5 \times 3} = \frac{9}{15}$$

Then convert 2⁄3 to 10⁄15:

$$\frac{2}{3} = \frac{2}{3} \times \frac{15 \div 3}{15 \div 3} = \frac{2}{3} \times \frac{5}{5} = \frac{2 \times 5}{3 \times 5} = \frac{10}{15}$$

To add the converted fractions, add the new numerators and place the result over the common denominator:

$$\frac{9}{15} + \frac{10}{15} = \frac{9 + 10}{15} = \frac{19}{15}$$

Reduce the fraction to its lowest terms:

$$\frac{19}{15} = 1\frac{4}{15}$$

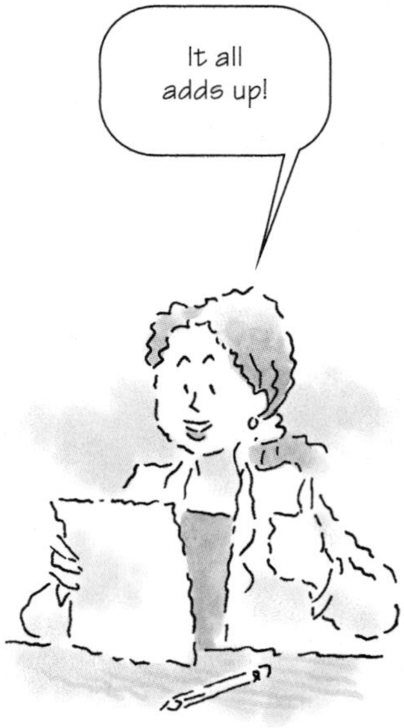

Subtracting fractions

Like addition, subtraction requires converting fractions to terms with common denominators.

Fraction subtraction

Here's an example of how to subtract one fraction from another. Follow the steps below to subtract 1⁄6 from 5⁄12.

Find the lowest common denominator — in this case, 12. The fraction 5⁄12 already has the lowest common denominator.

Convert the fraction 1⁄6 to a fraction with the lowest common denominator. To do this, multiply the fraction by the number 1 (in the form of a fraction).

$$\frac{1}{6} = \frac{1}{6} \times \frac{12 \div 6}{12 \div 6} = \frac{1}{6} \times \frac{2}{2} = \frac{1 \times 2}{6 \times 2} = \frac{2}{12}$$

Now, subtract the numerators and place the result over the common denominator:

$$\frac{5}{12} - \frac{2}{12} = \frac{5 - 2}{12} = \frac{3}{12}$$

Reduce the fraction to its lowest terms, if possible. The resulting fraction is your answer:

$$\frac{3}{12} = \frac{1}{4}$$

A second subtraction

To subtract 1⁄9 from 5⁄6, follow these steps:

Find the lowest common denominator—in this case, 18. (To find the lowest common denominator in this case, try prime factoring on your own.)

Convert the fractions to those with the lowest common denominator by multiplying each fraction by the number 1 (in the form of a fraction).

Convert 5⁄6 to 15⁄18:

$$\frac{5}{6} = \frac{5}{6} \times \frac{18 \div 6}{18 \div 6} = \frac{5}{6} \times \frac{3}{3} = \frac{5 \times 3}{6 \times 3} = \frac{15}{18}$$

Then convert 1⁄9 to 2⁄18:

$$\frac{1}{9} = \frac{1}{9} \times \frac{18 \div 9}{18 \div 9} = \frac{1}{9} \times \frac{2}{2} = \frac{1 \times 2}{9 \times 2} = \frac{2}{18}$$

Then subtract the numerators and place the result over the common denominator. Reduce the fraction to its lowest terms, if possible. In this case, the fraction can't be reduced:

$$\frac{15}{18} - \frac{2}{18} = \frac{15 - 2}{18} = \frac{13}{18}$$

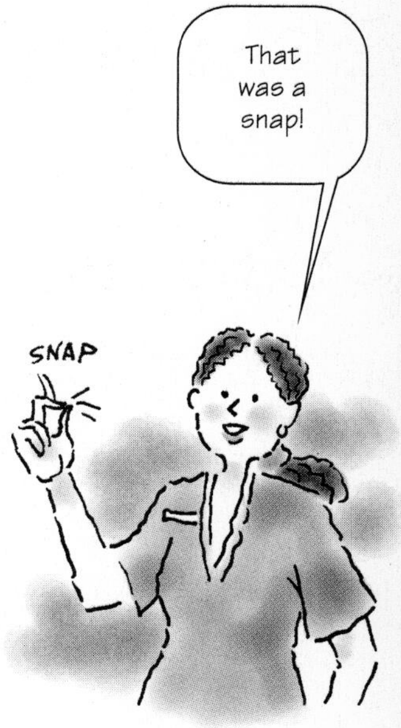

More subtraction action

To subtract 1⁄4 from 2⁄3, follow these steps:

Find the lowest common denominator — in this case, 12.

Convert the fractions to those with the lowest common denominator by multiplying each fraction by the number 1 (in the form of a fraction).

Convert 2⁄3 to 8⁄12:

$$\frac{2}{3} = \frac{2}{3} \times \frac{12 \div 3}{12 \div 3} = \frac{2}{3} \times \frac{4}{4} = \frac{2 \times 4}{3 \times 4} = \frac{8}{12}$$

Convert 1⁄4 to 3⁄12:

$$\frac{1}{4} = \frac{1}{4} \times \frac{12 \div 4}{12 \div 4} = \frac{1}{4} \times \frac{3}{3} = \frac{1 \times 3}{4 \times 3} = \frac{3}{12}$$

Subtract the numerators and place the result over the common denominator:

$$\frac{8}{12} - \frac{3}{12} = \frac{8 - 3}{12} = \frac{5}{12}$$

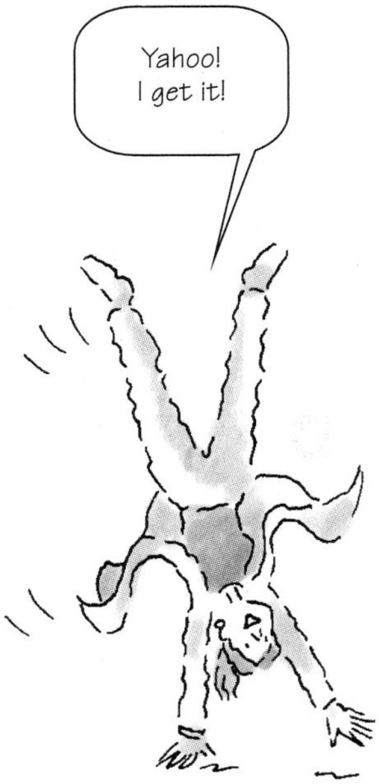

Multiplying fractions

Good news! There's no need to convert to common denominators when multiplying fractions. Simply multiply the numerators and denominators in turn to find the product.

For example, to multiply 4⁄7 by 5⁄8, multiply the numerators 4 and 5 and the denominators 7 and 8 to get a new fraction. Here's the calculation.

- Set up the equation:

$$\frac{4}{7} \times \frac{5}{8}$$

- Multiply the numerators and multiply the denominators:

$$\frac{4 \times 5}{7 \times 8} = \frac{20}{56}$$

- Reduce the answer to its lowest terms:

$$\frac{5}{14}$$

Let's see it again!

To multiply 5⁄6 by 1⁄3, multiply the numerators 5 and 1 and the denominators 6 and 3 to get the answer:

$$\frac{5}{6} \times \frac{1}{3} = \frac{5 \times 1}{6 \times 3} = \frac{5}{18}$$

A whole other matter

To multiply a fraction by a whole number, for example 1⁄9 by 4, follow these simple steps:

- First, convert the whole number 4 to the fraction 4⁄1.
- Then multiply the numerators and denominators. The complete calculation looks like this:

$$\frac{1}{9} \times 4 = \frac{1}{9} \times \frac{4}{1} = \frac{1 \times 4}{9 \times 1} = \frac{4}{9}$$

Divvying up the problem

Before you can divide numbers, you need to know what each part of a division problem is called. The division problem below can be written two different ways, but the terms remain the same.

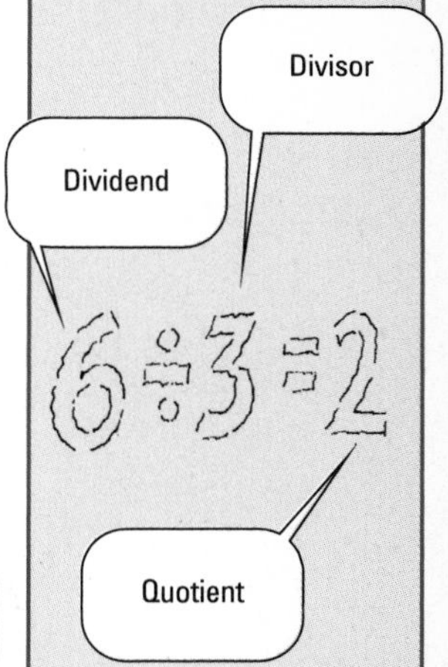

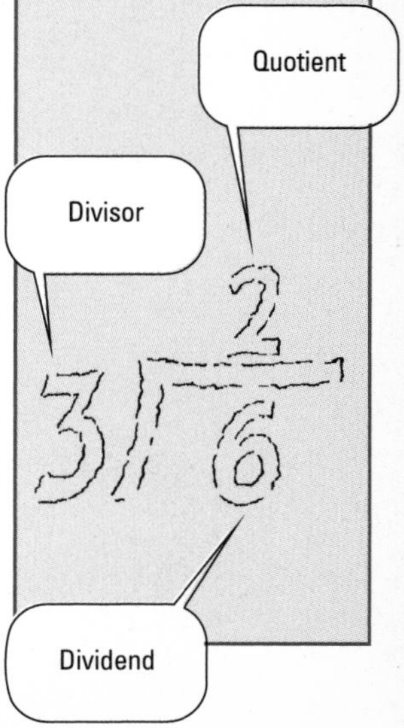

Dividing fractions

In division (as in multiplication), you don't need to convert the fractions. Division problems are usually written as two fractions separated by a division sign. The first fraction is the number to be divided (the *dividend*), and the second fraction is the number doing the dividing (the *divisor*); the answer is the *quotient*. (See *Divvying up the problem* for a quick review.)

To divide 5⁄7 by 2⁄3, first set up the problem:

This fraction is the dividend.

$$\frac{5}{7} \div \frac{2}{3}$$

This fraction is the divisor.

To divide fractions, multiply the dividend by the divisor's *reciprocal*, or the inverted divisor.

- To divide 5⁄7 by 2⁄3 (the divisor), first multiply 5⁄7 (the dividend) by 3⁄2 (the divisor's reciprocal):

$$\frac{5}{7} \div \frac{2}{3} = \frac{5}{7} \times \frac{3}{2}$$

Here's the divisor's reciprocal.

- Then complete the calculation and reduce the answer (the quotient) to its lowest terms:

$$\frac{5 \times 3}{7 \times 2} = \frac{15}{14} = 1\tfrac{1}{14}$$

A part divided by a whole

To divide a fraction by a whole number, use the same principle.

- To divide $\frac{3}{5}$ by 2, first convert the whole number 2 to the fraction $\frac{2}{1}$.

$$\frac{3}{5} \div 2 = \frac{3}{5} \div \frac{2}{1}$$

- Then multiply the dividend ($\frac{3}{5}$) by the reciprocal of the divisor ($\frac{1}{2}$). Reduce the answer to its lowest terms:

$$\frac{3}{5} \times \frac{1}{2} =$$

$$\frac{3 \times 1}{5 \times 2} =$$

$$\frac{3}{10}$$

In this case, the answer can't be further reduced.

Making things less complex

In complex fractions, the numerators and denominators are fractions themselves. Complex fractions can be simplified by following the rules for division of fractions. Think of the line separating the two fractions as a division sign. For example, follow the simple steps below to simplify the complex fraction:

$$\frac{1/3}{5/8}$$

First, rewrite the complex fraction as a division problem:

$$\frac{1/3}{5/8} = \frac{1}{3} \div \frac{5}{8}$$

Multiply the dividend ($\frac{1}{3}$) by the reciprocal of the divisor ($\frac{8}{5}$):

$$\frac{1}{3} \times \frac{8}{5}$$

Lastly, complete the calculation:

$$\frac{1 \times 8}{3 \times 5} = \frac{8}{15}$$

Real world problem

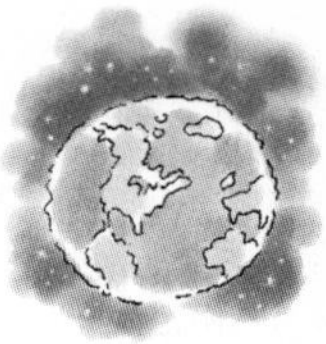

The nurse is totaling her patient's intake for her shift. In the past 8 hours, the patient drank ½ cup broth, ⅔ cup ginger ale, and ¾ cup water. How many cups of liquid has the patient had to drink?

Adding for a liquid solution

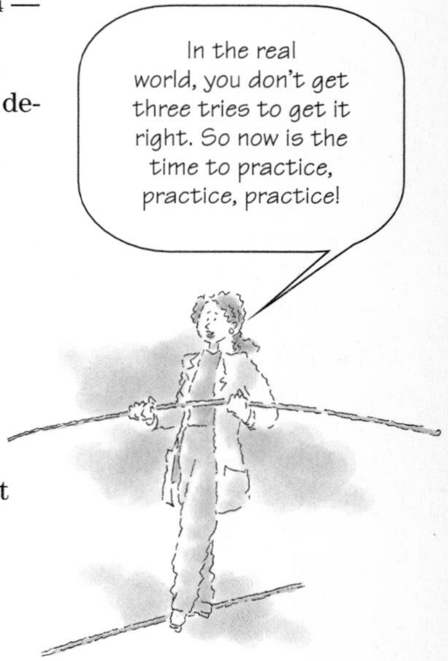

In the real world, you don't get three tries to get it right. So now is the time to practice, practice, practice!

To solve this problem, you need to add fractions.

• First, find the lowest common denominator for ½, ⅔, and ¾ — in this case, 12.

• Next, convert each fraction by multiplying each by 1 (in the form of a fraction) to yield fractions with the lowest common denominator:

$$\frac{1}{2} = \frac{1}{2} \times \frac{12 \div 2}{12 \div 2} = \frac{1}{2} \times \frac{6}{6} = \frac{1 \times 6}{2 \times 6} = \frac{6}{12}$$

$$\frac{2}{3} = \frac{2}{3} \times \frac{12 \div 3}{12 \div 3} = \frac{2}{3} \times \frac{4}{4} = \frac{2 \times 4}{3 \times 4} = \frac{8}{12}$$

$$\frac{3}{4} = \frac{3}{4} \times \frac{12 \div 4}{12 \div 4} = \frac{3}{4} \times \frac{3}{3} = \frac{3 \times 3}{4 \times 3} = \frac{9}{12}$$

• Lastly, add the converted fractions, and reduce to the lowest terms:

$$\frac{6}{12} + \frac{8}{12} + \frac{9}{12} = \frac{6 + 8 + 9}{12} = \frac{23}{12} = 1\frac{11}{12}$$

• The patient has had $1\frac{11}{12}$ cups of liquid to drink during the nurse's shift.

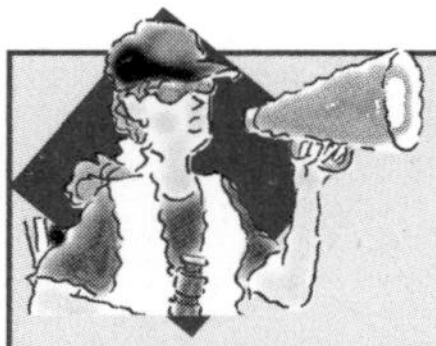

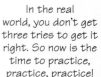

That's a wrap!

Fractions review

Here are some important facts about fractions you'll need to remember.

Fraction basics

• A fraction is a mathematical expression for parts of a whole.

• The denominator (bottom number) represents the total number of equal parts in the whole.

• The numerator (top number) represents the number of parts of the whole being considered.

Types of fractions

• *Common fraction:* both the numerator and denominator are whole numbers (such as ⅔)

• *Complex fraction:* the numerator and denominator are fractions (such as $\frac{2/7}{5/8}$)

(continued)

Fractions review *(continued)*

- *Proper fraction:* the numerator is smaller than the denominator (such as ¼)
- *Improper fraction:* the numerator is larger than the denominator (such as 8⁄3)

Converting to improper fractions
- Multiply the denominator by the whole number.
- Add the product to the numerator.
- The resulting sum is the new numerator.
- Leave the denominator as it is.

Reducing fractions
- Determine the largest common divisor.
- Divide the numerator and denominator by that number.

Common denominators
- Multiply all the denominators in a set of fractions to find the common denominator.
- The smallest multiple of the denominators is the lowest common denominator.
- Use prime factoring to determine the lowest common denominator.

Adding and subtracting fractions
- Always convert to fractions with common denominators first, then add or subtract the numerators and keep the denominator as it is.

Multiplying fractions
- Don't convert fractions to common denominators.
- Multiply the numerators and denominators in turn.

Dividing fractions
- Don't convert fractions to common denominators.
- Write them as two fractions separated by a division sign.
- Invert the divisor.
- Multiply the dividend by the inverted divisor (reciprocal).

Don't forget!
- Always reduce the final answer to its lowest terms.
- If the fraction is improper, convert to a mixed number.

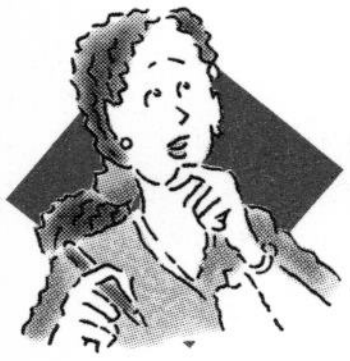

Quick quiz

1. The product of 2⁄3 × 5⁄7 is:

A. 14⁄15 .
B. 10⁄21.
C. 7⁄5.
D. 1⁄21.

Answer: B. To multiply two common fractions, multiply the numerators and then the denominators. The calculation looks like this:

$$\frac{2}{3} \times \frac{5}{7} = \frac{2 \times 5}{3 \times 7} = \frac{10}{21}$$

2. In the fraction $4/5$, the denominator is:
A. $5/4$.
B. $1\frac{1}{5}$.
C. 4.
D. 5.

Answer: D. The denominator is the bottom number of a fraction. The numerator is the top number.

3. When you reduce the fraction $8/24$ to its lowest terms, you get:
A. $2/6$.
B. $3/4$.
C. $1/3$.
D. $1/8$.

Answer: C. Both the numerator and the denominator are divisible by 8, leaving the reduced fraction $1/3$.

4. Which of the following is an improper fraction?
A. $9/17$
B. $11/2$
C. $1/3$
D. $3/4$

Answer: B. An improper fraction has a numerator that's larger than the denominator.

5. When adding the fractions $1/3$ and $1/2$, you get:
A. $2/5$.
B. $5/6$.
C. $3/6$.
D. $5/20$.

Answer: B. To add $1/2$ and $1/3$, first find the common denominator, which is 6. Convert the fractions to $3/6$ and $2/6$. Then add the numerators and place the result over the common denominator. The calculation looks like this:

$$\frac{1}{2} + \frac{1}{3} = \frac{3}{6} + \frac{2}{6} = \frac{3 + 2}{6} = \frac{5}{6}$$

6. Which of the following is a prime number?
A. 4
B. 5
C. 6
D. 8

Answer: B. The number 5 is a prime number because it can be divided only by itself and 1.

Scoring

☆☆☆ If you answered all six items correctly, wow! You're a number 1 math whiz (which is the same as a $2/2$, a $3/3$, or a $6/6$ math whiz).

☆☆ If you answered four or five items correctly, fantastic! You're a freewheeling fraction fiend.

☆ If you answered fewer than four items correctly, stick with it! You've shown great derring-do in dealing with dividends and divisors.

2

Decimals and percentages

Just the facts

In this chapter, you'll learn:

- what decimals and percentages are
- how to add, subtract, multiply, divide, and round off decimal fractions
- how to convert common fractions to decimal fractions and vice versa
- how to convert percentages to decimal fractions and common fractions and vice versa
- how to solve percentage problems.

A look at decimals and percentages

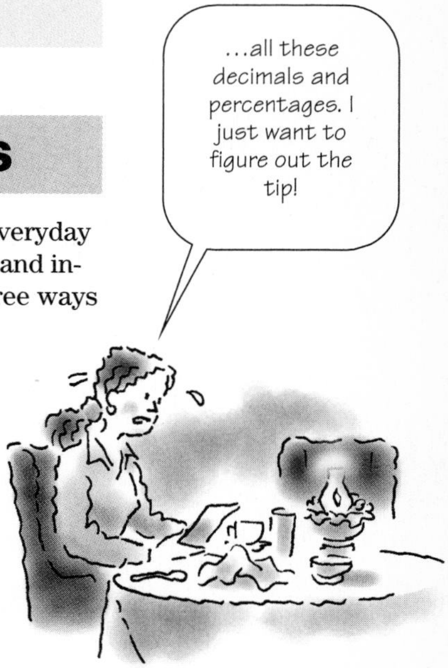

...all these decimals and percentages. I just want to figure out the tip!

For most people, decimals and percentages are a part of everyday life. Figuring a tip at a restaurant, balancing a checkbook, and interpreting the results of an election or a survey are just three ways people use decimals and percentages.

As a nurse, you also encounter decimals and percentages every day at work. The metric system, the most common system for measuring medications, is based on decimal numbers. You also use decimals and percentages when administering solutions such as 0.9% sodium chloride solution and drugs such as a 2.5% cream.

In the know

To administer medications accurately and efficiently, you must understand what decimals and percentages are and how to work with them in common calculations. You also need to know how to convert from percentages to decimal fractions and common fractions and then back to percentages. This chapter will sharpen your calculation skills and help you build confidence.

Deciphering decimals

A *decimal fraction* is a proper fraction in which the denominator is a power of 10, signified by a decimal point placed at the left of the numerator. An example of a decimal fraction is 0.2, which is the same as $\frac{2}{10}$.

In a *decimal number* — for example, 2.25 — the decimal point separates the whole number from the decimal fraction.

Look to the left...

Each number or place to the left of the decimal point represents a whole number that's a power of 10, starting with ones and working up to tens, hundreds, thousands, ten thousands, and so on.

...and then to the right

Each place to the right of the decimal point signifies a fraction whose denominator is a power of 10, starting with tenths and working up to hundredths, thousandths, ten thousandths, and so on. When working as a nurse, you'll rarely encounter decimal fractions beyond the thousandths. (See *Know your places.*)

Know your places

Based on its position relative to the decimal point, each decimal place represents a power of 10 or a fraction with a denominator that's a power of 10, as shown below.

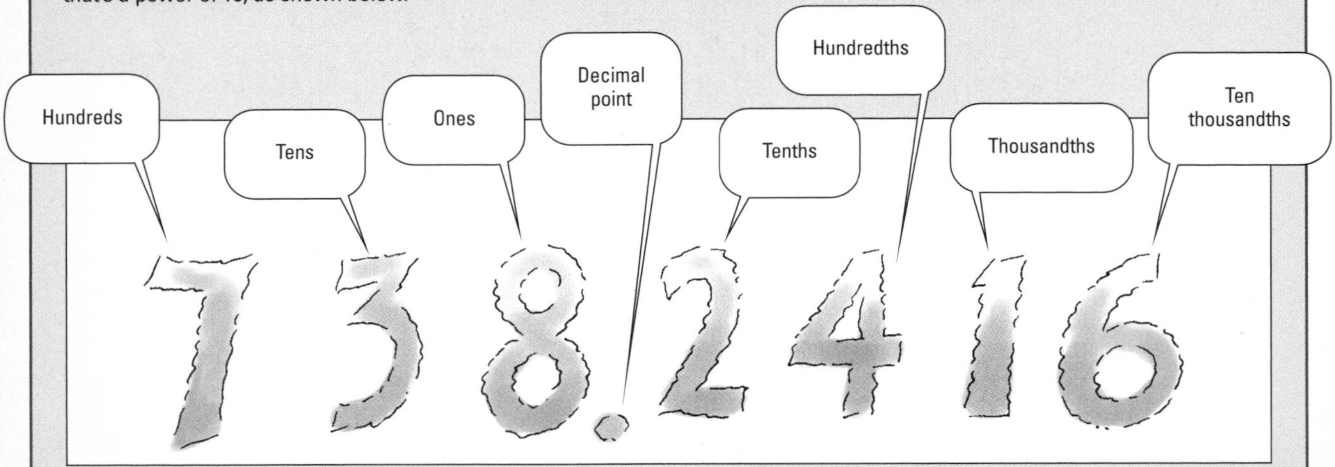

Getting to the point

When discussing money, people use the word *and* to signify the decimal point, for example, saying $5.20 as "5 dollars and 20 cents." However, when discussing decimal numbers in dosage calculations, use the word *point* to signify the decimal point. For example, say the number 5.2 as "5 point 2."

Zeroing in on zeros

Now that you've learned the basic terms used with decimal fractions, you're ready to review the decimal calculations most often performed by nurses. But first, review these two important rules:

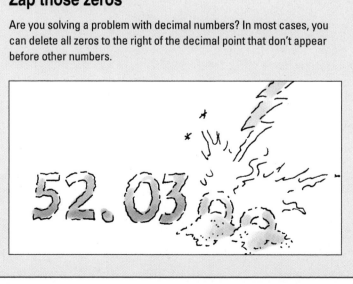

- After performing mathematical functions with decimal numbers, you may eliminate zeros to the right of the decimal point that don't appear before other numbers. (See *Zap those zeros.*) In other cases, you may wish to *add* zeros at the end of fractions (for example, as place holders). Deleting or adding zeros at the end of a decimal fraction doesn't change the value of the number.
- When writing answers to mathematical calculations and specifying drug dosages, always put a zero to the left of the decimal point if no other number appears there. This helps prevent errors. (See *Disappearing decimal alert,* page 30.)

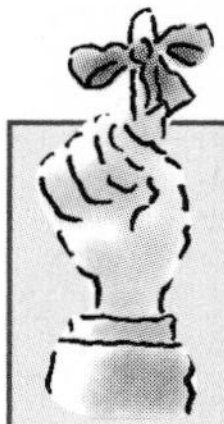

Memory jogger

To remember which zeros you can safely eliminate in a decimal number, think of the letters "l" and "r" in the words "left" and "right":

- ***Leave*** a zero to the **left** of the decimal point if no other number appears there and you need a place holder (as in 0.5 ml).
- ***Remove*** any trailing zeros to the **right** of the decimal point if no other number follows and you don't need a place holder (as in 7.5Ø mg).

Zap those zeros

Are you solving a problem with decimal numbers? In most cases, you can delete all zeros to the right of the decimal point that don't appear before other numbers.

Before you give that drug!

Disappearing decimal alert

Decimal points and zeros may be small items, but they're big deals in medication orders and administration records. When you get a drug order, study it closely. If a dose doesn't sound right, maybe a decimal point was left out or incorrectly placed.

For instance, an order that calls for ".5 mg lorazepam I.V." may be mistaken for "5 mg of lorazepam I.V." The correct way to write this order is to use a zero as a placeholder before the decimal point. The order would then become "0.5 mg lorazepam I.V."

Adding and subtracting decimal fractions

Before adding and subtracting decimal fractions, align the decimal points vertically to help you keep track of the decimal positions.

Placeholders, take your place

To maintain column alignment, add zeros as placeholders in decimal fractions.

Here's how to use zeros to align the decimal fractions 2.61, 0.315, and 4.8 before adding:

$$\begin{array}{r} 2.610 \\ 0.315 \\ +\ 4.800 \\ \hline 7.725 \end{array}$$

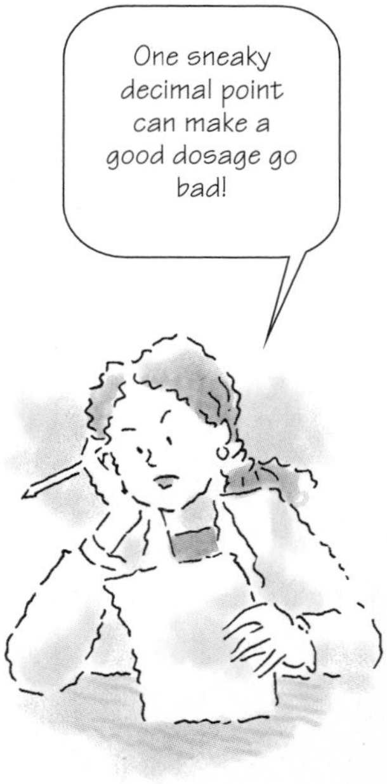

One sneaky decimal point can make a good dosage go bad!

Working it out

Here are two more examples of adding and subtracting decimal fractions. First, add 0.017, 4.8, and 1.22:

$$\begin{array}{r} 0.017 \\ 4.800 \\ +\ 1.220 \\ \hline 6.037 \end{array}$$

Next, subtract 0.05 from 4.726:

$$\begin{array}{r} 4.726 \\ -\ 0.050 \\ \hline 4.676 \end{array}$$

Multiplying decimal fractions

Aligning the decimal points isn't necessary before doing a multiplication problem with decimal fractions. Just leave the decimal points in their original positions and multiply the factors to find the product.

To determine where to place the decimal point in the final product, first add together the number of decimal places in both factors being multiplied. Then count out the same total number of places in the answer, starting from the right and moving to the left, and place the decimal point just to the left of the last place counted. Here's how you would multiply 2.7 and 0.81:

$$\begin{array}{r} 2.70 \\ \times\ 0.81 \\ \hline 2.1870 \end{array}$$

The decimal point goes here because there are four decimal places in the factors.

Multiple multiplication

Here are two more examples of multiplying decimal fractions. First, multiply 1.423 and 8.59:

$$\begin{array}{r} 1.423 \\ \times\ 8.59 \\ \hline 12.22357 \end{array}$$

Next, multiply 42.1 and 0.376:

$$\begin{array}{r} 42.1 \\ \times\ 0.376 \\ \hline 15.8296 \end{array}$$

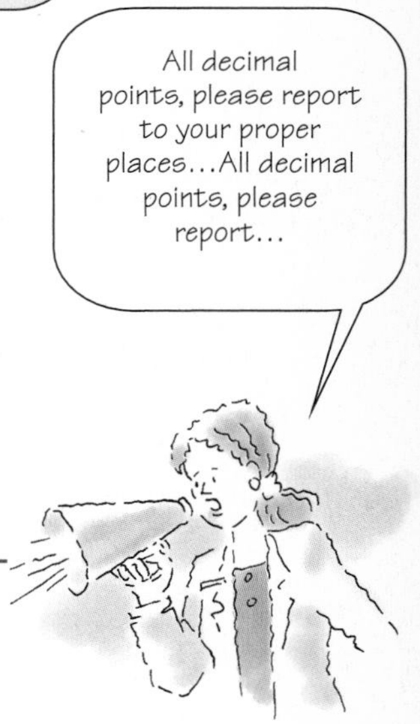

All decimal points, please report to your proper places...All decimal points, please report...

Dividing decimal fractions

When dividing decimal fractions, align the decimal points but don't add zeros as placeholders. *Remember:* The number to be divided is the *dividend*, the number that does the dividing is the *divisor*, and the answer is the *quotient*.

Whole-number divisors

Decimal point placement is easiest when the divisor is a whole number. Just place the decimal point in the quotient directly above the decimal point in the dividend and then work the problem. For example, here's how to divide 4.68 by 2:

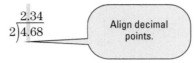

$$\begin{array}{r} 2.34 \\ 2\overline{)4.68} \end{array}$$

Align decimal points.

Revisiting decimal division

Here are two more examples of decimal point placement when the divisor is a whole number. First, divide 44.02 by 10:

$$\begin{array}{r} 4.402 \\ 10\overline{)44.020} \end{array}$$

Next, divide 9.093 by 3:

$$\begin{array}{r} 3.031 \\ 3\overline{)9.093} \end{array}$$

Align decimal points.

Decimal-fraction divisors

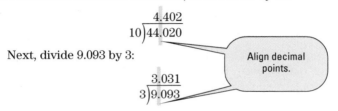

Of course, not every divisor is a whole number — some are decimal fractions. Dividing one decimal fraction into another requires moving the decimal points in both the divisor and the dividend. (See *Dividing decimal fractions.*)

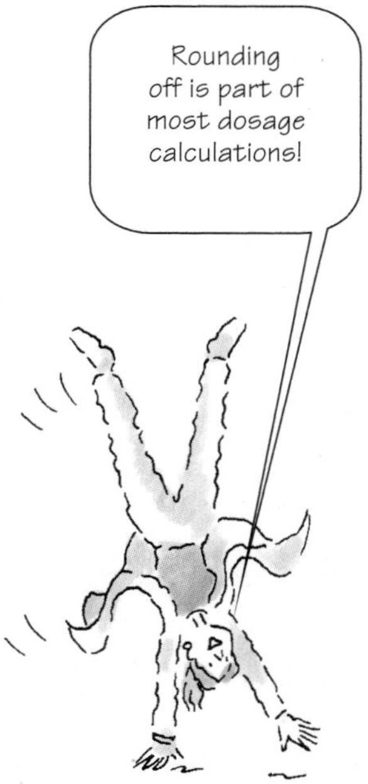

Rounding off is part of most dosage calculations!

Rounding off decimal fractions

Most of the instruments and measuring devices a nurse uses measure accurately only to a tenth or, at most, to a hundredth. So you'll need to round off decimal fractions — that is, convert long fractions to those with fewer decimal places. (See *Remember rounding*, page 34.)

Whittling decimals down

To round off a decimal fraction, follow these steps:

1. Suppose you want to round off the decimal fraction 0.4293. First, decide how many places to the right of the decimal point you want to keep. If you decide to round the number off to hundredths, you'll keep two places to the right of the decimal point and delete the rest (the 9 and the 3).

2. Now, look at the first number that you've deleted. Is this number 5 or greater than 5? If so, add 1 to the number in the

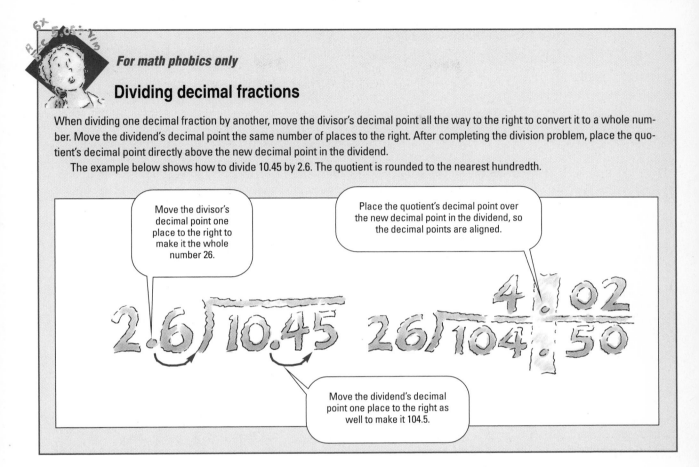

For math phobics only

Dividing decimal fractions

When dividing one decimal fraction by another, move the divisor's decimal point all the way to the right to convert it to a whole number. Move the dividend's decimal point the same number of places to the right. After completing the division problem, place the quotient's decimal point directly above the new decimal point in the dividend.

The example below shows how to divide 10.45 by 2.6. The quotient is rounded to the nearest hundredth.

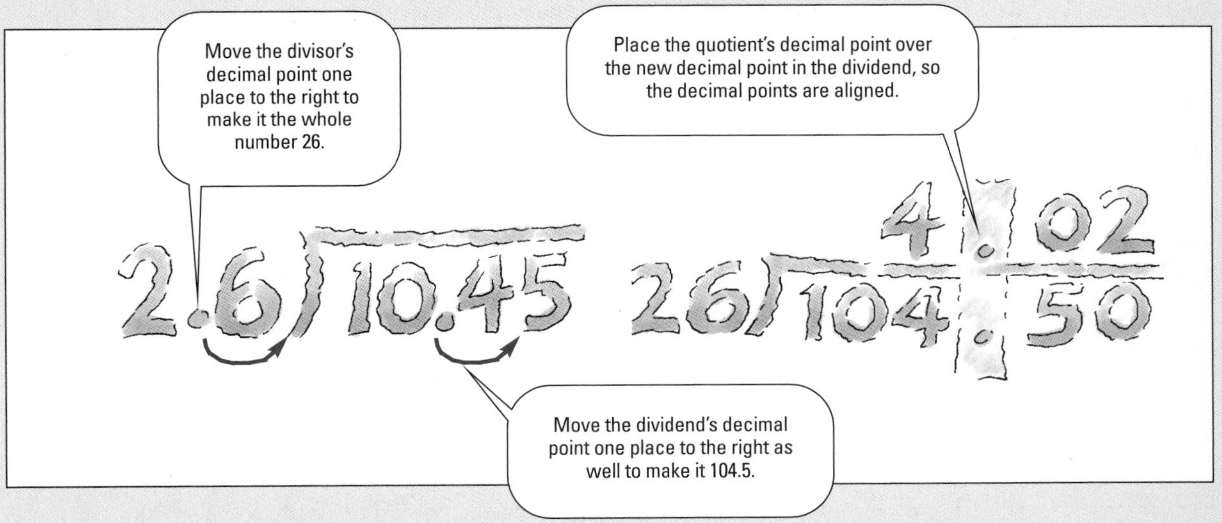

Move the divisor's decimal point one place to the right to make it the whole number 26.
Place the quotient's decimal point over the new decimal point in the dividend, so the decimal points are aligned.
2.6)10.45
4.02
26)104.50
Move the dividend's decimal point one place to the right as well to make it 104.5.

hundredths place — that is, to the number 2. Your rounded-off number is now 0.43.

Suppose the number that you delete is less than 5. Then don't add 1 to the number on the left. For example, to round off 1.9085 to the nearest tenth, identify the number in the tenths position (9) and delete all the numbers to the right of it (0, 8, and 5). Because the number directly to the right of 9 — the 0 — is less than 5, the number 9 stays the same. The number 1.9085 rounded off to the nearest tenth is 1.9.

A practice round

Try rounding off 14.723 to the nearest hundredth:

- First, decide what number is in the hundredths place (2) and delete all the numbers to the right of it (only the number 3).
- Because 3 is lower than 5, you don't add 1 to the 2. Thus, the rounded-off number is 14.72.

Now, round off 0.9875 to the nearest thousandth:

- The number in the thousandth place is 7. All numbers to the right of the 7 — the 5 — will be deleted.
- Because the number to be deleted is a 5, the 7 is rounded *up* to 8 (7 + 1). The rounded-off number is therefore 0.988.

Converting fractions

Many measuring devices have metric calibrations, so you'll often need to convert common fractions to decimal fractions. At times, you may also need to convert decimal fractions back into common fractions.

Converting common fractions to decimal fractions

Changing a common, proper fraction into a decimal fraction is simple. Just divide the numerator by the denominator. Add a zero as a placeholder to the left of the decimal point.

Commence converting

For example, here's how to convert $\frac{4}{10}$ to a decimal fraction:

$$\frac{4}{10} = 4 \div 10 = 10\overset{0.4}{\overline{)4.0}}$$

Keep on converting

Here are two more examples. First, convert $\frac{2}{5}$ to a decimal fraction:

$$\frac{2}{5} = 2 \div 5 = 5\overset{0.4}{\overline{)2.0}}$$

Next, convert $\frac{3}{8}$ to a decimal fraction:

$$\frac{3}{8} = 3 \div 8 = 8\overset{0.375}{\overline{)3.000}}$$

Converting mixed numbers to decimal fractions

How do you convert a mixed number to a decimal fraction? First, convert it to an improper fraction and then divide the numerator by the denominator, as shown above.

Remember rounding

When rounding, remember that 5 is the magic number. Check the number to the right of the decimal place that will be rounded off. If that number is 5 or greater, then add 1 to the place. If it's less than 5, leave the number alone.

For example, round off the following numbers to the nearest hundredths:

- 6.447
- 2.992
- 4.119

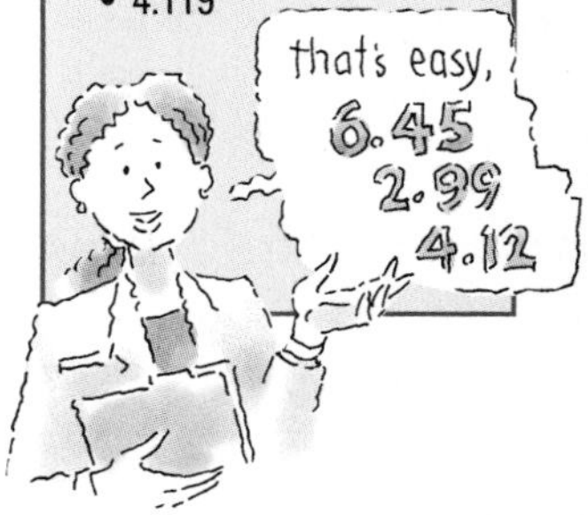

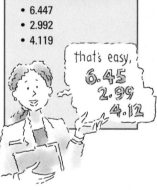

Mixing it up

Here's an example. To convert $4\frac{3}{4}$ to a decimal fraction, first convert the mixed number $4\frac{3}{4}$ to the improper fraction, $\frac{19}{4}$. Then divide 19 by 4 to find the decimal fraction:

$$4\tfrac{3}{4} = \tfrac{19}{4} = 19 \div 4 = \begin{array}{r} 4.75 \\ 4\overline{)19.00} \end{array}$$

Let's see that again

Here are two more calculations to try. First, convert $10\frac{7}{8}$ to a decimal fraction:

$$10\tfrac{7}{8} = \tfrac{87}{8} = 87 \div 8 = \begin{array}{r} 10.88 \\ 8\overline{)87.00} \end{array}$$

Note that the quotient above has been rounded off to the nearest hundredth.

Next, convert $1\frac{2}{9}$ to a decimal fraction:

$$1\tfrac{2}{9} = \tfrac{11}{9} = 11 \div 9 = \begin{array}{r} 1.22 \\ 9\overline{)11.00} \end{array}$$

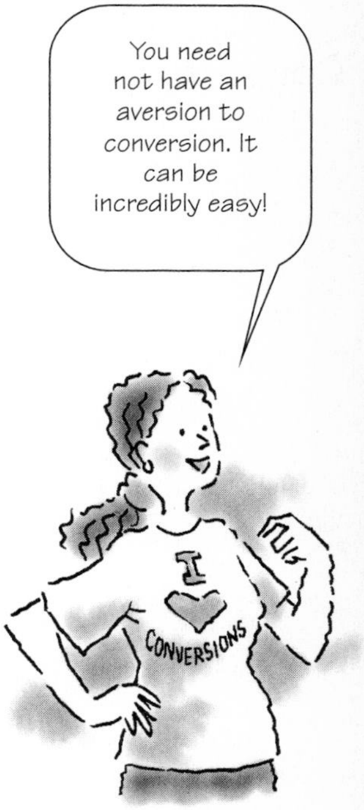

You need not have an aversion to conversion. It can be incredibly easy!
I ♥ CONVERSIONS

Converting decimal fractions to common fractions

To convert a decimal fraction to a common fraction, count the number of decimal places in the decimal fraction. This number reflects the number of zeros in the denominator of the common fraction.

For example, to convert the decimal fraction 0.33 into a common fraction, follow these steps:

1. Count the number of decimal places in 0.33. There are two decimal places, so the denominator of its common fraction is 100 because 100 has two zeros.
2. Remove the decimal point from 0.33 and use this number as the numerator. Reduce the fraction, if possible.

The calculation looks like this:

$$0.33 = \frac{33}{100}$$

This fraction can't be reduced further.

Practice, practice, practice

Try two more calculations. First, convert 0.413 to a common fraction. Here, the denominator is 1,000 because the decimal fraction (0.413) has three places after the decimal point.

The calculation looks like this:

$$0.413 = \frac{413}{1{,}000}$$

This fraction can't be reduced further.

Now convert 0.65 to a common fraction. The denominator is 100 because this decimal fraction has two places after the decimal point.

The calculation looks like this:

$$0.65 = \frac{65}{100} = \frac{13}{20}$$

Note that this fraction has been reduced to its lowest terms.

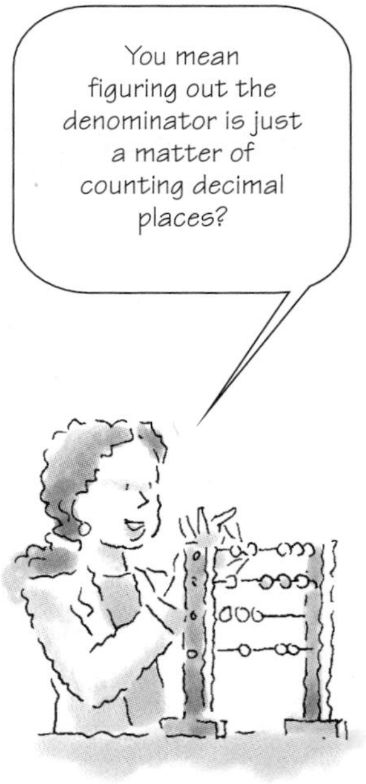

You mean figuring out the denominator is just a matter of counting decimal places?

Converting decimal fractions to mixed numbers

Use the same method as described previously to convert a decimal fraction to a mixed number (or to an improper fraction).

Mixed up but methodical

For example, to convert 5.75 to a fraction, use 100 as the denominator because 5.75 has two decimal places. Then convert the fraction to a mixed number.

The calculation looks like this:

$$5.75 = \frac{575}{100} = 5\,{}^{75}\!/_{100} = 5\,{}^{3}\!/_{4}$$

Note that this mixed number has been reduced to its lowest terms.

That was beautiful! Do it again!

Below are two more sample calculations. First, convert 3.25 to a fraction. Use 100 as the denominator because 3.25 has two decimal places. Then convert the fraction to a mixed number.

The calculation looks like this:

$$3.25 = \frac{325}{100} = 3\,{}^{25}\!/_{100} = 3\,{}^{1}\!/_{4}$$

Note that this mixed number has been reduced.

Once more and you got it!

Convert 1.9 to a fraction. Use 10 as the denominator because 1.9 has one decimal place. Then convert the fraction to a mixed number.

The calculation looks like this:

$$1.9 = \frac{19}{10} = 1\tfrac{9}{10}$$

Note that this mixed number can't be further reduced.

A point about percents

When you see %, the percent sign, think "for every hundred." Why? Because percentage means any quantity stated as parts per hundred. In other words, 75% is actually $\frac{75}{100}$ because the percent sign takes the place of the denominator 100.

Understanding percentages

Percentages are another way to express fractions and numerical relationships. The percent symbol may be used with a whole number such as 21%, a mixed number such as $34\frac{1}{2}$%, a decimal number such as 0.9%, or a fraction such as $\frac{1}{8}$%. (See *A point about percents.*)

From discounts to drug doses

You use percentages in everyday life when figuring department store discounts or restaurant tips. You also use them in nursing when calculating solutions and drug doses. Because percentages are such an important part of your work, you must know how to convert easily from percentages to decimal fractions and common fractions and vice versa.

Converting percentages to decimals

To change a percentage to a decimal fraction, remove the % sign and multiply the number in the percentage by $\frac{1}{100}$, or 0.01. For example, you would convert 84% and 35% to decimal fractions in this way:

$$84 \times 0.01 = 0.84$$

$$35 \times 0.01 = 0.35$$

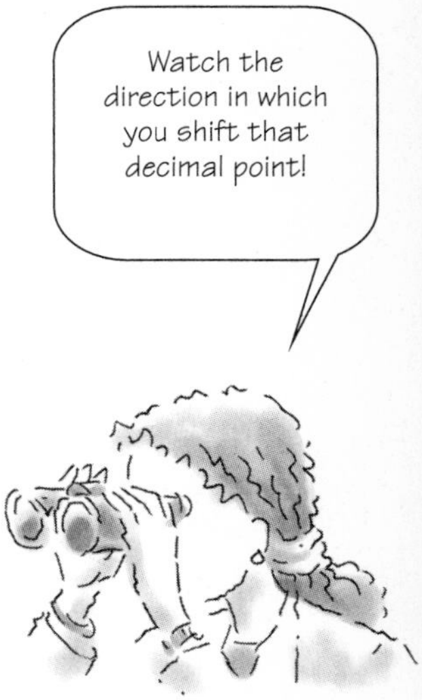

Watch the direction in which you shift that decimal point!

Watch that decimal point!

Make sure that you shift the decimal point in the right direction (to the left, when converting a percentage to a decimal); otherwise you could calculate a drug dose incorrectly. (See *From percentages to decimals [and back again]*, page 38.)

Converting percentages to common fractions

Suppose you want to convert 50% to a common fraction. To convert a percentage to a common fraction, follow these steps:

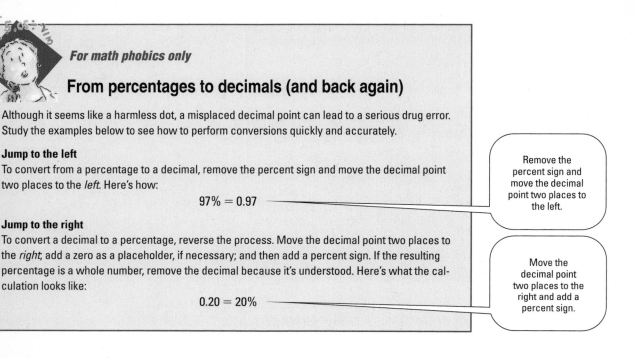

For math phobics only

From percentages to decimals (and back again)

Although it seems like a harmless dot, a misplaced decimal point can lead to a serious drug error. Study the examples below to see how to perform conversions quickly and accurately.

Jump to the left

To convert from a percentage to a decimal, remove the percent sign and move the decimal point two places to the *left*. Here's how:

$$97\% = 0.97$$

Remove the percent sign and move the decimal point two places to the left.

Jump to the right

To convert a decimal to a percentage, reverse the process. Move the decimal point two places to the *right*; add a zero as a placeholder, if necessary; and then add a percent sign. If the resulting percentage is a whole number, remove the decimal because it's understood. Here's what the calculation looks like:

$$0.20 = 20\%$$

Move the decimal point two places to the right and add a percent sign.

First, remove the percent sign and put the decimal point two places to the left, creating the decimal fraction 0.50:

$$50\% = 0.50$$

Next, convert 0.50 to a common fraction with a denominator that's a factor of 10. The result is $^{50}\!/_{100}$ because 0.50 has two decimal places:

$$0.50 = \frac{50}{100}$$

Lastly, reduce the fraction to its lowest terms, which is ½:

$$\frac{50}{100} = \frac{1}{2}$$

so,

$$50\% = \frac{1}{2}$$

Incredible! Do it again!

Here's another example. To convert 32.7% to a common fraction, remove the percent sign and put the decimal point two places to the left, creating the decimal fraction 0.327. Convert 0.327 to a common fraction using 1,000 as the denominator because 0.327 has three decimal places:

$$32.7\% = 0.327 = \frac{327}{1{,}000}$$

The result is $327/1{,}000$, a fraction that's already reduced to its lowest terms.

Again?

All right, here's one last example: To convert 20.05% to a common fraction, remove the percent sign and put the decimal point two places to the left, creating the decimal fraction 0.2005. Use 10,000 as the denominator because 0.2005 has four decimal places:

$$20.05\% = 0.2005 = \frac{2{,}005}{10{,}000} = \frac{401}{2{,}000}$$

The result is $2{,}005/10{,}000$, which becomes $401/2{,}000$ when reduced.

Converting common fractions to percentages

Converting a common fraction to a percentage involves two simple steps. Suppose you want to convert $2/5$ to a percentage. First, create a decimal fraction by dividing the numerator, 2, by the denominator, 5. You can do this by hand or with a calculator. (See *Thank heaven for calculators*.)

Thank heaven for calculators

A calculator can simplify converting a common fraction to a decimal fraction. For example, to convert a mixed number like $2\frac{4}{5}$ to a decimal fraction, first convert it to the improper fraction $14/5$. Then follow these steps on the calculator:

1. Enter the numerator, 14.
2. Press ÷.
3. Enter the denominator, 5.
4. Press = to obtain the converted number, 2.8.

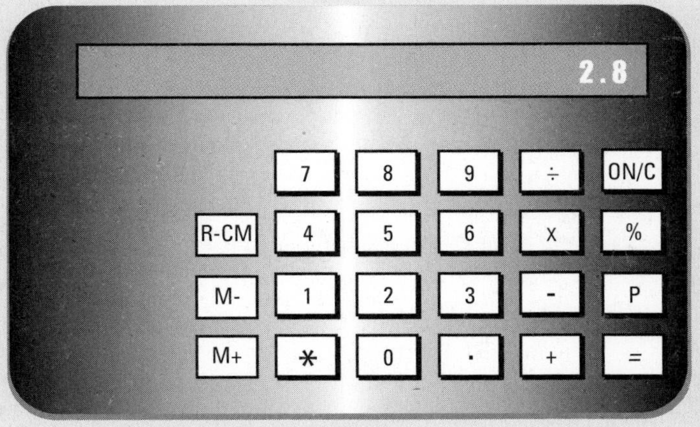

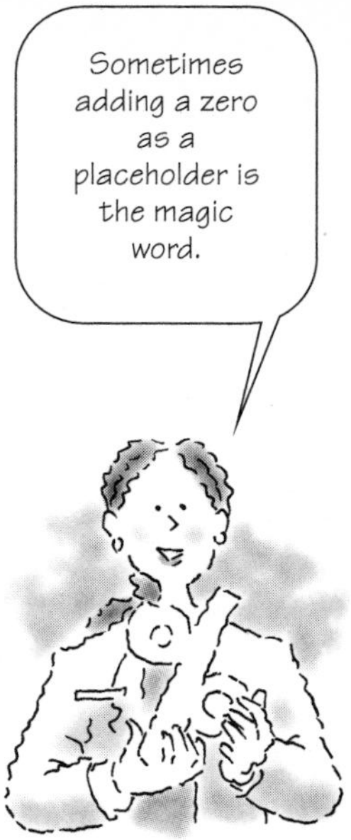

Sometimes adding a zero as a placeholder is the magic word.

The calculation looks like this:

$$\frac{2}{5} = 2 \div 5 = 5\overset{0.4}{\overline{)2.0}}$$

Next, convert the decimal fraction to a percentage by moving the decimal point two places to the right (you'll need to add a 0 as a placeholder) and then adding the percent sign.

Here's what the calculation looks like:

$$0.40 = 40\%$$

More practice to make you perfect

Here's a second example. To convert ⅓ to a percentage, create a decimal fraction by dividing 1 by 3. Round off the quotient to two decimal places:

$$\frac{1}{3} = 1 \div 3 = 0.333 = 0.33$$

Then convert the decimal fraction to a percentage by moving the decimal point two places to the right and adding the percent sign:

$$0.33 = 33\%$$

Once more to make sure

Here's a third example. To convert ⅜ to a percentage, create a decimal fraction by dividing 3 by 8:

$$\frac{3}{8} = 3 \div 8 = 0.375$$

Then convert the decimal fraction to a percentage by moving the decimal point two places to the right and adding the percent sign.

The result is:

$$0.375 = 37.5\%$$

Solving percentage problems

Solving percentage problems involves three types of calculations. They are:

- finding a percentage of a number
- finding what percentage one number is of another
- finding a number when a percentage of it is known. (See *Percentage problems: Watch the wording.*)

Percentage problems: Watch the wording

When a percentage problem is worded this way: "What is 25% of 80?" mentally change the *of* to a multiplication sign so the problem becomes "What is 25% (or, using a decimal fraction, .25) × 80?" Then continue with the calculation. (The answer is 20.)

If a problem is worded as "25 is what percentage of 80?" treat the *what* as a division sign so the problem becomes 25⁄80. Then continue with the calculation. (The answer is 0.3125, or 31.25%.)

You'll have an easier time solving these calculations if you follow a few simple guidelines.

Finding a percentage of a number

The question "What is 40% of 200?" is an example of the first type of calculation. To solve it, change the word *of* to a multiplication sign. This gives you:

$$40\% \times 200 = ?$$

Next, convert 40% to a decimal fraction by removing the percent sign and moving the decimal point two places to the left. This gives you:

$$40\% = 0.40$$

Then multiply the two numbers to get the answer, 80:

$$0.40 \times 200 = 80$$

40% of 200 is 80.

Practice time (again)

Now, try solving the problem, "What is 5% of 150?" First, restate it as a multiplication problem:

$$5\% \times 150 = ?$$

Next, convert 5% to the decimal fraction 0.05:

$$5\% = 0.05$$

Then multiply the two numbers to get the answer, 7.5:

$$0.05 \times 150 = 7.5$$

5% of 150 is 7.5.

Therefore, 7.5 is 5% of 150.

More practice (and you thought the piano was rough)

Here's one more example: "What is 7% of 300?" First, restate the question as a multiplication problem:

$$7\% \times 300 = ?$$

Convert 7% to the decimal fraction 0.07:

$$7\% = 0.07$$

Then multiply the two numbers to get the answer, 21:

$$0.07 \times 300 = 21$$

21 is 7% of 300.

Finding what percentage one number is of another

The question "10 is what percentage of 200?" is an example of this type of calculation. To solve it, restate the question as a division problem, with the number 10 as the dividend and the number 200 as the divisor. Here's how the calculation looks so far:

$$\begin{array}{r} 0.05 \\ 200\overline{)10.00} \end{array}$$

Now, move the decimal point in the quotient two places to the right and add a percent sign:

$$0.05 = 5\%$$

10 is 5% of 200.

Again (with a twist)

This type of problem can also be expressed in this way: "What percentage of 28 is 14?" To solve it, restate the question as a division problem by making 28 the divisor and 14 the dividend:

$$\begin{array}{r} 0.50 \\ 28\overline{)14.00} \end{array}$$

Then move the decimal point two places to the right and add a percent sign:

$$0.50 = 50\%$$

14 is 50% of 28.

One more time

Here's one last problem: "What percentage of 30 is 6?" First, restate the question as a division problem by making 30 the divisor and 6 the dividend:

$$\begin{array}{r} 0.20 \\ 30\overline{)6.00} \end{array}$$

Move the decimal point two places to the right and add a percent sign:

$$0.20 = 20\%$$

6 is 20% of 30.

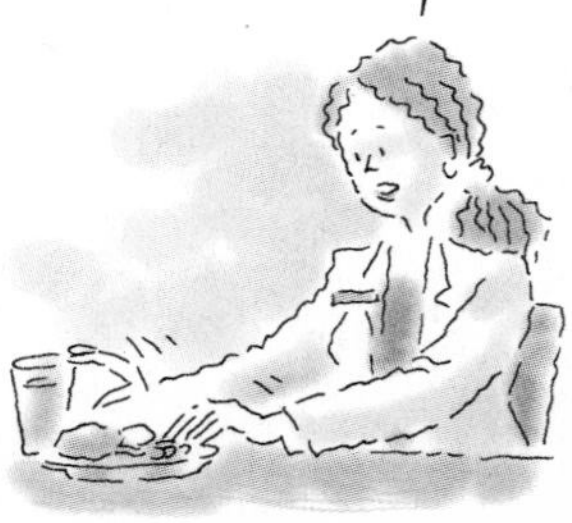
What to do with leftovers is always a challenge. In percentages, just make a common fraction.

What to do with the remainder

Sometimes, when determining what percentage one number is of another number, the divisor won't divide exactly into the dividend. In these cases, state the quotient as a mixed number by turning the remainder — the undivided part of the quotient — into a common fraction.

Here's how to do this using the problem, "3 is what percentage of 11?"

Restate the question as a division problem, making 11 the divisor and 3 the dividend. Work out the quotient to two places; then take the remainder, 3, and make it the numerator of a fraction with the divisor, 11, as the denominator.

Here's what the calculation looks like:

$$\begin{array}{r} 0.27 \\ 11\overline{)3.00} \\ \underline{2\,2} \\ 80 \\ \underline{77} \\ 3 \end{array}$$

The remainder as a common fraction is $3/11$.

Move the decimal point in the quotient two places to the right and add a percent sign. (The remaining fraction, $3/11$, is placed to the left of the percent sign.)

$$0.27 \text{ and } 3/11 = 27\,3/11\%$$

Back to practice

Let's try a second problem: "5 is what percent of 22?"

Restate the question as a division problem, leaving the remainder after two places as a common fraction:

$$\begin{array}{r} 0.22 \\ 22\overline{)5.00} \\ \underline{4\,4} \\ 60 \\ \underline{44} \\ 16 \end{array}$$

The remainder as a common fraction is $16/22$ (reduce to $8/11$).

Move the decimal point in the quotient two places to the right and add a percent sign:

$$0.22\,8/11 = 22\,8/11\%$$

Just can't get enough of those mixed number quotients

Here's the last example: "13 is what percentage of 45?" Restate the question as a division problem, leaving the remainder after two places as a common fraction:

$$\begin{array}{r} 0.28 \\ 45\overline{)13.00} \\ \underline{9\,0} \\ 4\,00 \\ \underline{3\,60} \\ 40 \end{array}$$

The remainder as a common fraction is $\frac{40}{45}$ (reduce to $\frac{8}{9}$).

Move the decimal point in the quotient two places to the right and add a percent sign:

$$0.28\tfrac{8}{9} = 28\tfrac{8}{9}\%$$

Finding a number when you know a percentage of it

The third type of problem, finding a number when you know a percentage of it, also requires division. For example, consider the following question: "70% of what number is 7?" Here's how to do this calculation.

First, convert 70% into a decimal fraction by removing the percent sign and moving the decimal point two places to the left:

$$70\% = 0.70$$

Next, divide 7 by 0.70. Move the decimal point two places to the right in both the divisor (to make it a whole number) and the dividend. The quotient is 10:

$$0.70\overline{)7.00\ 0} = 10.0$$

70% of 10 is 7.

Do you feel perfect yet?

Now try the problem "30% of what number is 90?" To solve it, convert 30% to a decimal fraction by removing the percent sign and moving the decimal point two places to the left:

$$30\% = 0.30$$

Then divide 90 by 0.30. Move the decimal point two places to the right in both the divisor (to make it a whole number) and the dividend. The quotient is 300.

$$0.30\overline{)90.000} = 300.0$$

30% of 300 is 90.

Now you're getting the hang of it!

Here's a third example: "70% of what number is 28?" To solve this problem, convert 70% to a decimal fraction by removing the percent sign and moving the decimal point two places to the left:

$$70\% = 0.70$$

Then divide 28 by 0.70. Move the decimal point two places to the right in both the divisor (to make it a whole number) and the dividend. The quotient is 40:

$$0.70\overline{)28.00\ 0}\quad = 40.0$$

70% of 40 is 28.

Real world problem

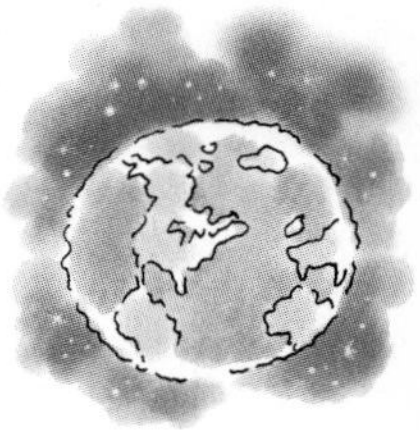

The patient received 600 ml of I.V. fluid out of 1,000 ml that was ordered. What percentage of I.V. fluid did the patient receive?

Devising the division

What you really want to find out in this problem is "600 is what percentage of 1,000?"

- First, restate it as a division problem, with 600 as the dividend and 1,000 as the divisor:

$$\begin{array}{r} 0.60 \\ 1000\overline{)600.00} \\ \underline{6000} \\ 00 \end{array}$$

- Next, move the decimal point in the quotient two places to the right and add a percent sign:

$$0.60 = 60\%$$

So, 600 is 60% of 1,000.

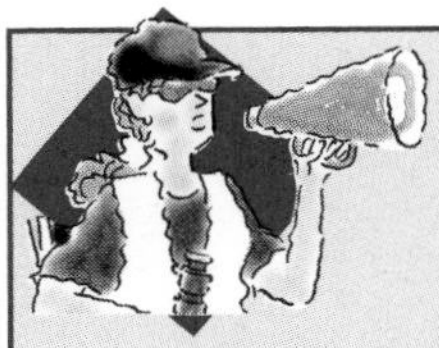

That's a wrap!

Decimals and percentages review

Keep in mind these important facts when working with decimals and percentages.

Decimals and percentages

- A decimal fraction is a proper fraction in which the denominator is a power of 10, signified by a decimal point placed at the left of the numerator.
- Each number or place to the left of the decimal point represents a whole number that's a power of 10.
- Each place to the right of the decimal point represents a fraction whose denominator is a power of 10.
- A percentage is any quantity stated as parts per hundred (the percent sign takes the place of the denominator 100).

Writing decimals

- Eliminate zeros to the right of the decimal point that don't appear before other numbers.

(continued)

Decimals and percentages review *(continued)*

• Always place a zero to the left of the decimal point if no other number appears there.

Adding and subtracting decimals

• Align the decimal points vertically.

• Use zeros to maintain column alignment.

Multiplying decimals

• Don't move decimal points.

• The number of decimal places in the product equals the sum of the decimal places in the numbers multiplied.

Dividing decimals

• When a whole number is the divisor, place the quotient's decimal point directly above the dividend's decimal point.

• When a decimal fraction is the divisor, move the divisor's decimal point to the right to convert to a whole number, then move the dividend's decimal point the same number of places to the right and, lastly, place the quotient's decimal point directly above the dividend's decimal point.

Rounding off decimals

• Check the number to the right of the decimal place that will be rounded off.

• If that number is less than 5, leave the number in the decimal place alone and delete the number less than 5.

• If that number is 5 or greater, add 1 to the decimal place and delete the number greater than 5.

Converting percentages to decimals

• Multiply the percentage number by $\frac{1}{100}$ (or 0.01).

• Or, shift the decimal two places to the left.

Converting decimals to percentages

• Divide the decimal fraction by $\frac{1}{100}$ (or 0.01).

• Or, shift the decimal two places to the right.

Converting percentages to common fractions

• Remove the percent sign.

• Move the decimal point two places to the left.

• Convert to a common fraction with a denominator that's a factor of 10.

Converting common fractions to percentages

• Divide the numerator by the denominator.

• Convert to a percentage by moving the decimal point two places to the right.

Finding a percentage of a number

• Restate as a multiplication problem by changing the word *of* to a multiplication sign.

• Convert the percentage to a decimal fraction.

• Multiply the two numbers.

Finding what percentage one number is of another

• Restate as a division problem.

• Convert the quotient to a percentage.

• If there's a remainder from the division problem, state the quotient as a mixed number by turning the remainder into a common fraction.

Finding a number when you know a percentage of it

• Convert the percentage into a decimal fraction.

• Divide the number by the decimal fraction.

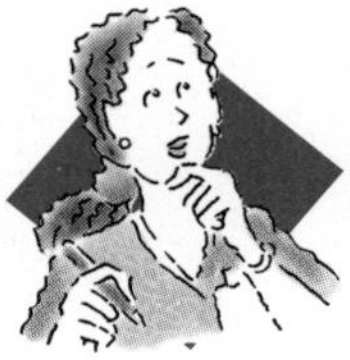

Quick quiz

1. What number is 16% of 79?

A. 0.20
B. 4.16
C. 4.93
D. 12.64

Answer: D. To solve this, restate the question as a multiplication problem. Convert 16% to a decimal fraction by removing the percent sign and moving the decimal point two places to the left. The decimal fraction is 0.16. Then multiply 0.16 by 79.

2. In the decimal fraction 1.2058, the tenths place is represented by what number?

A. 2
B. 0
C. 1
D. 5

Answer: A. The tenths place is to the immediate right of the decimal point.

3. When 3% is converted to a decimal fraction, it becomes what number?

A. 3.0
B. 0.30
C. 0.03
D. 0.33

Answer: C. Remove the percent sign and move the decimal point two places to the left.

4. Converting the common fraction ⅛ to a percentage yields which of the following?

A. 12.5%
B. 8%
C. ⅛%
D. 0.125%

Answer: A. To obtain 12.5, divide 1 by 8; then convert the answer to a percentage by moving the decimal point two places to the right and adding the percent sign.

5. The decimal fraction 1.9 divided by 3.2 yields what number?

A. 1.5
B. 0.59
C. 6.08
D. 10.55

Answer: B. To solve this, move the decimal points of both the divisor and the dividend one place to the right before dividing. Place the quotient's decimal point over the new decimal point in the dividend.

6. Multiplying 4.9 by 10.203 yields which product?
A. 49.9947
B. 49994.7
C. 0.499947
D. 499.947

Answer: A. When multiplying, the number of decimal places in the final product equals the sum of the decimal places in the numbers being multiplied. Count the decimal places starting from the right and place the decimal point there.

Scoring

☆☆☆ If you answered all six items correctly, that's 100% (or 6⁄6 or, if you prefer decimal fractions, 1.00).

☆☆ If you answered four or five items correctly, excellent! As they say, 4⁄6 to 5⁄6 ain't bad.

☆ If you answered fewer than four items correctly, here's what to do: Subtract the number you got right from 6 and add the result back to your score. Now you've got 100%. Reward yourself with a new calculator!

3

Ratios, fractions, proportions, and solving for X

Just the facts

In this chapter, you'll learn:

- definitions of ratios and proportions
- how to set up proportions using ratios and fractions
- how to solve for X in an equation
- how ratios, proportions, and solving for X relate to dosage calculations.

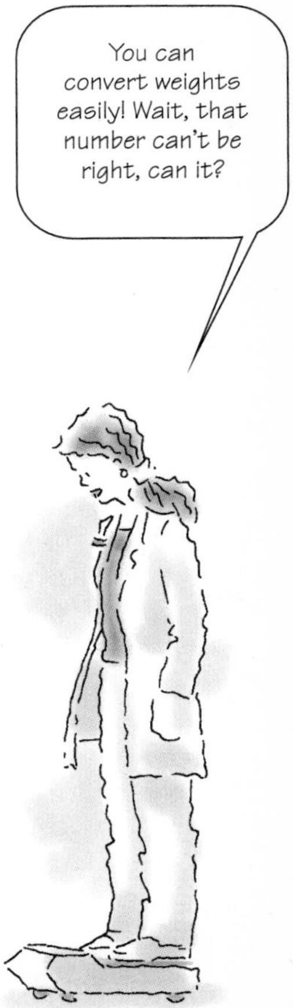
You can convert weights easily! Wait, that number can't be right, can it?

A look at numerical relationships

Ratios, fractions, and proportions describe relationships between numbers. Ratios use a colon between the numbers in the relationship, as in 4 : 9. Fractions use a slash between numbers in the relationship, as in 4⁄9.

Proportions are statements of equality between two ratios. For example, to show that 4 : 9 is equal to 8 : 18, you would write:

$$4:9::8:18$$

or

$$\frac{4}{9} = \frac{8}{18}$$

Three major problem solvers

When calculating dosages, you'll use ratios, fractions, and proportions frequently. You'll also use them to perform many other related tasks, such as calculating I.V. infusion rates, converting weights between systems of measurement and, in specialty settings, performing oxygenation and hemodynamic calculations. However, before you can use ratios, fractions, and proportions, you need to know how to develop and express them appropriately.

Ratios and fractions

Ratios and fractions are numerical ways to compare items.

Dare to compare

If 100 syringes come in 1 box, then the number of syringes compared to the number of boxes is 100 to 1. This can be written as the ratio 100 : 1 or as the fraction $^{100}/_{1}$.

Conversely, the number of boxes to syringes would be 1 : 100 or the fraction $^{1}/_{100}$, so pay attention to which item is mentioned first.

Twice more, with feeling

Here are two more examples.

If a hospital's critical care area requires 1 registered nurse for every 2 patients, then the relationship of registered nurses to patients is 1 to 2. You can express this with the ratio 1 : 2 or with the fraction $^{1}/_{2}$.

Suppose a vial has 8 mg of a drug in 1 ml of solution. By using a ratio, you can express this as 8 mg : 1 ml. By using a fraction, you can describe it as $^{8\text{ mg}}/_{1\text{ ml}}$.

Proportions

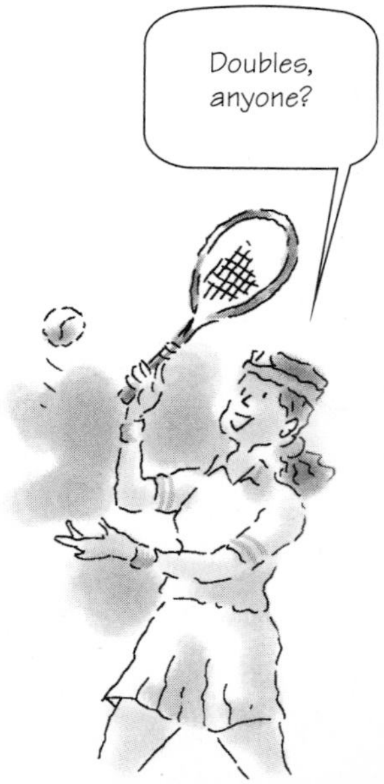

Any proportion that's expressed as two ratios also can be expressed as two fractions.

Using ratios in proportions

When using ratios in a proportion, separate them with double colons. Double colons represent equality between the two ratios.

For example, if the ratio of syringes to boxes is 100 : 1, then 200 syringes are provided in 2 boxes. This proportion can be written as:

$$100\text{ syringes} : 1\text{ box} :: 200\text{ syringes} : 2\text{ boxes}$$

or

$$100 : 1 :: 200 : 2$$

Proportion practice

Here's another example. If the critical care area has 1 nurse for every 2 patients, you can express this as the ratio 1 : 2. You can also say that this equals a ratio of 3 nurses for every 6 patients. In a proportion, you can express this relationship with the ratios:

1 nurse : 2 patients :: 3 nurses : 6 patients

or

1 : 2 :: 3 : 6

Another portion of proportions

Now, suppose you have a vial that contains 8 mg of a drug in 1 ml of a solution. You can state this as the ratio 8 mg : 1 ml, which equals 16 mg : 2 ml. This proportion can be expressed with ratios as follows:

8 mg : 1 ml :: 16 mg : 2 ml

or

8 : 1 :: 16 : 2

Using fractions in proportions

Any proportion that can be expressed with ratios can also be expressed with fractions. Here's how to do this using the previous examples.

If 100 syringes come in 1 box, this means that 200 syringes come in 2 boxes. Using fractions, you can write this proportion as:

$$\frac{100\text{ syringes}}{1\text{ box}} = \frac{200\text{ syringes}}{2\text{ boxes}}$$

or

$$\frac{100}{1} = \frac{200}{2}$$

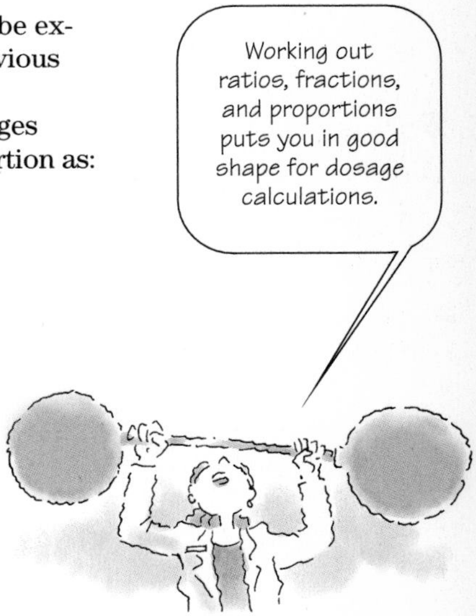

Working out ratios, fractions, and proportions puts you in good shape for dosage calculations.

Fraction action

If the critical care area has 1 nurse for every 2 patients, this means that it has 3 nurses for every 6 patients. Using fractions, you can express this relationship as:

$$\frac{1\text{ nurse}}{2\text{ patients}} = \frac{3\text{ nurses}}{6\text{ patients}}$$

or

$$\frac{1}{2} = \frac{3}{6}$$

Vial trial run

If there are 8 mg of a drug in 1 ml, this means there are 16 mg in 2 ml. This proportion can be expressed with fractions as:

$$\frac{8 \text{ mg}}{1 \text{ ml}} = \frac{16 \text{ mg}}{2 \text{ ml}}$$

or

$$\frac{8}{1} = \frac{16}{2}$$

Solving for *X*

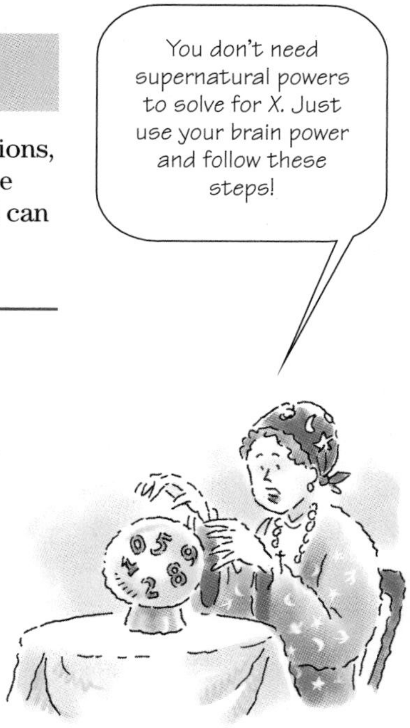

You don't need supernatural powers to solve for X. Just use your brain power and follow these steps!

We know that a proportion is a set of two equal ratios or fractions, but what if one ratio or fraction is incomplete? In this case, the unknown part of the ratio or fraction is represented by *X*. You can solve for *X* to determine the value of the unknown quantity.

Solving common-fraction equations

The method used to solve common-fraction equations forms the basis for solving other types of simple equations to find the value of *X*. For example, here's how to solve the common-fraction equation:

$$X = \frac{1}{5} \times \frac{3}{9}$$

1. Multiply the numerators:

$$1 \times 3 = 3$$

2. Multiply the denominators:

$$5 \times 9 = 45$$

3. Restate the equation with this new information:

$$X = \frac{1 \times 3}{5 \times 9} = \frac{3}{45}$$

Reduce the fraction by dividing the numerator and denominator by the lowest common denominator (3), to find that $X = \frac{1}{15}$.

$$X = \frac{3 \div 3}{45 \div 3} = \frac{1}{15}$$

Most dosage calculations require your answer to be in decimal form, so convert $\frac{1}{15}$ to a decimal fraction by dividing the numerator by the denominator. Round the answer off to the nearest hundredth. The final result is $X = 0.07$.

$$X = \frac{1}{15} = 1 \div 15 = 0.07$$

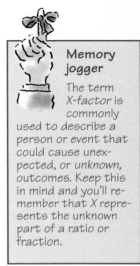

Memory jogger

The term *X-factor* is commonly used to describe a person or event that could cause unexpected, or unknown, outcomes. Keep this in mind and you'll remember that *X* represents the unknown part of a ratio or fraction.

Try this *X*-ample

Now, solve for *X* in the equation:

$$X = \frac{2}{3} \times \frac{5}{8}$$

Multiply the numerators:

$$2 \times 5 = 10$$

Multiply the denominators:

$$3 \times 8 = 24$$

Restate the equation with this new information:

$$X = \frac{2 \times 5}{3 \times 8} = \frac{10}{24}$$

Reduce the fraction by dividing the numerator and denominator by the lowest common denominator (2), to find that $X = \frac{5}{12}$.

$$X = \frac{10 \div 2}{24 \div 2} = \frac{5}{12}$$

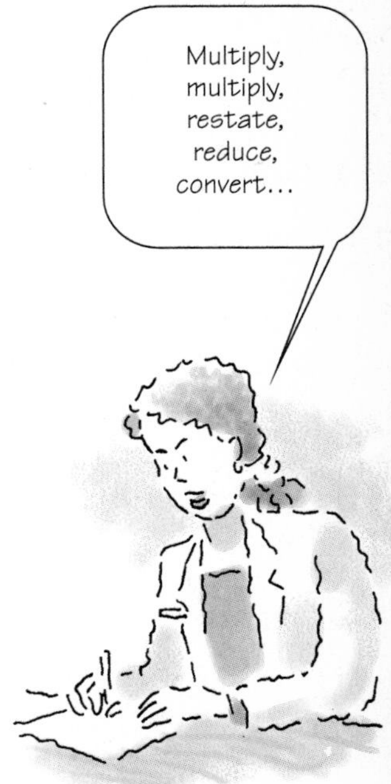
Multiply, multiply, restate, reduce, convert...

Convert $5/12$ to a decimal fraction by dividing the numerator by the denominator and then rounding it off. The final result is $X = 0.42$.

$$X = \frac{5}{12} = 5 \div 12 = 0.42$$

Here comes a curveball

This example has a twist—the whole number 3 is involved. (See *Making whole numbers fractions.*)

Here's how to solve for X in an equation with a whole number:

$$X = \frac{125}{500} \times 3$$

Convert the whole number 3 into the fraction $3/1$. The equation becomes:

$$X = \frac{125}{500} \times \frac{3}{1}$$

Next, reduce $125/500$ by dividing the numerator and denominator by the lowest common denominator (125) to get $1/4$. The equation becomes:

$$X = \frac{125 \div 125}{500 \div 125} \times \frac{3}{1}$$

or

$$X = \frac{1}{4} \times \frac{3}{1}$$

Then proceed as usual.

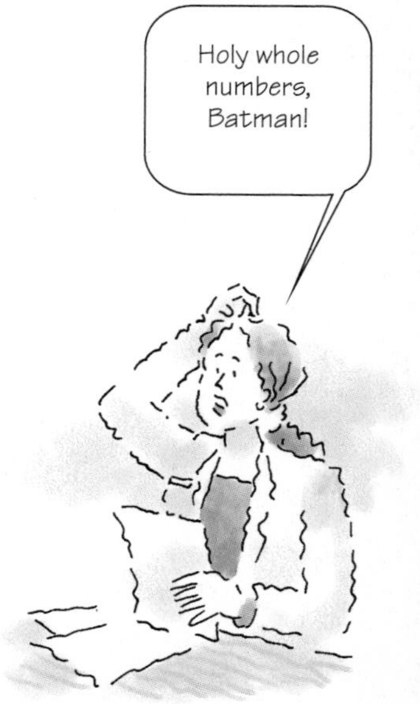
Holy whole numbers, Batman!

Multiply the numerators:

$$1 \times 3 = 3$$

Multiply the denominators:

$$4 \times 1 = 4$$

Restate the equation with this new information:

$$X = \frac{1 \times 3}{4 \times 1} = \frac{3}{4}$$

The fraction ¾ can't be reduced. Convert it to a decimal fraction by dividing the numerator by the denominator. The final result is $X = 0.75$.

$$X = \frac{3}{4} = 3 \div 4 = 0.75$$

For math phobics only

Making whole numbers fractions

You can change any whole number into a fraction by making the whole number the numerator and placing it over a 1, which is the denominator. The value of the number doesn't change.

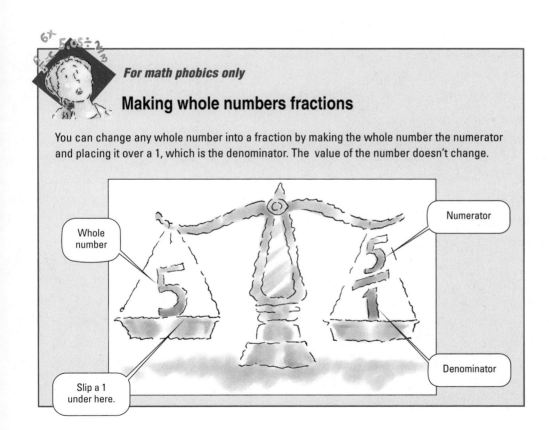

Solving decimal-fraction equations

To solve for X in equations with decimal fractions, use a method similar to that used in the previous examples. Here's how to solve for X in the equation:

$$X = \frac{0.05}{0.02} \times 3$$

Remove the decimal points from the fraction by moving them two spaces to the right. Then remove the zeros. The equation becomes:

$$X = \frac{5}{2} \times 3$$

Next, convert the whole number 3 to the fraction $3/1$. The equation becomes:

$$X = \frac{5}{2} \times \frac{3}{1}$$

Then multiply the numerators:

$$5 \times 3 = 15$$

Multiply the denominators:

$$2 \times 1 = 2$$

Restate the equation with this new information:

$$X = \frac{5 \times 3}{2 \times 1} = \frac{15}{2}$$

Convert the answer to decimal form by dividing 15 by 2. The final result is $X = 7.5$.

$$X = \frac{15}{2} = 15 \div 2 = 7.5$$

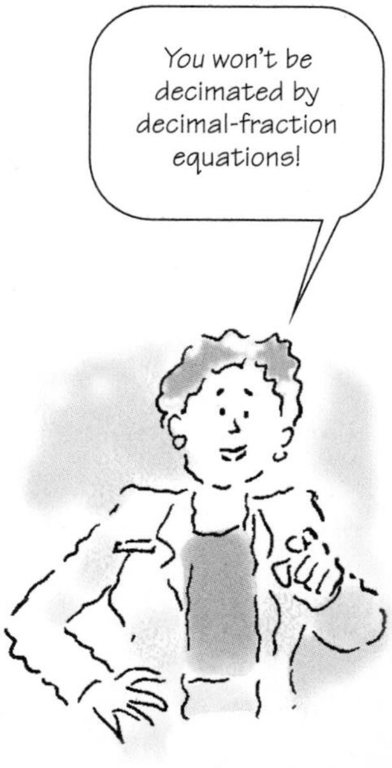

You won't be decimated by decimal-fraction equations!

X-tra credit

Here's another practice problem:

$$X = \frac{0.33}{0.11} \times 0.6$$

Remove the decimal points from the fraction by moving them two spaces to the right. Then remove the zeros. The equation becomes:

$$X = \frac{33}{11} \times 0.6$$

Convert the number 0.6 into the fraction $^{0.6}/_{1}$. The equation becomes:

$$X = \frac{33}{11} \times \frac{0.6}{1}$$

Multiply the numerators:

$$33 \times 0.6 = 19.8$$

Multiply the denominators:

$$11 \times 1 = 11$$

Restate the equation with this new information:

$$X = \frac{33 \times 0.6}{11 \times 1} = \frac{19.8}{11}$$

Convert the answer to decimal form by dividing 19.8 by 11. The final result is $X = 1.8$.

$$X = \frac{19.8}{11} = 19.8 \div 11 = 1.8$$

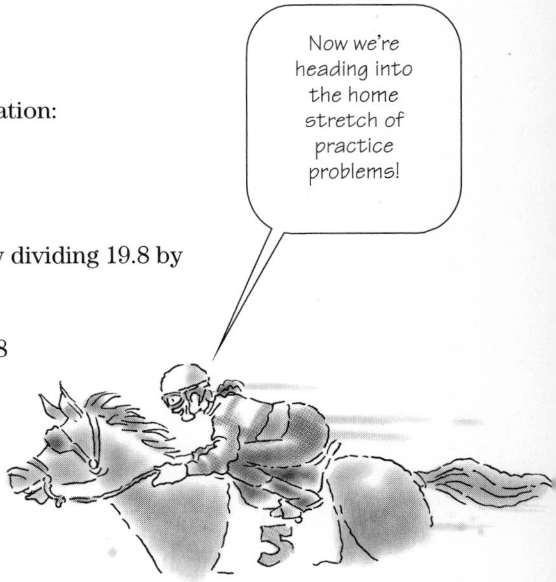

Now we're heading into the home stretch of practice problems!

X-tra, X-tra credit

Here's the last problem:

$$X = \frac{0.04}{0.05} \times 4$$

Remove the decimal points from the fraction by moving them two places to the right. Then delete the zeros. The equation becomes:

$$X = \frac{4}{5} \times 4$$

Turn 4 into the fraction 4⁄1. The equation becomes:

$$X = \frac{4}{5} \times \frac{4}{1}$$

Multiply the numerators:

$$4 \times 4 = 16$$

Multiply the denominators:

$$5 \times 1 = 5$$

Restate the equation with this new information:

$$X = \frac{4 \times 4}{5 \times 1} = \frac{16}{5}$$

Convert the answer to decimal form by dividing 16 by 5. The final answer is $X = 3.2$.

$$X = \frac{16}{5} = 16 \div 5 = 3.2$$

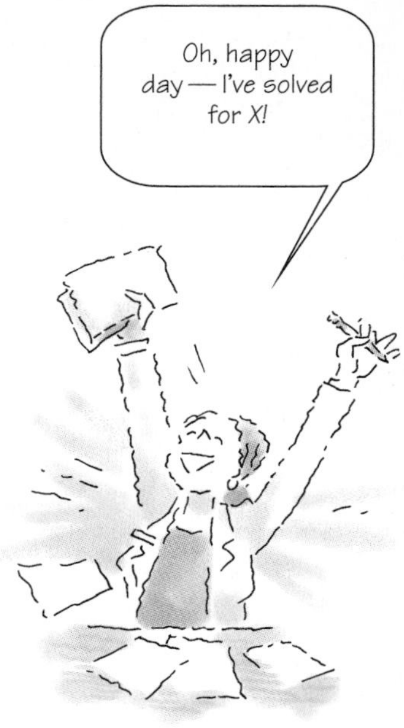

Oh, happy day — I've solved for X!

Solving proportion problems with ratios

A proportion can be written with ratios, as in:

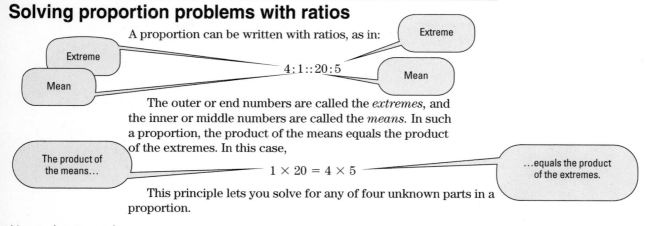

Extreme

Mean

$$4:1::20:5$$

Extreme

Mean

The outer or end numbers are called the *extremes*, and the inner or middle numbers are called the *means*. In such a proportion, the product of the means equals the product of the extremes. In this case,

The product of the means...

$$1 \times 20 = 4 \times 5$$

...equals the product of the extremes.

This principle lets you solve for any of four unknown parts in a proportion.

X marks another spot

Here's an example. Solve for *X* in the proportion:

$$4:8::8:X$$

Follow these steps:

Rewrite the problem so that the means and the extremes are multiplied:

$$8 \times 8 = 4 \times X$$

Obtain the products of the means and extremes and put them into an equation:

$$64 = 4X$$

Solve for *X* by dividing both sides by 4. Cancel the number (4) that appears in both the numerator and denominator. This isolates *X* on one side of the equation.

$$\frac{64}{4} = \frac{\cancel{4}X}{\cancel{4}}$$

Find *X*:

$$64 \div 4 = X$$

or

$$X = 16$$

Replace *X* with 16 and restate the proportion in ratios:

$$4:8::8:16$$

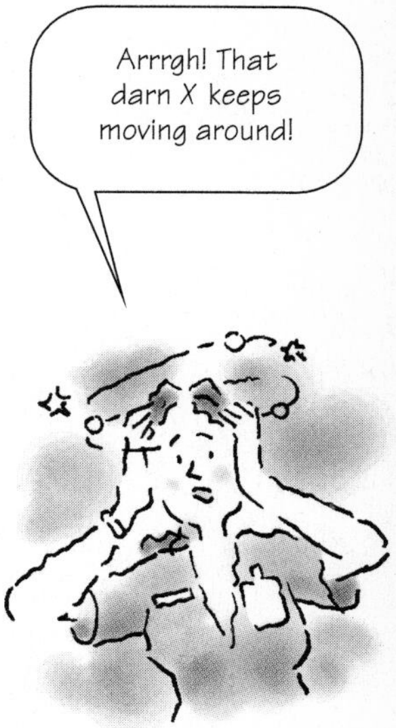
Arrrgh! That darn X keeps moving around!

X moves back to the front

Solve for *X* in the proportion:

$$X:12::6:24$$

Follow these steps:

Rewrite the problem so that the means and the extremes are multiplied:

$$12 \times 6 = X \times 24$$

Obtain the products of the means and extremes and put them into an equation:

$$72 = 24X$$

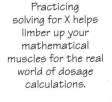

Solve for X by dividing both sides by 24. Cancel the number (24) that appears in both the numerator and denominator. This isolates X on one side of the equation:

$$\frac{72}{24} = \frac{\cancel{24}X}{\cancel{24}}$$

Find X:

$$72 \div 24 = X$$

or

$$X = 3$$

Replace X with 24 and restate the proportion in ratios:

$$3:12::6:24$$

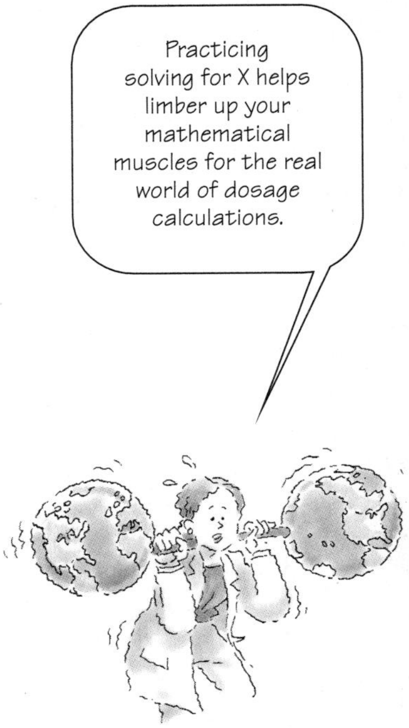

Practicing solving for X helps limber up your mathematical muscles for the real world of dosage calculations.

Another X-treme shift

Try one last problem, using this proportion:

$$10:20::X:40$$

Rewrite the problem so that the means and the extremes are multiplied:

$$20 \times X = 10 \times 40$$

Obtain the products of the means and extremes and put them into an equation:

$$20X = 400$$

Solve for X by dividing both sides by 20. Cancel the number (20) that appears in both the numerator and denominator. This isolates X on one side of the equation:

$$\frac{\cancel{20}X}{\cancel{20}} = \frac{400}{20}$$

Find X:

$$X = \frac{400}{20}$$

or

$$X = 20$$

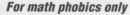

Replace X with 20 and restate the original proportion in ratios:

$$10:20::20:40$$

Solving proportion problems with fractions

Proportion problems may also be set up with fractions. In a proportion expressed as a fraction, cross products are equal—just as the means and extremes are equal in a proportion with ratios. (See *Cross product principle.*)

For math phobics only

Cross product principle

In a proportion expressed as fractions, cross products are equal. In other words, the numerator on the equation's left side multiplied by the denominator on the equation's right side equals the denominator on the equation's left side multiplied by the numerator on the equation's right side.

The above statement has a lot of words. The same meaning is communicated more simply in the illustration to the left below.

Applies to ratios as well

Note that the same principle applies to ratios. In a proportion expressed as ratios, the product of the **m**eans (numbers in the **m**iddle) equals the product of the **e**xtremes (numbers on the **e**nds). Consider the illustration to the right below.

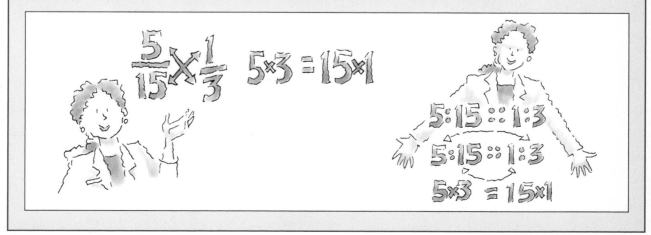

Using the cross products of a proportion, you can solve for any of four unknown parts. Once again, the position of the *X* doesn't matter because the cross products of a proportion are always equal. (See *Cross products to the rescue.*)

Keeping things in proportion

After studying the example in *Cross products to the rescue*, practice solving for *X* using this proportion:

$$\frac{3}{4} = \frac{9}{X}$$

Follow these steps:

1. Rewrite the problem so the cross products are multiplied:

$$3 \times X = 4 \times 9$$

2. Obtain the cross products and put them into an equation:

$$3X = 36$$

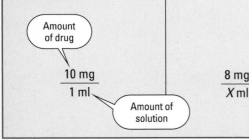

For math phobics only

Cross products to the rescue

Fractions can be used to describe the relative proportion of ingredients, for example, the amount of a drug relative to its solution.

Suppose you have a vial containing 10 mg/ml of morphine. You can write this fraction to describe it:

$$\frac{10 \text{ mg}}{1 \text{ ml}}$$

Amount of drug (10 mg) — Amount of solution (1 ml)

The plot thickens

Now suppose you need to administer 8 mg of morphine to your patient. How much of the solution should you use?

1. Write a second fraction using *X* to represent the amount of solution:

$$\frac{8 \text{ mg}}{X \text{ ml}}$$

An unknown quantity (*X* ml)

2. Set up the equation. Keep the fractions in the same relative proportion of drug to solution.

3. Rewrite the problem so cross products are multiplied:

$$\frac{10 \text{ mg}}{1 \text{ ml}} \quad \frac{8 \text{ mg}}{X \text{ ml}}$$

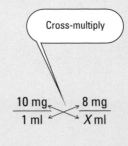

Cross-multiply

4. This gives you:

$$10X = 8$$

5. Solve for *X* by dividing both sides by 10, and you're left with:

$$X = \frac{8}{10}$$

6. Convert this to a decimal fraction because you'll be drawing up medication and need to work with a decimal:

$$X = 0.8 \text{ ml}$$

The answer!

This is how much of the morphine you should use.

Solve for *X* by dividing both sides by 3. Cancel the number (3) that appears in both the numerator and denominator. This isolates *X* on one side of the equation:

$$\frac{\cancel{3}X}{\cancel{3}} = \frac{36}{3}$$

Find *X*:

$$X = \frac{36}{3}$$

or

$$X = 12$$

Replace the *X* with 12 and restate the proportion in fractions:

$$\frac{3}{4} = \frac{9}{12}$$

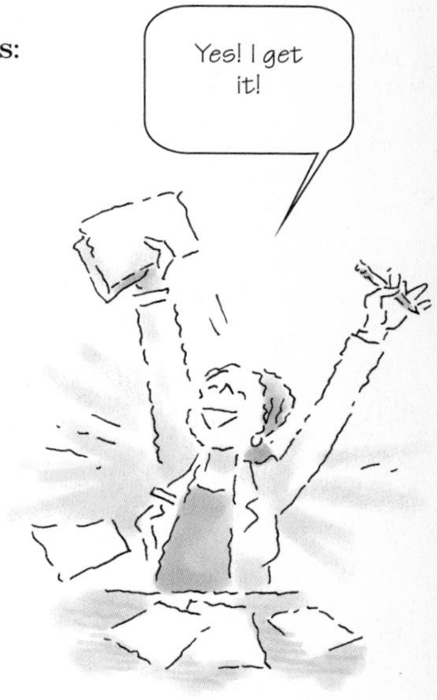

Final practice problem (Yippee!)

Solve one more problem:

$$\frac{12}{25} = \frac{X}{50}$$

Rewrite the problem so the cross products are multiplied:

$$12 \times 50 = 25 \times X$$

Obtain the cross products and put them into an equation:

$$600 = 25X$$

Solve for *X* by dividing both sides by 25:

$$\frac{600}{25} = \frac{\cancel{25}X}{\cancel{25}}$$

Find *X*:

$$X = 24$$

Replace *X* with 24 and restate the proportion in fractions:

$$\frac{12}{25} = \frac{24}{50}$$

Real world problems

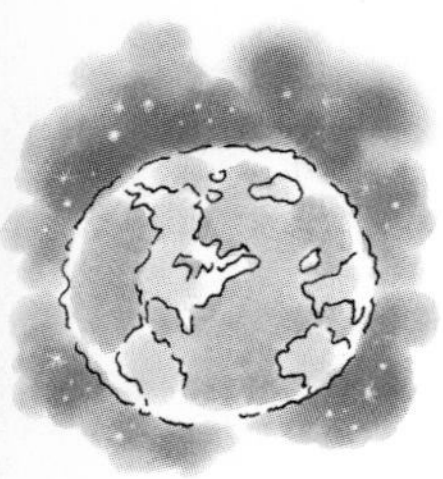

Next, you'll find three practical examples of proportions in everyday nursing practice.

How do you set up a proportion to solve a real world problem? Just place the known ratio on one side of the double colon and the unknown ratio on the other side. Make sure that the units of measure in each ratio are in the same positions on both sides of the proportion. (See *Write it down.*)

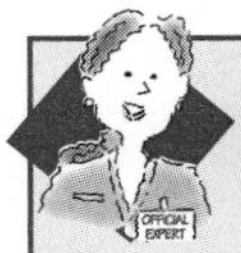

Advice from the experts

Write it down

When calculating dosages, you may be able to figure out some problems in your head. For instance, 4 mg in 2 ml is the same as 2 mg in 1 ml. If you're stumped, don't be shy about writing the proportion down on paper. Taking the time to see the numbers will help you avoid confusion and solve for *X* more quickly and accurately.

How much hydrogen peroxide?

Set up a proportion to find out how much hydrogen peroxide (H_2O_2) you should add to 1,000 ml of water (H_2O) to make a solution that contains 50 ml of H_2O_2 for every 100 ml of H_2O.

The ratio approach

To solve this problem using ratios, follow these steps:

1. Decide what part of the ratio is *X*. In this case, it's the amount of H_2O_2 in 1,000 ml of H_2O.

2. Set up the proportion so that similar parts of each ratio are in the same position:

$$X : 1{,}000 \text{ ml } H_2O :: 50 \text{ ml } H_2O_2 : 100 \text{ ml } H_2O$$

3. Multiply the means and the extremes and restate the problem as an equation:

$$1{,}000 \text{ ml } H_2O \times 50 \text{ ml } H_2O_2 = X \text{ ml } H_2O_2 \times 100 \text{ ml } H_2O$$

4. Solve for X by dividing both sides of the equation by 100 ml H_2O and canceling units that appear in both the numerator and denominator:

$$\frac{1{,}000 \cancel{\text{ ml } H_2O} \times 50 \text{ ml } H_2O_2}{100 \cancel{\text{ ml } H_2O}} = \frac{X \text{ ml } H_2O_2 \times \cancel{100 \text{ ml } H_2O}}{\cancel{100 \text{ ml } H_2O}}$$

5. Find *X:*

$$\frac{50{,}000 \text{ ml } H_2O_2}{100} = X$$

or

$$X = 500 \text{ ml } H_2O_2$$

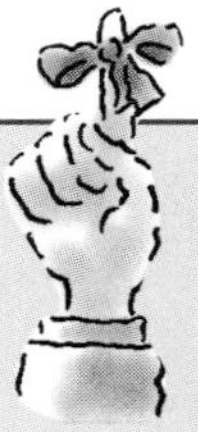

Memory jogger

When working with ratios, the product of the ***means*** always equals the product of the ***extremes***. To differentiate these terms, remember:

means (**m**iddle numbers)

extremes (**e**nd numbers)

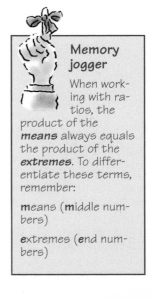

The fraction approach

If you set up a proportion with fractions, place similar units of measure for each fraction in the same position. Here's what the previous example looks like in fraction form:

$$\frac{X}{1{,}000 \text{ ml } H_2O} = \frac{50 \text{ ml } H_2O_2}{100 \text{ ml } H_2O}$$

Rewrite the equation by cross-multiplying the fractions:

$$X \times 100 \text{ ml } H_2O = 1{,}000 \text{ ml } H_2O \times 50 \text{ ml } H_2O_2$$

Solve for *X* by dividing both sides of the equation by 100 ml H_2O and canceling units that appear in both the numerator and denominator:

$$\frac{X \times \cancel{100 \text{ ml } H_2O}}{\cancel{100 \text{ ml } H_2O}} = \frac{1{,}000 \cancel{\text{ ml } H_2O} \times 50 \text{ ml } H_2O_2}{100 \cancel{\text{ ml } H_2O}}$$

Find *X*:

$$X = \frac{50{,}000 \text{ ml } H_2O_2}{100}$$

$$X = 500 \text{ ml } H_2O_2$$

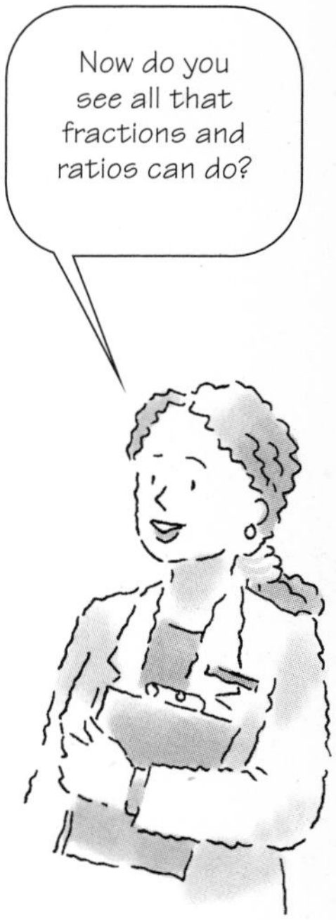

Now do you see all that fractions and ratios can do?

How many clinical instructors?

Set up another proportion problem with both ratios and fractions. If a school of nursing requires 1 clinical instructor for every 8 students, how many instructors are needed for a class of 24 students?

Resolving it with ratios

Use ratios first. Follow these steps:

Decide what part of the proportion is *X*. In this case, it's the number of instructors for 24 students.

Set up the proportion so that the units of measure (instructors and students) in each ratio are in the same position:

$$1 \text{ instructor} : 8 \text{ students} :: X : 24 \text{ students}$$

Multiply the means and the extremes and set up the equation:

$$8 \text{ students} \times X = 1 \text{ instructor} \times 24 \text{ students}$$

Solve for *X* by dividing both sides of the equation by 8 students and canceling units that appear in both the numerator and denominator:

$$\frac{\cancel{8\ \text{students}} \times X}{\cancel{8\ \text{students}}} = \frac{1\ \text{instructor} \times 24\ \cancel{\text{students}}}{8\ \cancel{\text{students}}}$$

$$X = \frac{24}{8}$$

Find *X*:

$$X = 3\ \text{instructors}$$

Figuring it out with fractions

If you prefer to solve the previous problem using fractions, follow these steps:

Set up the proportion so that the units of measure are in the same position in each fraction. Here's what the problem looks like in fraction form:

$$\frac{1\ \text{instructor}}{8\ \text{students}} = \frac{X}{24\ \text{students}}$$

Rewrite the equation by cross-multiplying the fractions:

$$1\ \text{instructor} \times 24\ \text{students} = X\ \text{instructors} \times 8\ \text{students}$$

Solve for *X* by dividing both sides of the equation by 8 students and canceling units that appear in both the numerator and denominator:

$$\frac{1\ \text{instructor} \times 24\ \cancel{\text{students}}}{8\ \cancel{\text{students}}} = \frac{X \times \cancel{8\ \text{students}}}{\cancel{8\ \text{students}}}$$

or

$$24 \div 8 = X\ \text{instructors}$$

Find *X*:

$$X = 3\ \text{instructors}$$

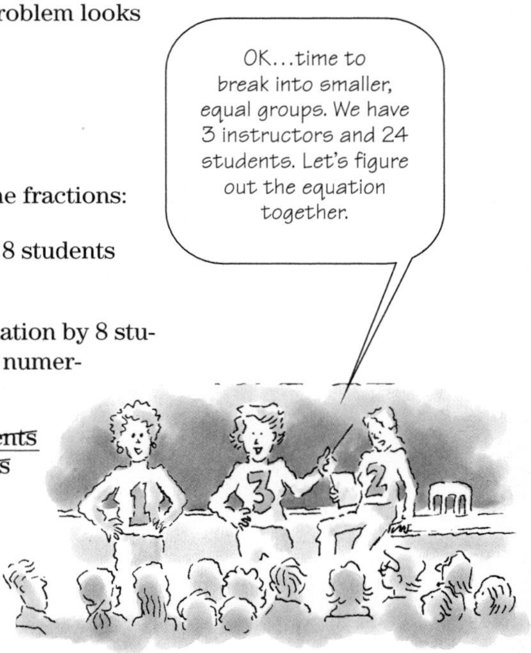
OK...time to break into smaller, equal groups. We have 3 instructors and 24 students. Let's figure out the equation together.

How many bags of I.V. fluid?

Here's one more problem. One case of I.V. fluid holds 20 bags. If your home care agency receives 6 cases, how many bags of I.V. fluid does it have?

The ratio rally

Solve this problem using ratios first. Follow these steps:

Decide what part of the ratio is X. In this case, it's the number of bags of I.V. fluid in 6 cases.

Set up the proportion so that the units of measure in each ratio are in the same position:

$$1 \text{ case} : 20 \text{ bags} :: 6 \text{ cases} : X$$

Multiply the means and the extremes and set up the equation:

$$20 \text{ bags} \times 6 \text{ cases} = X \text{ bags} \times 1 \text{ case}$$

Solve for X by dividing both sides of the equation by 1 case and canceling units that appear in both the numerator and denominator:

$$\frac{20 \text{ bags} \times 6 \cancel{\text{cases}}}{1 \cancel{\text{case}}} = \frac{X \times \cancel{1 \text{ case}}}{\cancel{1 \text{ case}}}$$

Find X.

$$120 \text{ bags} = X$$

The fraction finale

Now, use fractions to solve the problem. Here's what the equation looks like in fraction form:

$$\frac{1 \text{ case}}{20 \text{ bags}} = \frac{6 \text{ cases}}{X}$$

Rewrite the equation by cross-multiplying the fractions. Then solve for X by dividing each side of the equation by 1 case and canceling units that appear in both the numerator and denominator:

$$\frac{\cancel{1 \text{ case}} \times X}{\cancel{1 \text{ case}}} = \frac{6 \cancel{\text{cases}} \times 20 \text{ bags}}{1 \cancel{\text{case}}}$$

$$X = \frac{120}{1}$$

$$X = 120 \text{ bags}$$

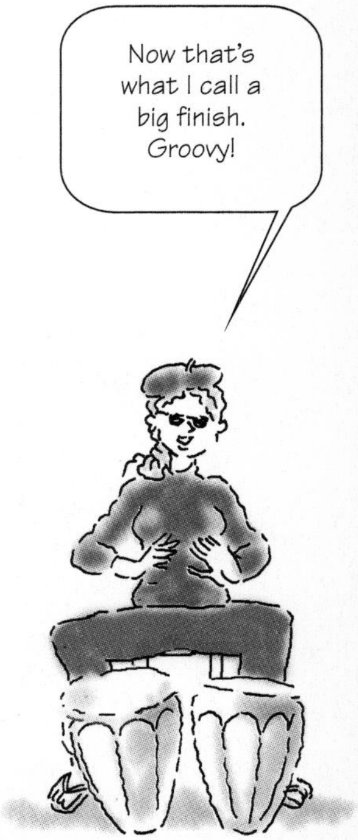

Now that's what I call a big finish. Groovy!

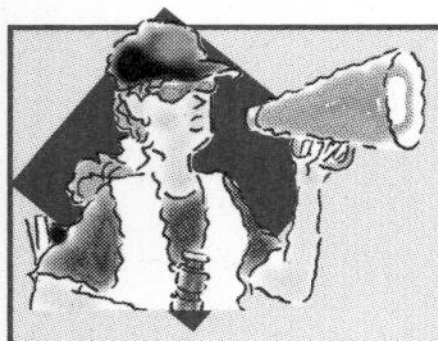

That's a wrap!

Ratios, fractions, proportions, and solving for *X* review

Some important facts about ratios, fractions, proportions, and solving for *X* are outlined below.

Numerical relationship basics

- *Ratio:* uses a colon between the numbers in a numerical relationship
- *Fraction:* uses a slash between numbers in a numerical relationship
- *Proportion:* a statement of equality between two ratios or two fractions

Solving common-fraction equations

- Multiply numerators.
- Multiply denominators.
- Restate the equation.
- Reduce the fraction.
- Convert the fraction to decimal form by dividing the numerator by the denominator.

Solving decimal-fraction equations

- Move the decimal points two spaces to the right.
- Remove the zeros.
- Convert the whole number to a fraction.
- Multiply the numerators.
- Multiply the denominators.
- Restate the equation.
- Convert the answer to decimal form by dividing the numerator by the denominator.

Solving proportions with ratios

- Means — middle numbers
- Extremes — end numbers
- Product of the means = product of the extremes
- Isolate *X* on one side of the equation.
- Solve for *X*.

Solving proportions with fractions

- Cross products of a proportion are always equal.
- Multiply the cross products.
- Put the cross products into the equation, and isolate *X* on one side of the equation.
- Solve for *X*.

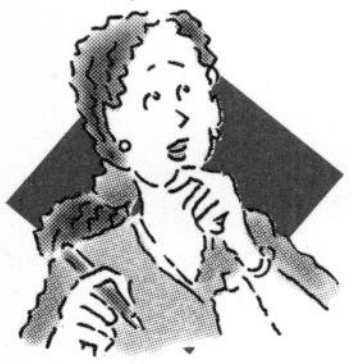

Quick quiz

1. Which is an example of a proportion?

A. 4 : 5 :: 8 : 12
B. 6 : 1 :: 18 : 3
C. 7 : 1 :: 14 : 7
D. 3 : 8 :: 2 : 6

Answer: B. In a proportion, the ratios are equal.

2. The proportion 1 : 5 :: 2 : 10 can be restated in fraction form as which of the following?

A. $\frac{1}{5} = \frac{2}{10}$
B. $\frac{5}{1} = \frac{2}{10}$
C. $\frac{2}{5} = \frac{1}{10}$
D. $\frac{5}{2} = \frac{10}{1}$

Answer: A. Make the ratios on both sides into fractions by substituting slashes for colons.

3. If there are 50 mg of a drug in 5 ml of solution, the amount of drug in 15 ml of solution is:

A. 10 mg.
B. 150 mg.
C. 75 mg.
D. 100 mg.

Answer: B. Substitute *X* for the amount of drug in 15 ml of solution and then set up a proportion with ratios or fractions.

4. The amount of salt you should add to 32 oz of water to make a solution with ½ (0.5) tsp of salt for every 8 oz of water is:

A. 2 tsp.
B. 4 tsp.
C. 1 tsp.
D. 3 tsp.

Answer: A. Substitute *X* for the amount of salt in 32 oz of water and then set up a proportion with ratios or fractions.

5. A physician prescribes 0.125 mg of a drug. The vial you have from the pharmacy contains 0.25 mg per ml of solution. How many ml of the solution should you administer?

A. 1 ml
B. 2 ml
C. 0.5 ml
D. 1.5 ml

Answer: C. Substitute *X* for the amount of solution needed to administer 0.125 mg of the drug and then set up a proportion with ratios or fractions.

6. A physician prescribes 40 mg of the drug furosemide (Lasix). The vial sent by the pharmacy contains 10 mg per ml of solution. How many ml of solution should you administer?

A. 1 ml
B. 2 ml
C. 3 ml
D. 4 ml

Answer: D. Substitute *X* for the amount of solution needed to administer 40 mg of the drug and then set up a proportion with ratios or fractions.

Scoring

☆☆☆ If you answered all six items correctly, wow! You're a whiz at relationships (numerical relationships, that is).

☆☆ If you answered four or five items correctly, all right! You have everything in proportion.

☆ If you answered fewer than four items correctly, a quick review will get your numbers back on track!

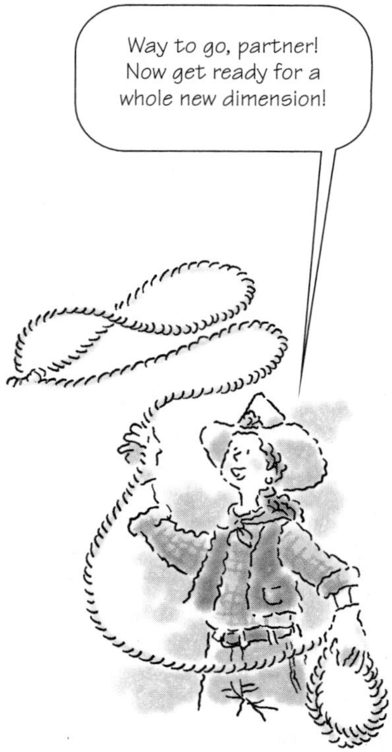

Way to go, partner! Now get ready for a whole new dimension!

4

Dimensional analysis

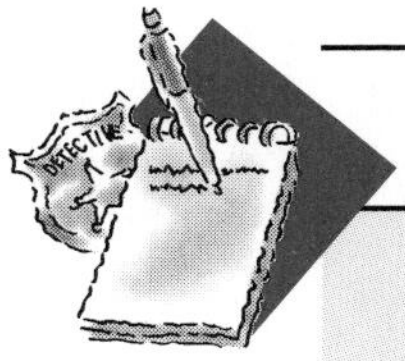

Just the facts

In this chapter, you'll learn:

- what dimensional analysis is
- how to set up an equation using dimensional analysis
- how to identify conversion factors
- how to solve dosage calculations using dimensional analysis.

A look at dimensional analysis

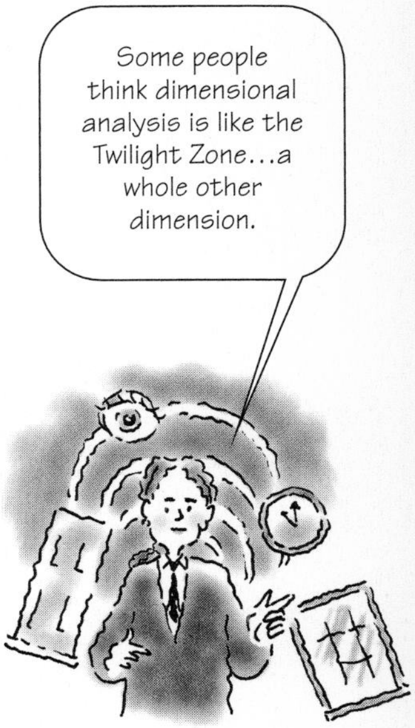
Some people think dimensional analysis is like the Twilight Zone...a whole other dimension.

Dimensional analysis, also known as *factor analysis* or *factor labeling*, is an alternative way of solving mathematical problems. It's a basic and easy approach to calculating drug dosages because it eliminates the need to memorize formulas. Only one equation is required to determine each answer.

Factors are the main actors

When using dimensional analysis, a series of ratios, called *factors*, are arranged in a fractional equation. Each factor, written as a fraction, consists of two quantities of measurement that are related to each other in a given problem. Dimensional analysis uses the same terms as fractions, specifically the terms *numerator* and *denominator*.

Setting the stage

Let's say you want to change 48″ to feet. The problem is written as follows:

$$48'' = X \text{ feet}$$

Some problems contain all of the information needed to identify the factors, set up the equation, and find the solution. Other problems, such as this one, require a conversion factor.

Conversion factors

Conversion factors are equivalents between two measurement systems or units of measurement. For example, 1 day equals 24 hours. In this case, day and hour are units of measurement and, when stated as 1 day = 24 hours, they're equivalent. This conversion factor can be used to solve problems involving the measure of time. There are many commonly used conversion factors. (See *Common conversion factors.*)

Putting it into practice

In the previous problem of how many feet are in 48″, use the conversion factor 12″ equals 1′.

Because the quantities and unit of measurement are equivalent, they can serve as the numerator or denominator. The conversion can be written as:

$$\frac{12}{1}$$

or

$$\frac{1}{12}$$

Setting up the equation

Solving a problem using dimensional analysis is like climbing a staircase — it requires steps. Six simple steps need to be followed to solve any problem. (See *Following the steps.*)

Stepping up to the problem

Let's take it one step at a time:

1. Given quantity — This is the beginning point of the problem. Identify the given quantity in the problem. In this case,

48″

2. Wanted quantity — This is the answer to the problem. Identify the wanted quantity in the problem as an unknown unit. In this problem it's :

X feet

3. Conversion factors — Again, these are the equivalents that are necessary to convert between systems. The conversion factor for this problem is :

12″ = 1′

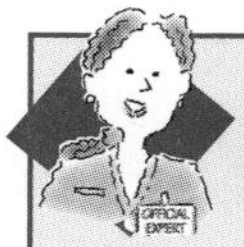

Advice from the experts

Common conversion factors

Keep this chart handy for quick reference to breeze through problems that call for these common conversions.

1 kg	=	2.2 lb
16 oz	=	1 lb
8 oz	=	1 cup
1 oz	=	30 ml
1 tsp	=	5 ml
1 grain	=	60 mg
12″	=	1′
3′	=	1 yd

Advice from the experts

Following the steps

Remember these steps when calculating an equation using dimensional analysis, and you'll soon be standing on top of a solution.

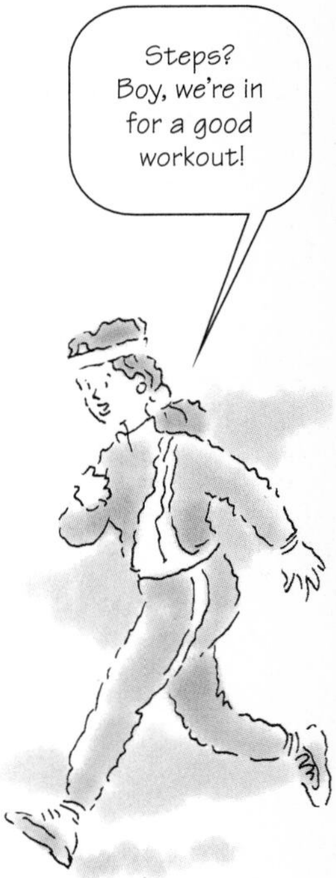

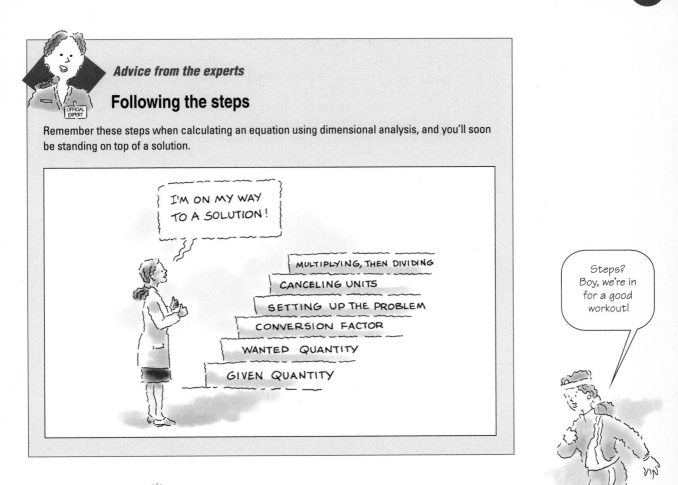

Set up the problem using necessary equivalents as conversion factors. When setting up equations, make sure that units you want canceled out appear in both a numerator and a denominator. If an unwanted unit appears in two numerators, for example, you won't be able to cancel it. In this example, you want to cancel the inches and get the answer in feet. To do this, you must multiply 48″ by a fraction that has inches in the denominator and feet in the numerator. The problem should be set up as:

$$\frac{48 \text{ inches}}{1} \times \frac{1 \text{ foot}}{12 \text{ inches}}$$

Just as with any type of mathematical problem, you'll cancel units that appear in both the numerator and denominator to isolate the unit you're seeking. In this case, you'll cancel inches, thereby isolating feet, which is the desired measurement. The step will look like this:

$$\frac{48\ \cancel{\text{inches}}}{1} \times \frac{1\ \text{foot}}{12\ \cancel{\text{inches}}}$$

Multiply the numerators, multiply the denominators, and divide the product of the numerators by the product of the denominators to reach the wanted quantity.

$$\frac{48}{1} \times \frac{1\ \text{foot}}{12} = \frac{48 \times 1\ \text{foot}}{1 \times 12} = \frac{48\ \text{feet}}{12} = 4\ \text{feet}$$

There are 4′ in 48″.

Let's step to it again!

Now try to solve another problem using dimensional analysis. A package weighs 38 oz. How many pounds does it weigh?

- Identify the given:

$$38\ \text{oz}$$

- Identify the wanted:

$$X\ \text{pounds}$$

- Identify the conversion factor:

$$1\ \text{lb} = 16\ \text{oz}$$

- Set up the equation:

$$\frac{38\ \text{oz}}{1} \times \frac{1\ \text{lb}}{16\ \text{oz}}$$

- Cancel units that appear in both the numerator and the denominator:

$$\frac{38\ \cancel{\text{oz}}}{1} \times \frac{1\ \text{lb}}{16\ \cancel{\text{oz}}}$$

- Multiply the numerators and denominators and divide the products:

$$\frac{38 \times 1\ \text{lb}}{1 \times 16} = \frac{38\ \text{lb}}{16} = 2.4\ \text{lb}$$

There are 2.4 lb in 38 oz.

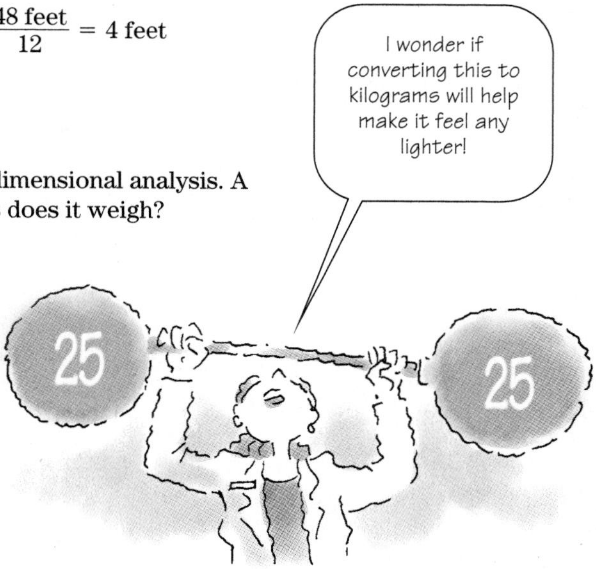

I wonder if converting this to kilograms will help make it feel any lighter!
25
25

Feel the conversion burn!

Now see how we can use dimensional analysis to take this same example a little further. If the same package weighs 38 oz, what does it weigh in kilograms?

- Identify the given:

38 oz

- Identify the wanted:

X kilograms

- Identify the conversion factors (in this case, there are two):

1 lb = 16 oz

1 kg = 2.2 lb

- Set up the equation:

$$\frac{38 \text{ oz}}{1} \times \frac{1 \text{ lb}}{16 \text{ oz}} \times \frac{1 \text{ kg}}{2.2 \text{ lb}}$$

- Cancel units that appear in both the numerator and the denominator:

$$\frac{38 \cancel{\text{oz}}}{1} \times \frac{1 \cancel{\text{lb}}}{16 \cancel{\text{oz}}} \times \frac{1 \text{ kg}}{2.2 \cancel{\text{lb}}}$$

- Multiply the numerators and denominators and divide the products:

$$\frac{38 \times 1 \times 1 \text{ kg}}{1 \times 16 \times 2.2} = \frac{38 \text{ kg}}{35.2} = 1.08 \text{ kg}$$

There are 1.08 kg in 38 oz.

Let's cool down...with one more rep!

Getting a good workout? Try one more to keep in peak shape. If you drank 64 oz of juice, how many cups of juice did you drink?

- Identify the given:

64 oz

- Identify the wanted:

X cups

- Identify the conversion factor:

8 oz = 1 cup

- Set up the equation:

$$\frac{64 \text{ oz}}{1} \times \frac{1 \text{ cup}}{8 \text{ oz}}$$

- Cancel units that appear in both the numerator and the denominator:

$$\frac{64\ \cancel{\text{oz}}}{1} \times \frac{1\ \text{cup}}{8\ \cancel{\text{oz}}}$$

- Multiply the numerators and denominators and divide the products:

$$\frac{64 \times 1\ \text{cup}}{1 \times 8} = \frac{64\ \text{cups}}{8} = 8\ \text{cups}$$

There are 8 cups in 64 oz.

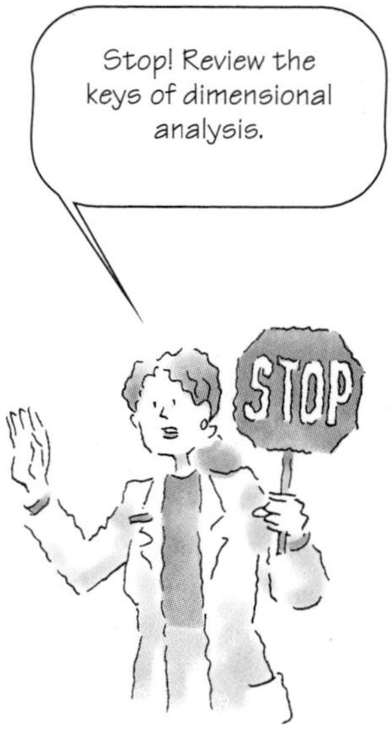

Stop! Review the keys of dimensional analysis.
STOP

Take a breath and let's review

Now that you've made it through the steps again, let's pause to study some key ideas. Dimensional analysis is a method of problem solving that can be used whenever two quantities are directly proportional to each other. One of the quantities can be converted to another unit of measurement by using common equivalents or conversion factors. The problem is treated as an equation using fractions. (See *Quick guide to dimensional analysis.*)

Now on your feet and do it again!

Apply the concepts you just reviewed above. Tom is recovering from arthroscopic surgery. As part of his rehabilitation, he walks one-half of a mile each day. If he usually walks at a pace of 1.5 miles per hour, how long will it take Tom to complete his walk?

- Identify the given:

$$0.5\ \text{miles}$$

- Identify the wanted:

$$X\ \text{hours}$$

- Identify the conversion factor:

$$1.5\ \text{miles} = 1\ \text{hour}$$

- Set up the equation:

$$\frac{0.5\ \text{miles}}{1} \times \frac{1\ \text{hour}}{1.5\ \text{miles}}$$

- Cancel units that appear in both the numerator and the denominator:

$$\frac{0.5\ \cancel{\text{miles}}}{1} \times \frac{1\ \text{hour}}{1.5\ \cancel{\text{miles}}}$$

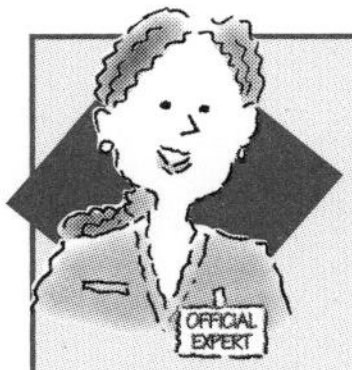

Advice from the experts

Quick guide to dimensional analysis

Need to calculate a dosage? Need to figure out a drip rate? Don't panic! Just follow this step-by-step guide to dimensional analysis to come up with the number you need quickly and accurately.

Step 1: Given
Identify the given quantity in the problem.

Step 2: Wanted
Identify the wanted quantity in the problem (the unknown unit, or the answer to the problem).

Step 3: Conversion factor
Write down the equivalents that are necessary to convert between systems.

Step 4: The problem
Set up the fractions so that the units you need to cancel appear as both a numerator and a denominator. Units can't be canceled if they appear only as numerators or only as denominators.

Step 5: Unwanted units
Cancel unwanted units that appear in the numerator and denominator to isolate the unit you're seeking for the answer.

Step 6: Multiply, multiply, and divide
This is where you use math to solve the problem. Multiply the numerators, multiply the denominators, and divide the products.

Fun with dimensional analysis!
Now try this sample problem using the steps identified above.

A doctor prescribes 75 mg of a drug. The pharmacy stocks a solution containing the drug at a concentration of 100 mg/ml. What dose should you give in milliliters?

- *Step 1:* Given = 75 mg
- *Step 2:* Wanted = *X* ml
- *Step 3:* Conversion factor: 100 mg = 1 ml
- *Step 4:* Set up the equation (Remember that units you want canceled should be positioned in both a numerator and a denominator.):

$$\frac{75\text{ mg}}{1} \times \frac{1\text{ ml}}{100\text{ mg}}$$

- *Step 5:* Cancel unwanted units:

$$\frac{75\ \cancel{\text{mg}}}{1} \times \frac{1\text{ ml}}{100\ \cancel{\text{mg}}}$$

- *Step 6:* Multiply, multiply, and divide:

$$\frac{75 \times 1\text{ ml}}{1 \times 100} = \frac{75}{100} = 0.75\text{ ml of the solution}$$

More fun!
Here's one more:

The doctor prescribes 250 mg of amoxicillin (Amoxil), which comes in a suspension of 25 mg/ml. You need to give the dose in teaspoons (tsp). How many teaspoons of the suspension should you give?

- *Step 1:* Given = 250 mg
- *Step 2:* Wanted = *X* tsp
- *Step 3:* Conversion factors (Remember, some conversion factors you should know by memory, such as 1 tsp = 5 ml.): 25 mg = 1 ml; 1 tsp = 5 ml
- *Step 4:* Set up the equation:

$$\frac{1\text{ tsp}}{5\text{ ml}} \times \frac{1\text{ ml}}{25\text{ mg}} \times \frac{250\text{ mg}}{1}$$

- *Step 5:* Cancel unwanted units:

$$\frac{1\text{ tsp}}{5\ \cancel{\text{ml}}} \times \frac{1\ \cancel{\text{ml}}}{25\ \cancel{\text{mg}}} \times \frac{250\ \cancel{\text{mg}}}{1}$$

- *Step 6:* Multiply, multiply, and divide:

$$\frac{1\text{ tsp} \times 1 \times 250}{5 \times 25 \times 1} = \frac{250\text{ tsp}}{125} = 2\text{ tsp of the suspension}$$

- Multiply the numerators and denominators and divide the products:

$$\frac{0.5 \times 1 \text{ hour}}{1 \times 1.5} = \frac{0.5 \text{ hours}}{1.5} = 0.33 \text{ hours}$$

It will take Tom 0.33 hours to complete his walk.

Real world problems

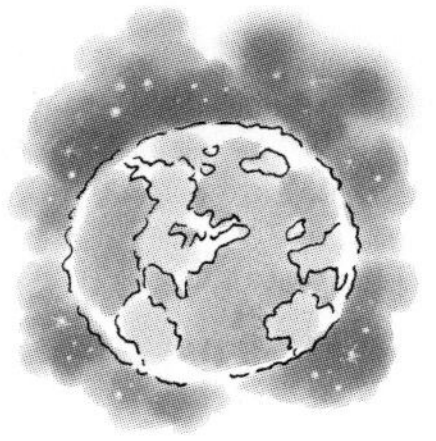

A patient is ordered to receive 70 mg of enoxaparin (Lovenox). It's available in vials that contain 30 mg per 0.3 ml. How much should be prepared?

- Begin by identifying the given quantity:

$$70 \text{ mg}$$

- Then isolate what you're looking for:

$$X \text{ ml}$$

- Know your conversion factor:

$$30 \text{ mg} = 0.3 \text{ ml}$$

- Set up the equation:

$$\frac{70 \text{ mg}}{1} \times \frac{0.3 \text{ ml}}{30 \text{ mg}}$$

- Identify and cancel units that appear in both the numerator and the denominator:

$$\frac{70 \cancel{\text{mg}}}{1} \times \frac{0.3 \text{ ml}}{30 \cancel{\text{mg}}}$$

- Lastly, multiply the numerators and denominators and divide the products:

$$\frac{70 \times 0.3 \text{ ml}}{1 \times 30} = \frac{21 \text{ ml}}{30} = 0.7 \text{ ml}$$

The patient would receive 0.7 ml of Lovenox.

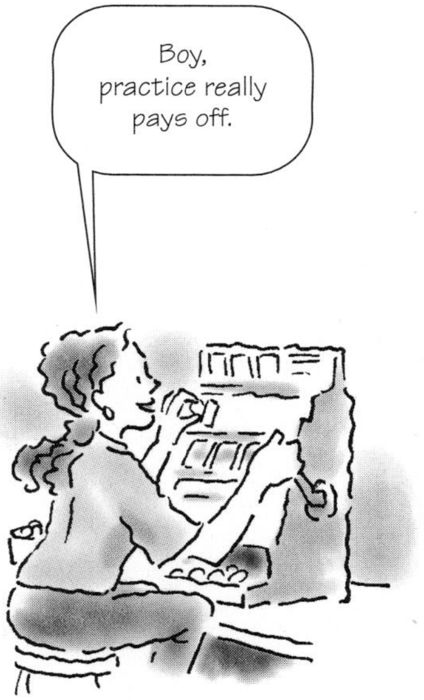
Boy, practice really pays off.

Solve for Synthroid

A patient is to receive 50 mcg of levothyroxine (Synthroid). The drug is available as 200 mcg per 5 ml. How many milliliters should the nurse prepare?

- The given quantity:

$$50 \text{ mcg}$$

- The wanted quantity:

$$X \text{ ml}$$

- The conversion factor:

$$200 \text{ mcg} = 5 \text{ ml}$$

- Set up the equation:

$$\frac{50 \text{ mcg}}{1} \times \frac{5 \text{ ml}}{200 \text{ mcg}}$$

- Cancel units that appear in both the numerator and the denominator:

$$\frac{50\ \cancel{\text{mcg}}}{1} \times \frac{5 \text{ ml}}{200\ \cancel{\text{mcg}}}$$

- Then multiply the numerators and denominators and divide the products:

$$\frac{50 \times 5 \text{ ml}}{1 \times 200} = \frac{250 \text{ ml}}{200} = 1.3 \text{ ml}$$

The nurse should prepare 1.3 ml of Synthroid.

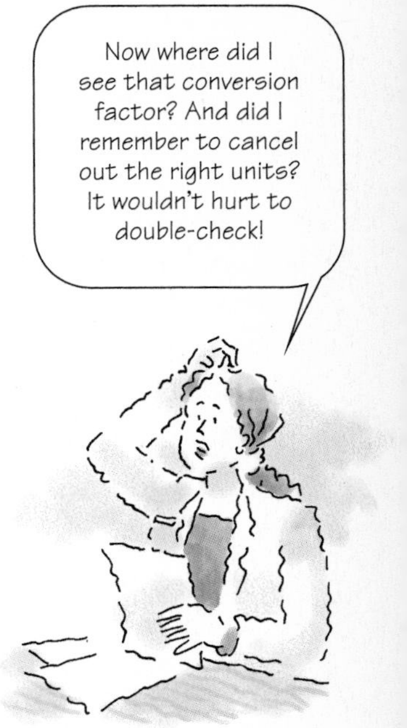

Now where did I see that conversion factor? And did I remember to cancel out the right units? It wouldn't hurt to double-check!

How much heparin?

The doctor prescribes 10,000 units of heparin added to 500 ml of D_5W at 1,200 units/hour. How many drops per minute should you administer if the I.V. tubing delivers 10 gtt/ml?

- The given quantities (in this case there are three):

$$\text{1st quantity: } \frac{10 \text{ gtt}}{1 \text{ ml}}$$

$$\text{2nd quantity: } \frac{500 \text{ ml}}{10{,}000 \text{ units}}$$

$$\text{3rd quantity: } \frac{1{,}200 \text{ units}}{1 \text{ hour}}$$

- The wanted quantity:

$$X \text{ gtt/minute}$$

- The conversion factor:

$$\frac{1 \text{ hour}}{60 \text{ minutes}}$$

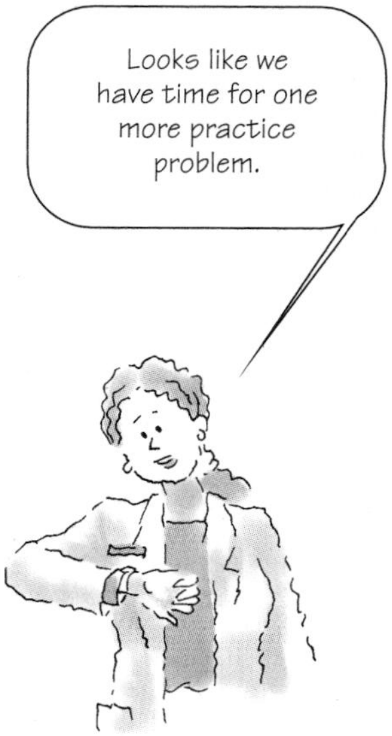

Looks like we have time for one more practice problem.

- Set up the equation:

$$\frac{10\text{ gtt}}{1\text{ ml}} \times \frac{500\text{ ml}}{10{,}000\text{ units}} \times \frac{1{,}200\text{ units}}{1\text{ hour}} \times \frac{1\text{ hour}}{60\text{ minutes}}$$

- Cancel units that appear in both the numerator and the denominator:

$$\frac{10\text{ gtt}}{1\ \cancel{\text{ml}}} \times \frac{500\ \cancel{\text{ml}}}{10{,}000\ \cancel{\text{units}}} \times \frac{1{,}200\ \cancel{\text{units}}}{1\ \cancel{\text{hour}}} \times \frac{1\ \cancel{\text{hour}}}{60\text{ minutes}}$$

- Then multiply the numerators and denominators and divide the products:

$$\frac{10 \times 500 \times 1{,}200\text{ gtt}}{10{,}000 \times 60\text{ minutes}} = \frac{6{,}000{,}000\text{ gtt}}{600{,}000\text{ minutes}} = 10\text{ gtt/minute}$$

You should administer the heparin at a rate of 10 gtt/minute.

Learning Lasix lingo

Let's try one more problem. Your patient is to receive 20 mg of furosemide (Lasix) oral solution. The bottle is labeled 40 mg per 5 ml. How many milliliters will the patient receive?

- The given quantity:

$$20\text{ mg}$$

- The wanted quantity:

$$X\text{ ml}$$

- The conversion factor:

$$40\text{ mg} = 5\text{ ml}$$

- Set up the equation:

$$\frac{20\text{ mg}}{1} \times \frac{5\text{ ml}}{40\text{ mg}}$$

- Cancel units that appear in both the numerator and the denominator:

$$\frac{20\ \cancel{\text{mg}}}{1} \times \frac{5\text{ ml}}{40\ \cancel{\text{mg}}}$$

- Multiply the numerators and denominators and divide the products:

$$\frac{20 \times 5\text{ ml}}{1 \times 40} = \frac{100\text{ ml}}{40} = 2.5\text{ ml}$$

The patient would receive 2.5 ml of Lasix oral solution.

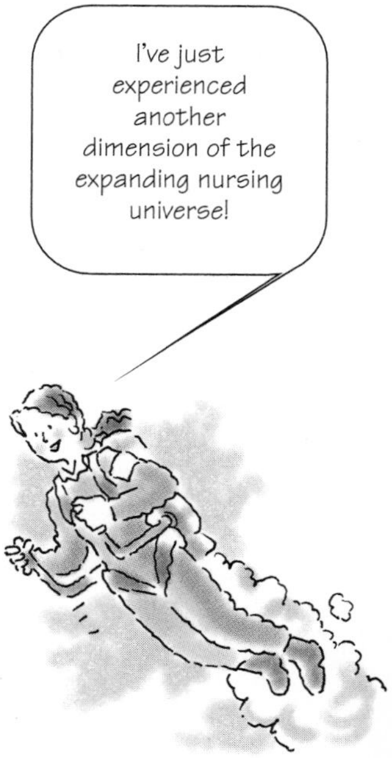

I've just experienced another dimension of the expanding nursing universe!

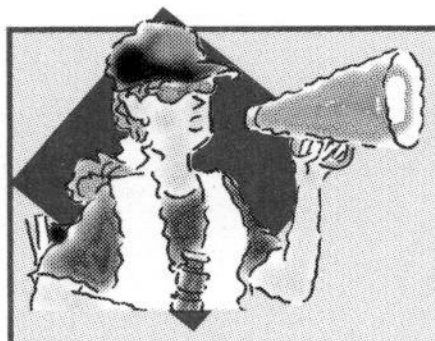

That's a wrap!

Dimensional analysis review

Remember these important facts about dimensional analysis for dosage calculations.

Dimensional analysis basics
- Use whenever two quantities are directly proportional to each other.
- Use common equivalents or conversion factors to convert to the same unit of measurement.
- Set up the problem using fractions.

Performing dimensional analysis—6 steps
- Determine the given quantity.
- Determine the wanted quantity.
- Select conversion factors.
- Set up the problem.
- Cancel unwanted units.
- Multiply the numerators, multiply the denominators, and divide the products.

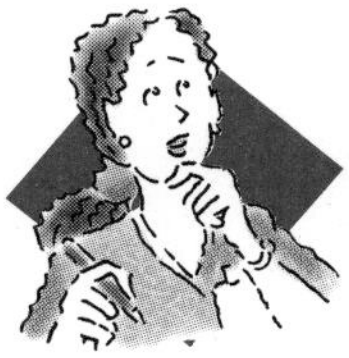

Quick quiz

1. When using dimensional analysis, factors are written as:
A. fractions.
B. whole numbers.
C. percentages.
D. ratios.

Answer: A. Factors are always written as common fractions. When a problem includes a quantity and its unit of measurement is unrelated to any other factor in the problem, that quantity serves as the numerator of the fraction, and 1 (which is implied) becomes the denominator.

2. Conversion factors in a dimensional analysis equation are:
A. identified as the given quantity and the wanted quantity.
B. equivalents necessary to convert between two systems.
C. always placed as numerators.
D. always placed as denominators.

Answer: B. Conversion factors involve equivalent measurements that allow for conversion between different systems.

3. Dimensional analysis involves calculations that can be solved:
A. in three simple steps.
B. in a single equation.
C. using formulas that must be memorized.
D. using common denominators.

Answer: B. Although dimensional analysis uses a step-by-step approach, the problem can be simplified in one single equation.

4. Your patient is 60″ tall. How much is this in feet?
- A. 6′
- B. 6′ 3″
- C. 5′
- D. 5′ 3″

Answer: C. Use the conversion factor 12″ equals 1′. Then set up the equation and follow the steps:

$$\frac{60 \text{ \sout{inches}}}{1} \times \frac{1 \text{ foot}}{12 \text{ \sout{inches}}}$$

$$\frac{60 \times 1 \text{ foot}}{1 \times 12} = \frac{60 \text{ feet}}{12} = 5 \text{ feet}$$

5. How many pounds are in 48 oz?
- A. 4 lb
- B. 6 lb
- C. 5 lb
- D. 3 lb

Answer: D. Use the conversion factor 16 oz equals 1 lb to solve:

$$\frac{48 \text{ \sout{oz}}}{1} \times \frac{1 \text{ lb}}{16 \text{ \sout{oz}}}$$

$$\frac{48 \times 1 \text{ lb}}{1 \times 16} = \frac{48 \text{ lb}}{16} = 3 \text{ lb}$$

Scoring

☆☆☆ If you answered all five items correctly, congratulations! You've added an impressive dimension to your intellect!

☆☆ If you answered three or four items correctly, label yourself a factor to be reckoned with. Don't convert to lazy ways; keep up the good work!

☆ If you answered fewer than three items correctly, please retrace your steps to discover where you went wrong. You'll soon be the equivalent of an expert!

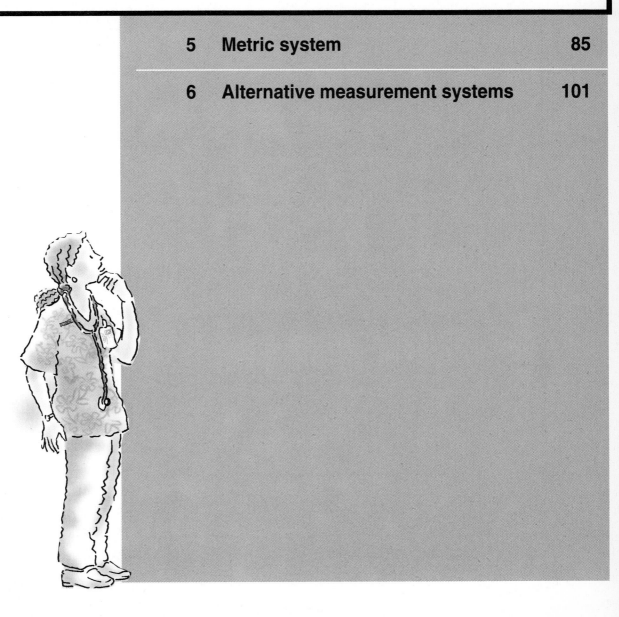

Part II Measurement systems

5

Metric system

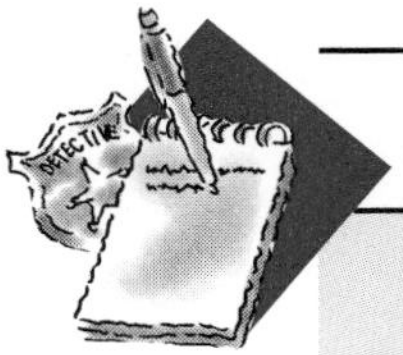

Just the facts

In this chapter, you'll learn:

- metric units of measure
- how to convert measurements from one metric unit to another
- how to solve basic arithmetic problems in metric units
- how to calculate drug dosages using the metric system.

A look at the metric system

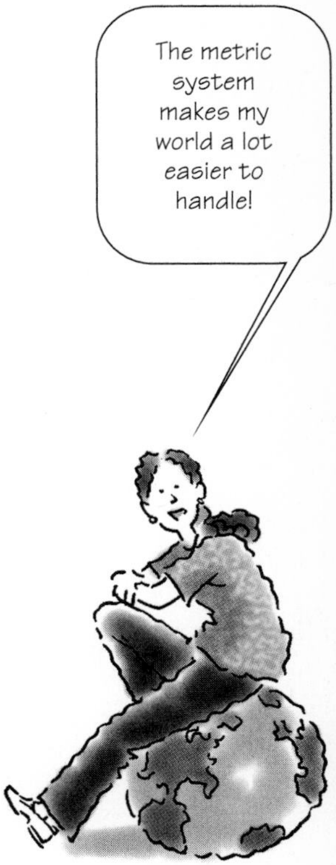

The metric system makes my world a lot easier to handle!

Today, most nations of the world rely on the metric system of measurement. It's also the most widely used system for measuring amounts of drugs.

The metric system is a decimal system. That means it's based on the number 10 and multiples and subdivisions of 10. The metric system offers three advantages over other systems:

- It eliminates common fractions.
- It simplifies the calculation of large and small units.
- It simplifies the calculation of drug doses. (See *Tips for going metric*, page 86.)

Beginning with the basics

The three basic units of measurement in the metric system (along with the abbreviation for each) are the meter (m), liter (L), and gram (g):

- The meter is the basic unit of length.
- The liter is the basic unit of volume — it's equivalent to 1/10 of a cubic meter.
- The gram is the basic unit of weight — it represents the weight of 1 cubic centimeter (cm^3 or cc) of water at 4° C (39.2° F).

What's in a name?

All other units of measure are based on these three major units. When you see the root word *meter*, *liter*, or *gram* within a measurement, you can easily tell if you're measuring length, volume, or weight.

For example, centi*meter* (cm) and milli*meter* (mm) are units of length, centi*liter* (cl) and milli*liter* (ml) are units of volume, and kilo*gram* (kg) and milli*gram* (mg) are units of weight.

Measure for measure

Three devices — the metric ruler, the metric graduate, and metric weights — are used to measure meters, liters, and grams. (See *Measuring meters, liters, and grams.*)

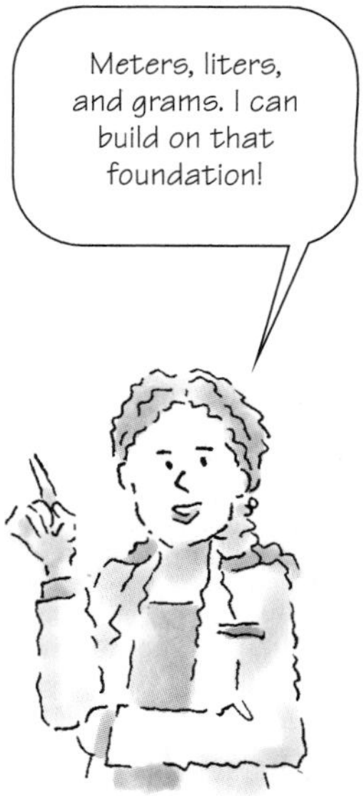
Meters, liters, and grams. I can build on that foundation!

Building on the basics

Multiples and subdivisions of meters, liters, and grams are indicated by using a prefix before the basic unit. Each prefix that's used in the metric system represents a multiple or subdivision of 10.

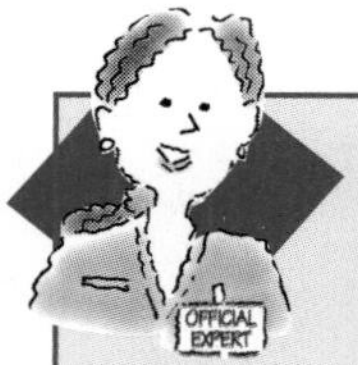
OFFICIAL EXPERT

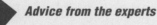

Advice from the experts

Tips for going metric

Remember these tips when using the metric system.

Tip	Example
Use the correct abbreviation for each unit of measurement. The abbreviation always follows a number that represents a quantity.	Five kilograms is abbreviated as 5 kg. Five and one-half milligrams is abbreviated as 5.5 mg.
Use decimal fractions to represent a part of a whole.	2.5 mg represents 2 milligrams plus five out of ten parts of 1 milligram.
Place a zero before the decimal point for amounts that are less than 1.	0.5 mg, 0.2 ml, and 0.65 mcg are less than 1.
Eliminate extra zeros so they aren't misread.	Use 5 mg (not 5.0 mg) and 0.5 ml (not 0.500 ml).

Consider the gram. The most common multiple of a gram is the *kilo*gram, which is 1,000 times greater than the gram. The most common subdivision of a gram is the *milli*gram, which represents 1/1,000 of a gram, or 0.001 g.

Keeping it brief

Any metric measurement can be represented by a number and an abbreviation that represents the unit of measure. The abbreviation stands for the basic unit of measure — gram (g), meter (m), liter (L) — and the prefix, such as kilo (k), centi (c), and milli (m). For example, *kg* stands for kilogram, *cm* for centimeter, and *ml* for milliliter. (See *What a little prefix can do*, page 88.)

A cubic curiosity

The metric system also includes one unusual unit of volume — the cubic centimeter (cc). Because a cubic centimeter occupies the same space as 1 ml of liquid, the two units of volume are considered equal and may be used interchangeably. However, cubic cen-

Measuring meters, liters, and grams

What tools do you need to measure meters, liters, and grams? The appropriate measuring devices, of course. A metric ruler, which resembles a yardstick, is used to measure length. A metric graduate can be used to measure the volume of a fluid in liters. (An enclosed chamber, such as a cylinder with a tight-fitting lid, is needed to measure a volume of gas.) A set of metric weights can be used with a metric balance to measure weight in grams.

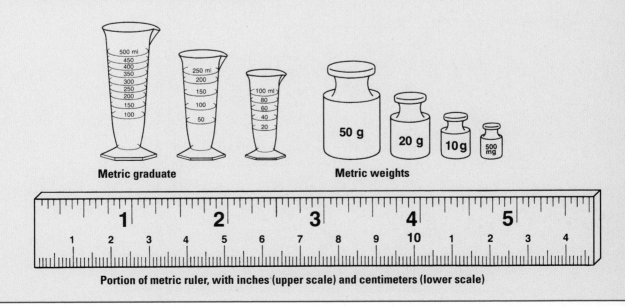

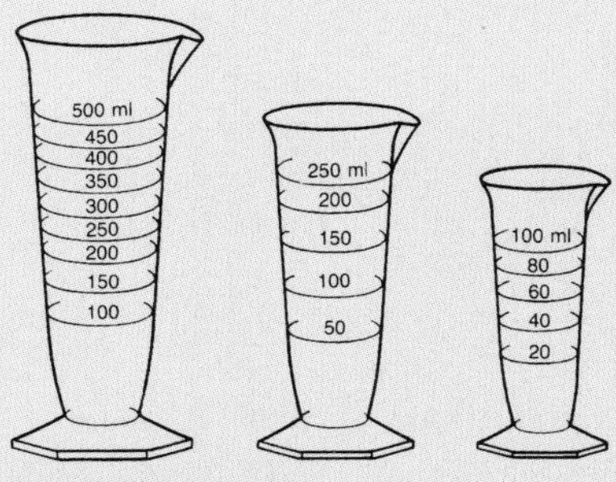

Metric graduate

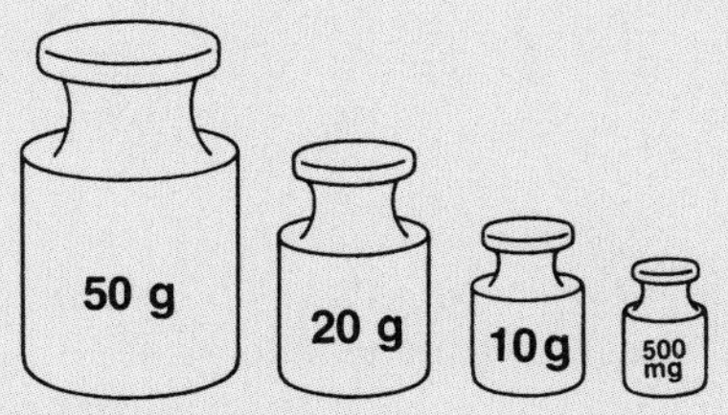

Metric weights

Portion of metric ruler, with inches (upper scale) and centimeters (lower scale)

What a little prefix can do

In the metric system, the addition of a prefix to one of the basic units of measure indicates a multiple or subdivision of that unit. Here's a list of prefixes, abbreviations, and multiples and subdivisions of each unit.

Prefix	Abbreviation	Multiples and subdivisions
kilo	k	1,000
hecto	h	100
deka	dk	10
deci	d	0.1 (1⁄10)
centi	c	0.01 (1⁄100)
milli	m	0.001 (1⁄1,000)
micro	mc	0.000001 (1⁄1,000,000)
nano	n	0.000000001 (1⁄1,000,000,000)
pico	p	0.000000000001 (1⁄1,000,000,000,000)

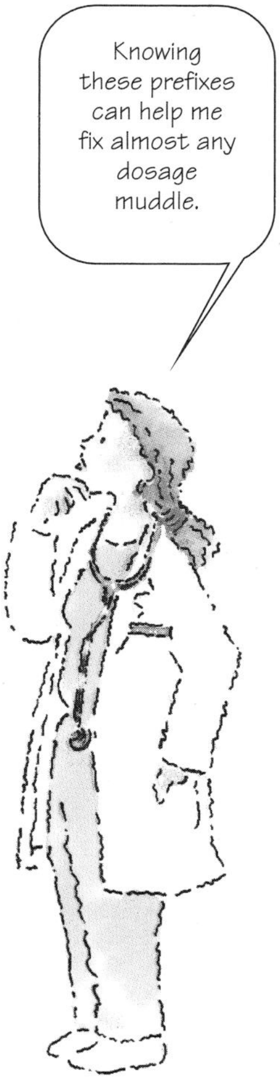

Knowing these prefixes can help me fix almost any dosage muddle.

timeters usually refer to gas volumes, and milliliters usually describe liquid volumes.

Failing to meet standards

The International Bureau of Weights and Measures adopted the International System of Units in 1960 to promote the standard use of metric abbreviations and prevent errors in drug transcriptions. Unfortunately, some health care providers still use the old abbreviations.

So stay alert for nonstandard abbreviations, especially l instead of L to represent liters, and gm or GM instead of g to represent grams. As a precaution, some nurses and doctors use L in all liter-related abbreviations, such as mL and dL. However, this isn't required.

Metric conversions

Because the metric system is decimal based, converting from one metric unit to another is easy. To convert a smaller unit to a larger

Insta-metric conversion table

Want a quick and easy way to jump back and forth between different metric measures? Just use the fantastic "insta-metric" table below. Make a copy of it to post in a conspicuous spot on your unit. Always remember, a milliliter is to a liter as a microgram is to a milligram.

Liquids	Solids
1 ml = 1 cm^3 (or cc)	1,000 mcg = 1 mg
1,000 ml = 1 L	1,000 mg = 1 g
100 cl = 1 L	100 cg = 1 g
10 dl = 1 L	10 dg = 1 g
10 L = 1 dkl	10 g = 1 dkg
100 L = 1 hl	100 g = 1 hg
1,000 L = 1 kl	1,000 g = 1 kg

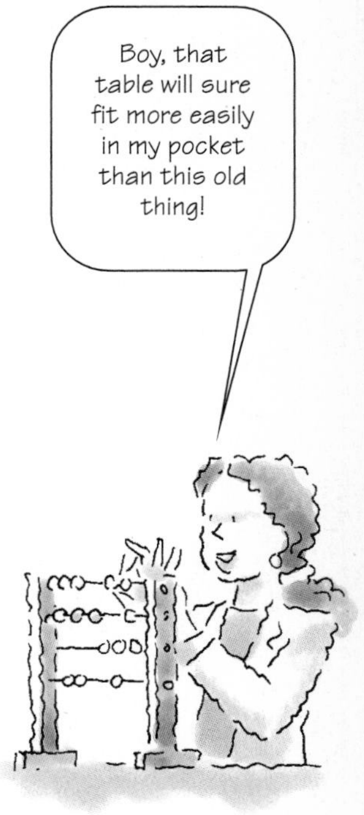

Boy, that table will sure fit more easily in my pocket than this old thing!

unit, move the decimal point to the left. To convert a larger unit to a smaller unit, move the decimal point to the right.

Because all metric units are multiples or subdivisions of the major units, you can also convert a smaller unit to a larger unit by dividing by the appropriate multiple or multiplying by the appropriate subdivision. To convert a larger unit to a smaller unit, multiply by the appropriate multiple or divide by the appropriate subdivision.

Turning the tables on measurements

Luckily, there are tables you can turn to for help in quickly converting measurements. (See *Insta-metric conversion table* and *Amazing metric decimal place finder*, page 90.)

Converting meters to kilometers

Suppose you want to convert 15 meters (m) to kilometers (km). There are two ways to get this done.

Dancing decimal

Using the *Amazing metric decimal place finder*, page 90, you can follow these steps:

Amazing metric decimal place finder

When performing metric conversions, use the following scale as a guide to decimal placement. Each bar represents one decimal place.

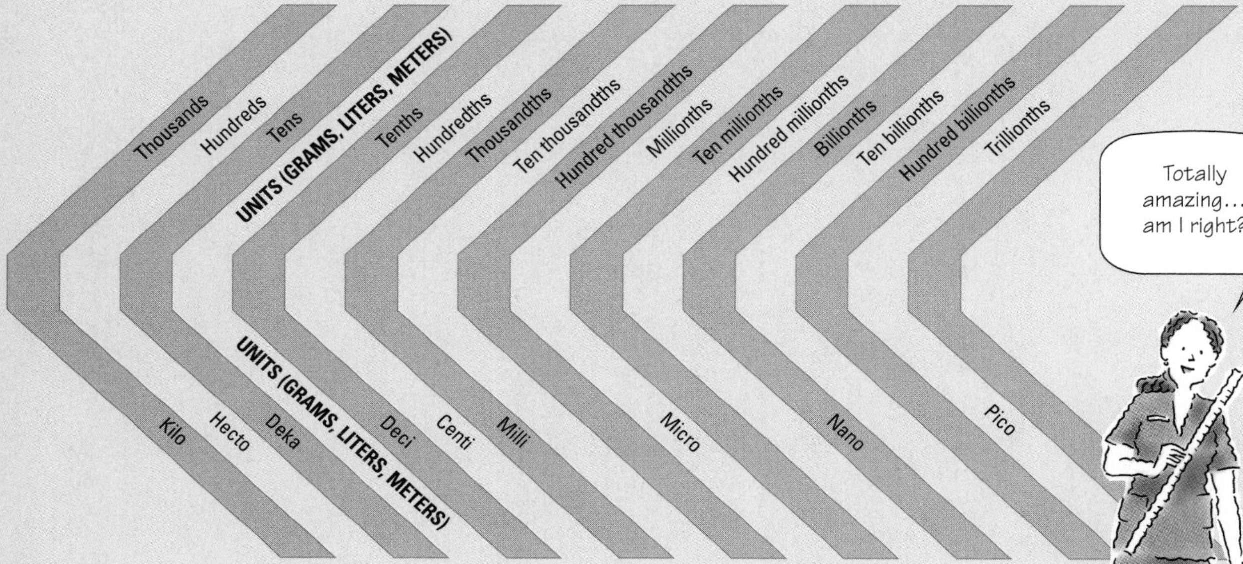

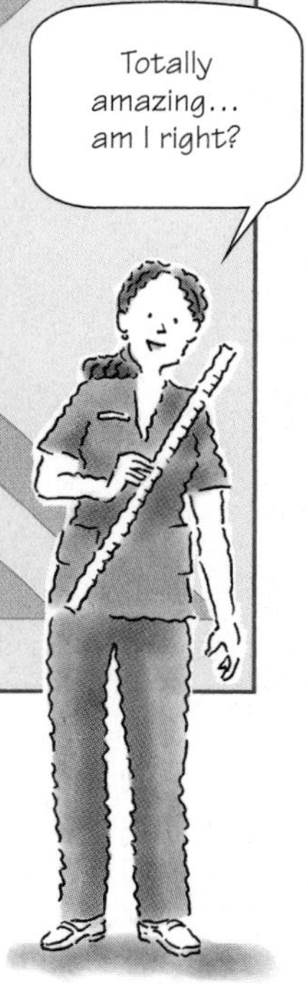

☝ Count the number of places to the right or left of *meters* it takes to reach *kilo*. You'll see that *kilo* is *three* places to the left, indicating that a kilometer is 1,000 times larger than a meter (note the three zeros in 1,000).

✌ Move the decimal point in 15.0 three places to the *left*, creating the number 0.015. So, 15 m = 0.015 km. *Remember to place a zero in front of the decimal point to draw attention to the decimal point's presence.*

On another road to conversion

Another way to complete this conversion is to use the chart in *What a little prefix can do*, page 88. First, find *kilo*. You'll see that it indicates a multiple of 1,000. When using this chart to go from smaller units to larger units (as you're doing with meters to kilometers), you divide by the multiple.

Here's why: 1 meter multiplied by 1,000 equals 1 km. Think of driving in Europe or Canada, where road distance is measured in kilometers; if you drive 1 m of a 1-km road, you're $\frac{1}{1,000}$ of the way there. Therefore, 1 m equals $\frac{1}{1,000}$ km.

To convert 15 m to kilometers, divide by 1,000. You might want to set up a simple equation:

$$X = \frac{15\text{ m}}{1,000}$$

$$X = 0.015\text{ km}$$

So, 15 m = 0.015 km, or 15 thousandths of a kilometer.

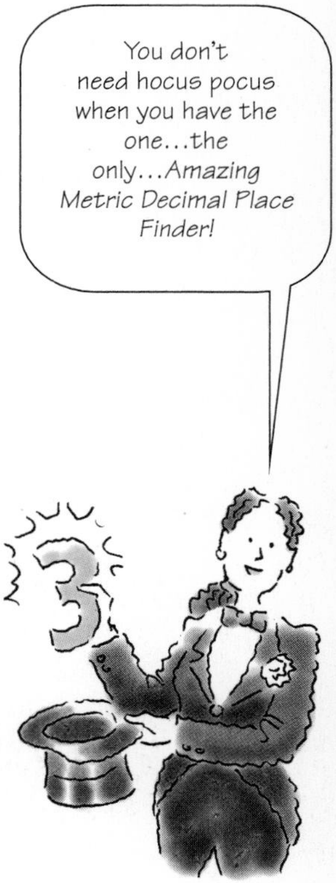
You don't need hocus pocus when you have the one...the only...Amazing Metric Decimal Place Finder!

Converting grams to milligrams

Now let's say that you want to convert 5 g to milligrams. Again, you can use one of two methods.

Decimal dances again

Using the *Amazing metric decimal place finder*, follow these steps:

1. Count the number of places to the right or left of *grams* it takes to reach *milli.* You'll see that *milli* is three places to the right, indicating that a milligram is 1,000 times smaller than a gram (note the three zeros in 1,000).
2. Move the decimal point in 5.0 three places to the right, creating the number 5,000. So 5 g = 5,000 mg.

The multiplying subdivision

Or, as before, the chart in *What a little prefix can do*, page 88, can help you complete your conversion. This time, find *milli.* You'll see that its subdivision is 0.001, or $\frac{1}{1,000}$. When using this table to go from a larger unit to a smaller unit (such as grams to milligrams), divide by the subdivision. Here's why: 1 milligram is $\frac{1}{1,000}$ of a gram. Therefore, 1 g equals 1,000 mg. If you divide 1 g by the subdivision ($\frac{1}{1,000}$), you get 1,000 mg (dividing by $\frac{1}{1,000}$ is the same as multiplying by 1,000). So to convert 5 g to milligrams, divide 5 g by $\frac{1}{1,000}$ (or multiply it by 1,000).

$$X = \frac{5\text{ g}}{\frac{1}{1,000}}$$

$$X = 5\text{ g} \times 1,000$$

$$X = 5,000\text{ mg}$$

As you can see, 5 g = 5,000 mg.

Converting centiliters to liters

How do you convert 350 cl to liters? Here's how using both charts.

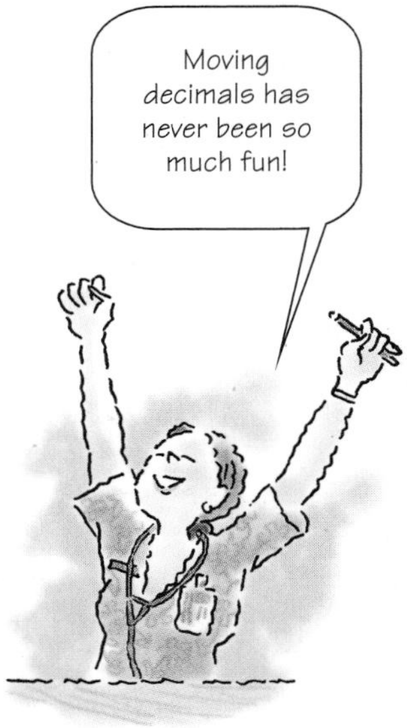

Moving decimals has never been so much fun!

Dancing decimal never rests

Using the *Amazing metric decimal place finder*, page 90, follow these steps:

1. Count the number of places to the right or left of *centi* it takes to reach *liters*. You'll see that *liters* is two places to the left, indicating that a liter is 100 times larger than a centiliter.

2. To show this, move the decimal point in 350.0 two places to the left, creating the number 3.5. So, 350 cl = 3.5 L.

Another vision of subdivision

Now refer to the chart in *What a little prefix can do*, page 88. First, find *centi*. You'll see that its subdivision is 0.01 or $\frac{1}{100}$. When using this chart to go from a smaller unit to a larger one (centiliters to liters), you multiply by the subdivision.

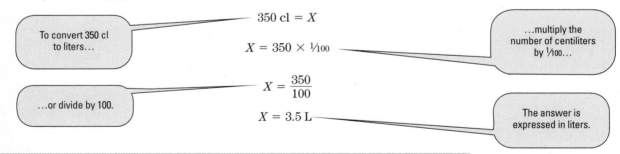

Here's why: 1 L equals 100 cl. Therefore, 1 centiliter is $\frac{1}{100}$ L (or 1 liter divided by 100). To convert 350 cl to liters, multiply 350 cl by $\frac{1}{100}$ (which is the same as dividing by 100) to get 3.5 L.

To convert 350 cl to liters...

$$350 \text{ cl} = X$$

...multiply the number of centiliters by $\frac{1}{100}$...

$$X = 350 \times \frac{1}{100}$$

...or divide by 100.

$$X = \frac{350}{100}$$

The answer is expressed in liters.

$$X = 3.5 \text{ L}$$

Solving for *X*

Another way to convert between metric units is by solving for *X*. The following examples show how to solve for *X* in three clinical situations. If you don't like fractions, see *Overcoming fear of fractions*, on page 93.

How much does that baby weigh?

An infant weighs 6.5 kg. How much does he weigh in grams? To solve the problem, follow these steps:

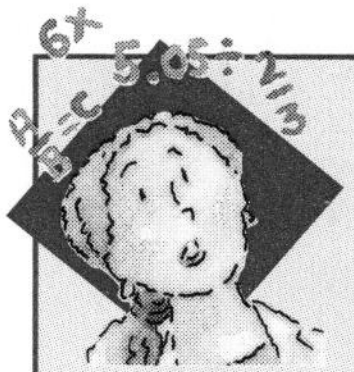

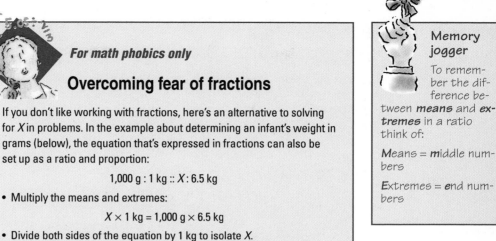

For math phobics only

Overcoming fear of fractions

If you don't like working with fractions, here's an alternative to solving for X in problems. In the example about determining an infant's weight in grams (below), the equation that's expressed in fractions can also be set up as a ratio and proportion:

$$1{,}000 \text{ g} : 1 \text{ kg} :: X : 6.5 \text{ kg}$$

- Multiply the means and extremes:

$$X \times 1 \text{ kg} = 1{,}000 \text{ g} \times 6.5 \text{ kg}$$

- Divide both sides of the equation by 1 kg to isolate X.
- Cancel units that appear in both the numerator and denominator.

$$X = 6{,}500 \text{ g}$$

The infant weighs 6,500 g.

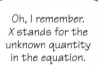

Memory jogger

To remember the difference between **means** and **extremes** in a ratio think of:

Means = **m**iddle numbers

Extremes = **e**nd numbers

First, refer to the *Insta-metric conversion table*, page 89. You'll see that 1,000 g equals 1 kg.

Now set up the following equation, substituting X for the unknown weight in grams:

$$\frac{1{,}000 \text{ g}}{1 \text{ kg}} = \frac{X}{6.5 \text{ kg}}$$

Cross-multiply the fractions:

$$\frac{1{,}000 \text{ g}}{1 \text{ kg}} \quad \times \quad \frac{X}{6.5 \text{ kg}}$$

$$X \times 1 \text{ kg} = 6.5 \text{ kg} \times 1{,}000 \text{ g}$$

Divide both sides of the equation by 1 kg to isolate X. Cancel units that appear in both the numerator and denominator:

$$\frac{X \times \cancel{1 \text{ kg}}}{\cancel{1 \text{ kg}}} = \frac{6.5 \cancel{\text{kg}} \times 1{,}000 \text{ g}}{1 \cancel{\text{kg}}}$$

$$X = 6{,}500 \text{ g}$$

The infant weighs 6,500 g.

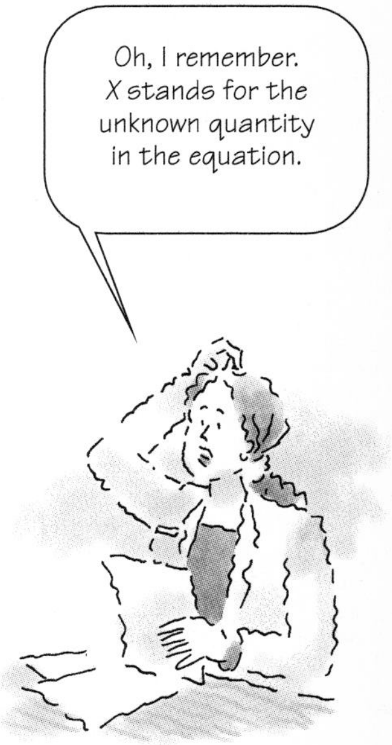

Oh, I remember. X stands for the unknown quantity in the equation.

How much I.V. fluid?

If a patient received 0.375 L of lactated Ringer's solution, how many milliliters did he receive?

- Refer to the *Insta-metric conversion table*, page 89. You'll see that 1 L is equal to 1,000 ml.
- Now set up the following equation, substituting *X* for the unknown amount of I.V. solution in milliliters:

$$\frac{1\text{ L}}{1{,}000\text{ ml}} = \frac{0.375\text{ L}}{X}$$

- Cross-multiply the fractions:

$$\frac{1\text{ L}}{1{,}000\text{ ml}} \times \frac{0.375\text{ L}}{X}$$

$$X \times 1\text{ L} = 0.375\text{ L} \times 1{,}000\text{ ml}$$

- Divide both sides of the equation by 1 L to isolate *X*. Cancel units that appear in both the numerator and denominator:

$$\frac{X \times \cancel{1\text{ L}}}{\cancel{1\text{ L}}} = \frac{0.375\ \cancel{\text{L}} \times 1{,}000\text{ ml}}{1\ \cancel{\text{L}}}$$

$$X = 375\text{ ml}$$

The patient received 375 ml of I.V. fluid.

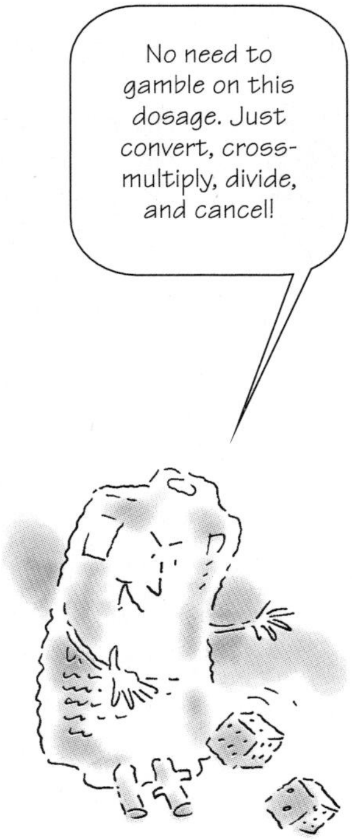

No need to gamble on this dosage. Just convert, cross-multiply, divide, and cancel!

How much medication?

A nurse administered 2 g of ceftriaxone (Rocephin). How many milligrams of this medication did the patient receive?

- Refer to the *Insta-metric conversion table*, page 89. You'll see that 1 g is equal to 1,000 mg.
- Now set up the following equation, substituting *X* for the unknown amount of medication in milligrams:

$$\frac{1\text{ g}}{1{,}000\text{ mg}} = \frac{2\text{ g}}{X}$$

- Cross-multiply the fractions:

$$\frac{1\text{ g}}{1{,}000\text{ mg}} \times \frac{2\text{ g}}{X}$$

$$X \times 1\text{ g} = 2\text{ g} \times 1{,}000\text{ mg}$$

- Divide each side of the equation by 1 g, to isolate *X*. Cancel units that appear in both the numerator and denominator:

$$\frac{X \times \cancel{1\text{ g}}}{\cancel{1\text{ g}}} = \frac{2\ \cancel{\text{g}} \times 1{,}000\text{ mg}}{1\ \cancel{\text{g}}}$$

$$X = 2{,}000\text{ mg}$$

The patient received 2,000 mg of Rocephin.

Dosage drill

Test your math skills with this drill.

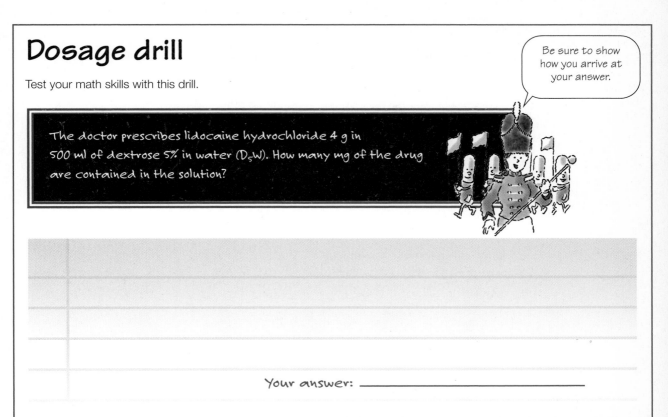

Be sure to show how you arrive at your answer.

The doctor prescribes lidocaine hydrochloride 4 g in 500 ml of dextrose 5% in water (D_5W). How many mg of the drug are contained in the solution?

Your answer: ____________________

To determine the correct answer, first refer to the *Insta-metric conversion table,* page 89. You'll see that 1 g is equal to 1,000 mg. Next, set up an equation, substituting *X* for the unknown amount of medication in milligrams.

$$\frac{1\text{ g}}{1{,}000\text{ mg}} = \frac{4\text{ g}}{X}$$

Now cross-multiply the fractions.

$$X \times 1\text{ g} = 4\text{ g} \times 1{,}000\text{ mg}$$

Divide each side of the equation by 1 g to isolate *X*. Cancel units that appear in both the numerator and denominator.

$$\frac{X \times \cancel{1\text{g}}}{\cancel{1\text{g}}} = \frac{4\,\cancel{\text{g}} \times 1{,}000\text{ m}}{\cancel{1\text{g}}}$$

$$X = 4{,}000\text{ mg}$$

The solution contains 4,000 mg of lidocaine hydrochloride.

Metric mathematics

To add, subtract, multiply, or divide different metric units, first convert all quantities to the same unit. Unless the problem calls for an answer in a specific unit, use the common unit that's easiest for you to work with and then perform the arithmetic.

For example, suppose you want to add 2 kg, 202 mg, and 222 g, expressing the total in grams. Here's how to do this:

1. First, convert all the measurements to grams. (Refer to the *Insta-metric conversion table*, page 89.)
2. 1 kg equals 1,000 g. Therefore, you can multiply 2 kg by 1,000 to get 2,000 g.
3. 1,000 mg equals 1 g and 1 mg equals $\frac{1}{1,000}$ g. Therefore, you can divide 202 mg by 1,000 to get 0.202 g.
4. Now do the addition:

$$2,000 + 0.202 + 222 = 2,222.202 \text{ g}$$

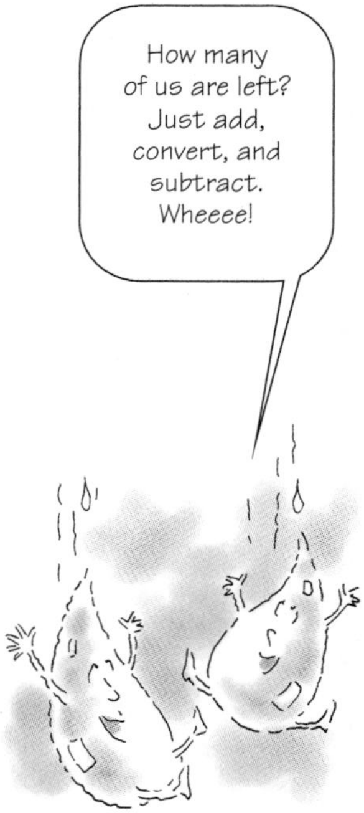

How many of us are left? Just add, convert, and subtract. Wheeee!

Real world problems

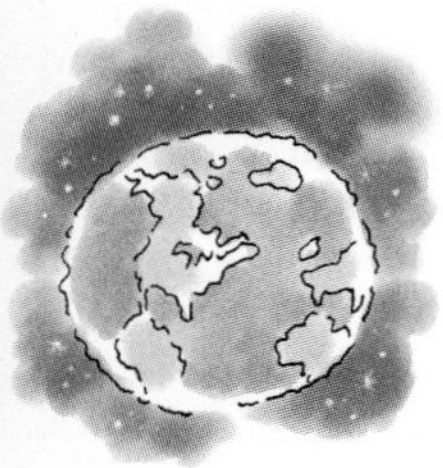

A patient with a 1 L bag of I.V. fluid received 500 ml of fluid over the first shift, 225 ml over the second shift, and 150 ml over the third shift. How many milliliters of fluid remain in the I.V. bag?

- First, determine how much fluid the patient received. To do this, add:

$$500 + 225 + 150 = 875 \text{ ml}$$

- Because you're trying to determine the number of milliliters remaining, you need to convert only 1 L to milliliters. Refer to the *Insta-metric conversion table*, page 89, where you'll see that 1 L = 1,000 ml.
- Lastly, compute the amount of fluid remaining in the I.V. bag by subtracting 875 ml from 1,000 ml. The answer is 125 ml.

A tantalizing tablet tabulation!

A patient is to receive 5 g of erythromycin (Erythrocin) before intestinal surgery. If erythromycin is available in 500-mg tablets, how many tablets should be administered?

- First, convert all the measures to the same units. Because you're trying to determine the number of 500-mg tablets to administer, convert 5 g to milligrams. Refer to the *Insta-metric conversion table*, page 89, where you'll see that 1 g is equal to 1,000 mg.
- To find how many milligrams are in 5 g, set up this proportion using fractions:

$$\frac{1{,}000\text{ mg}}{1\text{ g}} = \frac{X}{5\text{ g}}$$

- Then cross-multiply the fractions and divide each side of the resulting equation by 1 g to solve for X:

$$\frac{1{,}000\text{ mg}}{1\text{ g}} \times \frac{X}{5\text{ g}}$$

$$X \times 1\text{ g} = 1{,}000\text{ mg} \times 5\text{ g}$$

$$\frac{X \times \cancel{1\text{ g}}}{\cancel{1\text{ g}}} = \frac{1{,}000\text{ mg} \times 5\text{ }\cancel{\text{g}}}{1\text{ }\cancel{\text{g}}}$$

$$X = 5{,}000\text{ mg}$$

- You find that X is 5,000 mg.
- To determine the number of 500-mg tablets that need to be administered to provide 5,000 mg, set up another proportion using fractions:

$$\frac{500\text{ mg}}{1\text{ tablet}} = \frac{5{,}000\text{ mg}}{X}$$

- Cross-multiply the fractions and divide each side of the resulting equation by 500 mg to solve for X:

$$\frac{500\text{ mg}}{1\text{ tablet}} \times \frac{5{,}000\text{ mg}}{X}$$

$$X \times 500\text{ mg} = 5{,}000\text{ mg} \times 1\text{ tablet}$$

$$\frac{X \times \cancel{500\text{ mg}}}{\cancel{500\text{ mg}}} = \frac{1\text{ tablet} \times 5{,}000\text{ }\cancel{\text{mg}}}{500\text{ }\cancel{\text{mg}}}$$

$$X = 10\text{ tablets}$$

- You find that X is 10 tablets.

You should administer 10 tablets of erythromycin. (See *Did I get it right?*)

Did I get it right?

There may be times when you work out a dosage calculation and your answer doesn't strike you as being correct. Try verifying your answer by inserting it for *X* in the equation and doing the calculations. Both sides of the equation should be equal. As an example, let's use the previous problem about erythromycin tablets:

In this problem $X = 10$ tablets, so let's substitute that in the equation for *X*:

$$\frac{500\text{ mg}}{1\text{ tablet}} = \frac{5{,}000\text{ mg}}{10\text{ tablets}}$$

$$\frac{500\text{ mg}}{1\text{ tablet}} \times \frac{5{,}000\text{ mg}}{10\text{ tablets}}$$

$$10\text{ tablets} \times 500\text{ mg} = 5{,}000\text{ mg} \times 1\text{ tablet}$$

$$\frac{10\text{ tablets} \times \cancel{500\text{ mg}}}{\cancel{500\text{ mg}}} = \frac{1\text{ tablet} \times 5{,}000\text{ }\cancel{\text{mg}}}{500\text{ }\cancel{\text{mg}}}$$

$$10\text{ tablets} = 10\text{ tablets}$$

As you can see, both sides of the equation are equal. Congratulations! You got it right!

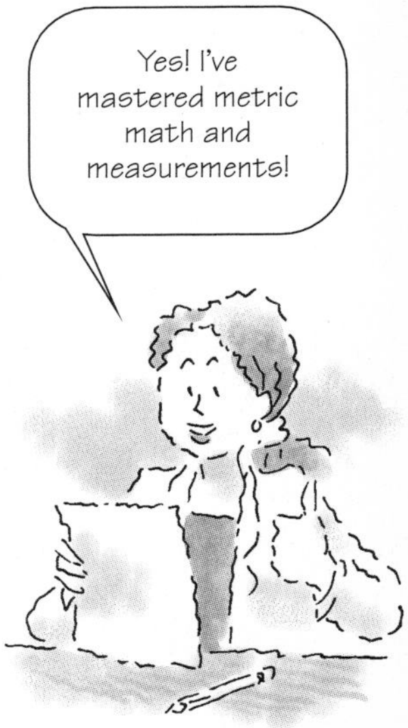
Yes! I've mastered metric math and measurements!

Dosage drill

Test your math skills with this drill.

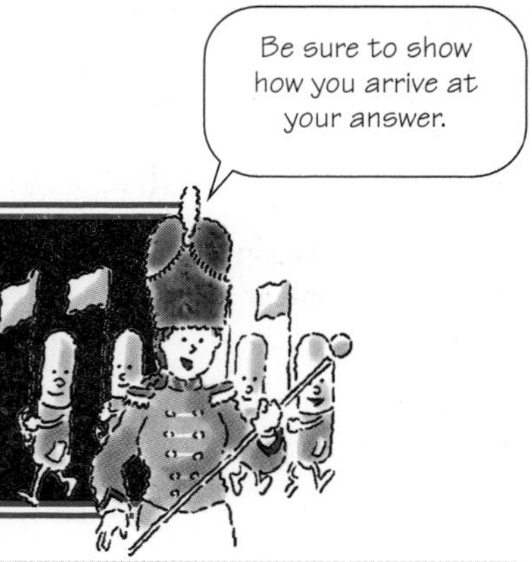
Be sure to show how you arrive at your answer.

A patient is prescribed a single dose of tinidazole (Tindamax) 2 g P.O. for treatment of trichomoniasis. If tinidazole is available in 500-mg tablets, how many tablets should the patient receive?

Your answer: ____________________

To find the answer, first refer to the *Insta-metric conversion table,* page 89. You'll see that 1 g is equal to 1,000 mg. Now, set up an equation substituting *X* for the unknown amount of milligrams.

$$\frac{1\text{ g}}{1{,}000\text{ mg}} = \frac{2\text{ g}}{X}$$

Cross-multiply the fractions.

$$X \times 1\text{ g} = 2\text{ g} \times 1{,}000\text{ mg}$$

Divide each side of the equation by 1 g to isolate *X*. Cancel units that appear in both the numerator and denominator:

$$\frac{X \times \cancel{1\text{ g}}}{\cancel{1\text{ g}}} = \frac{2\text{ }\cancel{\text{g}} \times 1{,}000\text{ mg}}{1\text{ }\cancel{\text{g}}}$$

$$X = 2{,}000\text{ mg}$$

To determine how many 500-mg tablets the patient should receive to provide the 2,000-mg dose, set up the following equation.

$$\frac{500\text{ mg}}{1\text{ tablet}} = \frac{2{,}000\text{ mg}}{X}$$

Cross-multiply the fractions.

$$X \times 500\text{ mg} = 2{,}000\text{ mg} \times 1\text{ tablet}$$

$$\frac{X \times \cancel{500\text{ mg}}}{\cancel{500\text{ mg}}} = \frac{1\text{ tablet} \times 2{,}000\text{ }\cancel{\text{mg}}}{500\text{ }\cancel{\text{mg}}}$$

$$X = 4\text{ tablets}$$

The patient should receive 4 tablets.

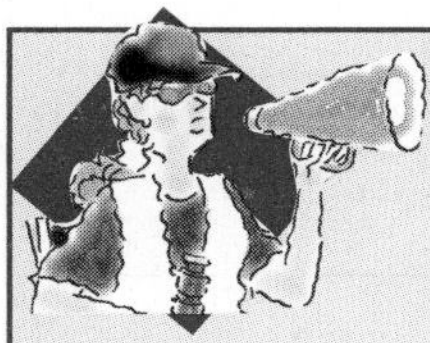

That's a wrap!

Metric system review

Knowing these important facts about the metric system will make your calculations incredibly easy!

Metric basics

- It's the most widely used system for measuring amounts of drugs.
- It's a decimal system (based on the number 10 and its multiples and subdivisions).
- Three basic units of measurement are used in the metric system:
  - *meter,* basic unit of length
  - *liter,* basic unit of volume
  - *gram,* basic unit of weight.
- Multiples and subdivisions of meters, liters, and grams are indicated by using a prefix before the basic unit, such as *kilo, centi,* or *milli.*

Metric conversions

- To convert a smaller unit to a larger unit:
  - move the decimal point to the left
  - OR divide by the appropriate multiple
  - OR multiply by the appropriate subdivision.
- To convert a larger unit to a smaller unit:
  - move the decimal point to the right
  - OR multiply by the appropriate multiple
  - OR divide by the appropriate subdivision.

Solving for *X*

- Set up an equation, substituting *X* for the unknown you're trying to determine.
- Cross-multiply the fractions.
- Divide both sides to isolate *X* on one side.
- Cancel units that appear in both the numerator and denominator.
- Do the math!

Metric math

- First, convert all quantities to the same unit.
- Use the common unit that's easiest (unless the problem calls for a specific unit).
- Do the math!

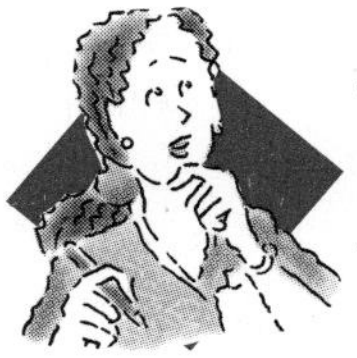

Quick quiz

1. According to the International System of Units, the correct abbreviation for gram is:

A. gm.
B. g.
C. Gm.
D. GM.

Answer: B. The standard abbreviation for gram is g.

2. The number of milligrams in 3,120 mcg is:

A. 3,120,000 mg.
B. 0.312 mg.
C. 31.2 mg.
D. 3.12 mg.

Answer: D. Locate *milli* and *micro* on the *Amazing metric decimal place finder*, page 90, count the number of places *milli* is to the left of *micro*, then move the decimal point three places to the left.

3. The total volume in milliliters of 312 ml, 3.12 L, and 312 L is:
- A. 327.12 ml.
- B. 315,432 ml.
- C. 31,543.2 L.
- D. 3,154 ml.

Answer: B. Convert all the measures to milliliters and then add all three numbers.

4. The measure that's equivalent to a milliliter (ml) is:
- A. cubic centimeter.
- B. kiloliter.
- C. hectoliter.
- D. centimeter.

Answer: A. A ml of liquid occupies a cubic centimeter of space.

5. The weight in grams of a baby who weighs 5.2 kg is:
- A. 5.2 g.
- B. 5.02 g.
- C. 50.2 g.
- D. 5,200 g.

Answer: D. Knowing that 1 kg is equal to 1,000 g, set up an equation with *X* grams as the unknown quantity and multiply 5.2 kg by 1,000 g/kg.

6. The number of milliliters left in a 4-L bag of normal saline solution after you remove 50 ml, 250 ml, 2.5 L, and 750 ml is:
- A. 3,550 ml.
- B. 450 ml.
- C. 50 ml.
- D. 40 ml.

Answer: B. Convert all the measurements to milliliters, add the last four numbers to find out how many milliliters were removed from the bag, then subtract this number from the amount of fluid in the bag.

Scoring

☆☆☆ If you answered all six items correctly, give yourself 6 points! If each point equalled a gram, you would have 6 grams, or 60 decigrams, or 600 centigrams…

☆☆ If you answered five items correctly, dig those decimals! You're a metric master.

☆ If you answered fewer than five items correctly, leapin' milliliters! Review the chapter and you'll soon be doing a hecto of a good job.

6

Alternative measurement systems

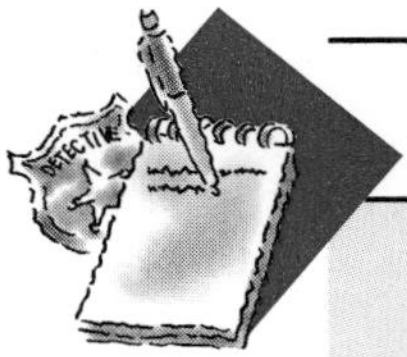

Just the facts

In this chapter, you'll learn:

- ♦ what the apothecaries' system is and how it works
- ♦ what the household system is and how it works
- ♦ what the avoirdupois system is and how it works
- ♦ what the unit system is and how it works
- ♦ what the milliequivalent system is and how it works
- ♦ how to perform common conversions.

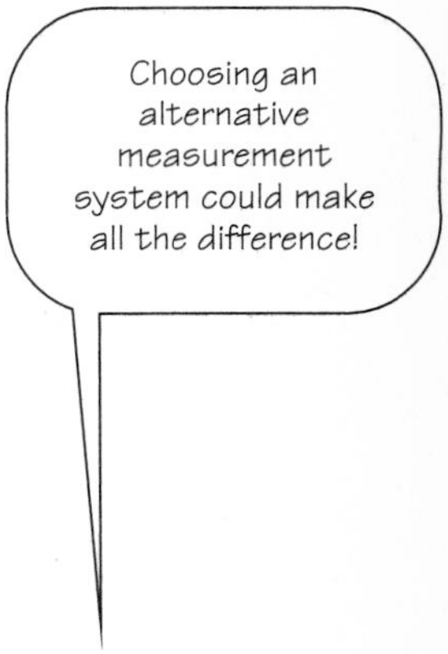

Choosing an alternative measurement system could make all the difference!

A look at alternative systems

Although the metric system is most commonly used in clinical settings, you'll work with other systems from time to time. These systems include the apothecaries', household, avoirdupois, unit, and milliequivalent systems.

When the alternative is the answer...

When would you use these other systems? For example, you might:

- receive a drug order written using the apothecaries' system
- teach a patient to use a measuring device calibrated in the household system
- use the avoirdupois system to calculate a dose that's based on a patient's weight.

You can prepare yourself for these occasions by familiarizing yourself with alternative measurement systems.

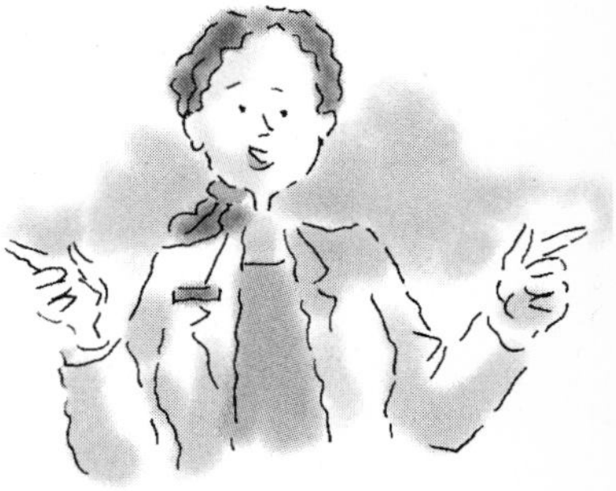

Apothecaries' system

Doctors and pharmacists used the apothecaries' system before the metric system was introduced. Since widespread adoption of the metric system, use of this older system has declined. Even though the apothecaries' system is rarely seen anymore, you should still be familiar with it.

Basic minims and grains

Unlike the metric system, which is used to measure length, volume, and weight, the apothecaries' system is used to measure only liquid volume and solid weight. The basic unit for measuring liquid volume is the minim, and the basic unit for measuring solid weight is the grain.

Think water and wheat

One way to remember these units is to visualize the minim as about the size of a drop of water, which weighs about the same as a grain of wheat. The following mathematical statement sums up this relationship:

$$1 \text{ drop} = 1 \text{ minim} = 1 \text{ grain}$$

Other units of measure in the apothecaries' system build on these two basic units. Many of these units are also common household measurements. (See *Ye olde apothecaries' system.*)

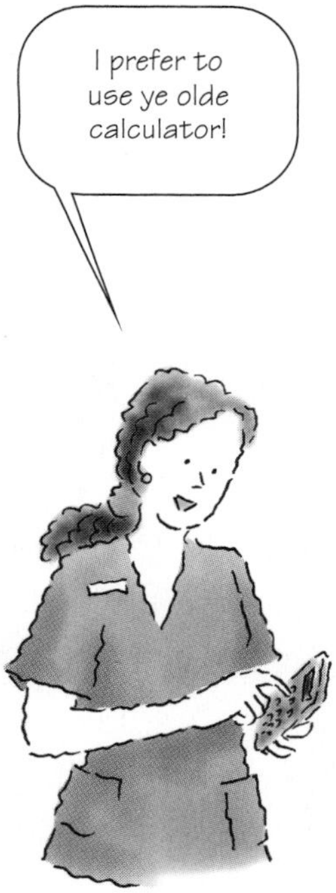
I prefer to use ye olde calculator!

The dram-a of conversions

Measurements of liquids and solids that are expressed in the apothecaries' system can easily be converted from one unit of measure to another. Here are a few examples:

- How many fluidrams are in 60 minims? From the table shown in *Ye olde apothecaries' system*, you can see that 60 minims equal 1 fluidram.
- How many quarts are in 1 gallon? One gallon equals 4 quarts of fluid.
- How many drams are in 30 grains? Because 60 grains equal 1 dram, 30 grains equal ½ dram.

Roman numerals

Some doctors and pharmacists express apothecaries' system dosages in Arabic numerals followed by units of measure.

Ye olde apothecaries' system

The apothecaries' system uses the following units to measure liquid volume and solid weight.

Liquid volume	
	60 minims (m) = 1 fluidram
	8 fluidrams = 1 fluid ounce (oz)
	16 fluid oz = 1 pint (pt)
	2 pt = 1 quart (qt)
	4 qt = 1 gallon (gal)
Solid weight	
	60 grains (gr) = 1 dram
	8 drams = 1 oz
	12 oz = 1 pound (lb)

However, the apothecaries' system traditionally uses Roman numerals. (See *The road to Roman numerals*, page 104.)

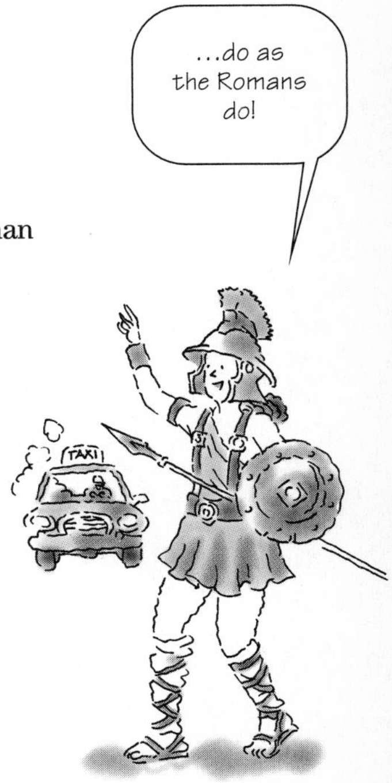

When in Rome...

When used in pharmacologic applications, Roman numerals ss (½) through x (10) are usually written in lower case. When Roman numerals are used, the unit of measure goes before the numeral. For example, 5 grains is written *grains v.* Fractions of less than ½ are written as common fractions using Arabic numerals. Other quantities are expressed by combining letters according to two general rules.

- When a smaller numeral precedes a larger numeral, subtract the smaller numeral from the larger numeral. For example:

$$IX = 10 - 1 = 9$$

- When a smaller numeral follows a larger numeral, add the numerals. For example:

$$XI = 10 + 1 = 11$$

The road to Roman numerals

Here's a handy review of Roman numerals.

½ = ss	11 = XI	40 = XL
1 = I	12 = XII	50 = L
2 = II	13 = XIII	60 = LX
3 = III	14 = XIV	70 = LXX
4 = IV	15 = XV	80 = LXXX
5 = V	16 = XVI	90 = XC
6 = VI	17 = XVII	100 = C
7 = VII	18 = XVIII	500 = D
8 = VIII	19 = XIX	1,000 = M
9 = IX	20 = XX	
10 = X	30 = XXX	

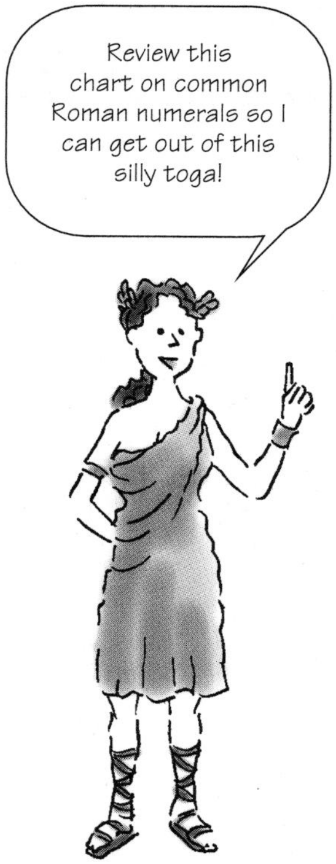

Review this chart on common Roman numerals so I can get out of this silly toga!

Breaking up is easy to do

To convert an Arabic numeral to a Roman numeral, first break the Arabic numeral into its component parts; then translate each part into Roman numerals. For example:

36 = 30 + 6 = XXX + VI = XXXVI

Roman numeral conversions

Now that you understand how Roman numerals work, convert the numbers below.

- Write 53 using Roman numerals:

  53 = 50 + 3 = L + III = LIII

- Write CXXVI using Arabic numerals:

  CXXVI = C + X + X + VI = 100 + 10 + 10 + 6 = 126

- Write 1,558 using Roman numerals:

  1,558 = 1,000 + 500 + 50 + 8 = M + D + L + VIII = MDLVIII

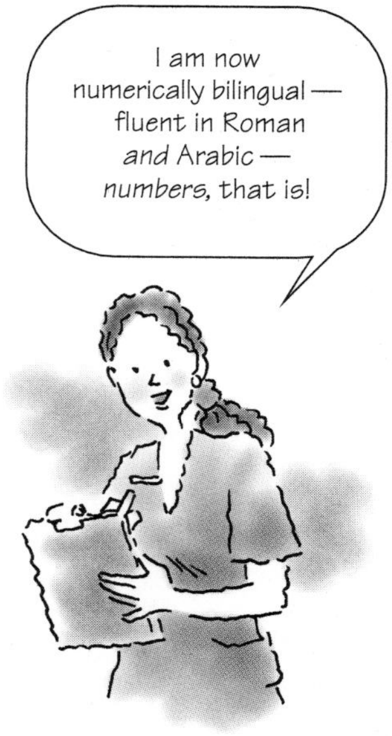

I am now numerically bilingual — fluent in Roman and Arabic — numbers, that is!

Household system

The household system of measurement uses droppers, teaspoons, tablespoons, and cups to measure liquid medication doses. However, because these measuring devices aren't all alike, the household system is useful only for approximate measurements. For exact measurements, use the metric system. (See *Making sure the cup doesn't runneth over.*)

To measure prescribed drug doses at home, teach the patient the household system. (See *A spoonful of sugar*, page 106.)

Household system conversions

The examples that follow show how to convert measurements using the household system.

Making sure the cup doesn't runneth over

Will your patient be taking medication at home? If so, teach him to use the devices below to help ensure accurate measurements.

Medication cup

A medication cup is calibrated in household, metric, and apothecaries' systems. Tell the patient to set the cup on a counter or flat surface and to check the fluid measurement at eye level.

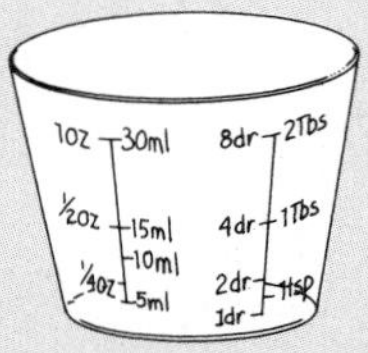

Dropper

A dropper is calibrated in household or metric systems or in terms of medication strength or concentration. Advise the patient to hold the dropper at eye level to check the fluid measurement.

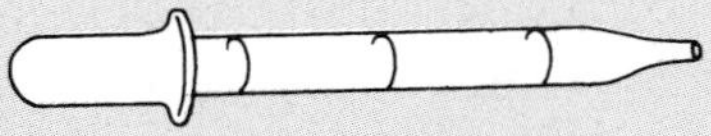

Hollow-handle spoon

A hollow-handle spoon is calibrated in teaspoons and tablespoons. Teach the patient to check the dose after filling by holding the spoon upright at eye level. Instruct him to administer the medication by tilting the spoon until the medicine fills the bowl of the spoon and then placing the spoon in his mouth.

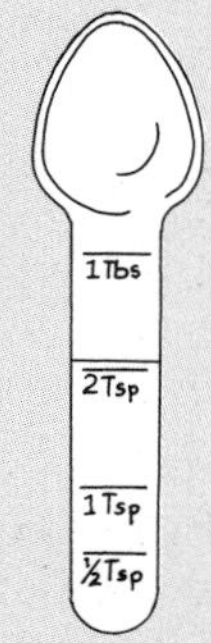

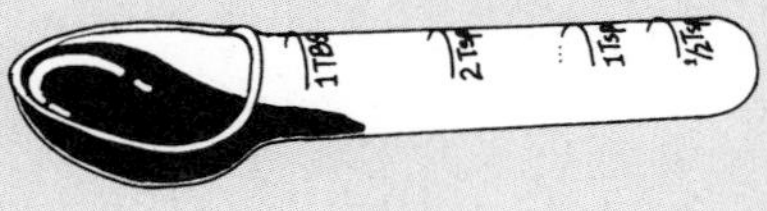

Cough syrup conundrum

The doctor has ordered 120 drops (gtt) of an expectorant cough syrup every 6 hours for your patient. The drug label gives instructions in teaspoons. How many teaspoons should you administer?

- There are 60 gtt of liquid in 1 teaspoon (tsp). To find out how many teaspoons are in 120 gtt, set up the following equation, using X as the unknown quantity:

$$\frac{60 \text{ gtt}}{1 \text{ tsp}} = \frac{120 \text{ gtt}}{X}$$

- Cross-multiply the fractions:

$$X \times 60 \text{ gtt} = 1 \text{ tsp} \times 120 \text{ gtt}$$

- Solve for X by dividing both sides of the equation by 60 gtt and canceling units that appear in both the numerator and denominator:

$$\frac{X \times \cancel{60 \text{ gtt}}}{\cancel{60 \text{ gtt}}} = \frac{1 \text{ tsp} \times 120 \cancel{\text{gtt}}}{60 \cancel{\text{gtt}}}$$

$$X = \frac{1 \text{ tsp} \times 120}{60}$$

$$X = 2 \text{ tsp}$$

The patient should receive 2 tsp of cough syrup.

Broth brain buster

Your patient is on a clear liquid diet. For lunch he drank 6 tablespoons (tbs) of chicken broth. How many ounces did he consume?

- There are 2 tbs of liquid in 1 ounce (oz). To find out how many ounces are in 6 tbs, set up the following equation, using X as the unknown quantity:

$$\frac{2 \text{ tbs}}{1 \text{ oz}} = \frac{6 \text{ tbs}}{X}$$

- Cross-multiply the fractions:

$$X \times 2 \text{ tbs} = 1 \text{ oz} \times 6 \text{ tbs}$$

- Find X by dividing each side of the equation by 2 tbs and canceling units that appear in both the numerator and denominator:

$$\frac{X \times \cancel{2 \text{ tbs}}}{\cancel{2 \text{ tbs}}} = \frac{1 \text{ oz} \times 6 \cancel{\text{tbs}}}{2 \cancel{\text{tbs}}}$$

$$X = 3 \text{ oz}$$

The patient consumed 3 oz of chicken broth.

A spoonful of sugar

Mary Poppins was no pharmacist, but she knew how to make the medicine go down. She recommended a spoonful of sugar. The question is, how much is in a spoonful?

Here's a rundown of the most commonly used household units of measure and their equivalent liquid volumes. *Note:* Don't use the abbreviations "t" for teaspoon and "T" for tablespoon because it's easy to make errors when writing them quickly.

60 drops (gtt) = 1 teaspoon (tsp)

3 tsp = 1 tablespoon (tbs)

2 tbs = 1 ounce (oz)

8 oz = 1 cup

16 oz (2 cups) = 1 pint (pt)

2 pt = 1 quart (qt)

4 qt = 1 gallon (gal)

Dosage drill

Test your math skills with this drill.

Be sure to show how you arrive at your answer.

The doctor has ordered acetaminophen (Tylenol) 2 tablespoons (tbs) by mouth every 4 hours, as needed for temperature greater than 101.5° F (38.6° C). The drug label gives instructions in teaspoons (tsp). How many tsp should you administer?

Your answer: ____________________

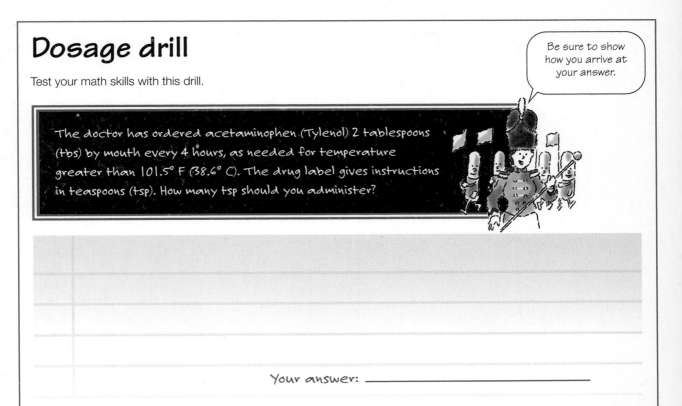

To find the answer, remember there are 3 tsp of liquid in 1 tbs. Set up the following equation to find out how many tsp are in 2 tbs:

$$\frac{3\text{ tsp}}{1\text{ tbs}} = \frac{X}{2\text{ tbs}}$$

Cross-multiply the fractions.

$$1\text{ tbs} \times X = 3\text{ tsp} \times 2\text{ tbs}$$

Divide each side of the equation by 1 tbs to isolate *X*. Cancel units that appear in both the numerator and denominator:

$$\frac{X \times \cancel{1\text{ tbs}}}{\cancel{1\text{ tbs}}} = \frac{3\text{ tsp} \times 2\,\cancel{\text{tbs}}}{1\,\cancel{\text{tbs}}}$$

$$X = 6\text{ tsp}$$

You should administer 6 tsp of acetaminophen.

Milk of magnesia mystery

Your patient is to receive 4 tbs of milk of magnesia. This is equal to how many teaspoons?

- There are 3 tsp of liquid in 1 tbs. To find out how many teaspoons are in 4 tbs, set up the following equation using *X* as the unknown quantity:

$$\frac{3 \text{ tsp}}{1 \text{ tbs}} = \frac{X}{4 \text{ tbs}}$$

- Solve for *X* by cross-multiplying the fractions, dividing each side of the equation by 1 tbs, and canceling units that appear in both the numerator and denominator:

$$\frac{X \times \cancel{1 \text{ tbs}}}{\cancel{1 \text{ tbs}}} = \frac{3 \text{ tsp} \times 4 \cancel{\text{tbs}}}{1 \cancel{\text{tbs}}}$$

$$X = 12 \text{ tsp}$$

The patient gets 12 tsp of milk of magnesia.

Avoirdupois system

This difficult-to-pronounce system of measurement (av-wah-doo-PWAH) is used for ordering and purchasing some pharmaceutical products and for weighing patients.

In this system, which means *goods sold by weight,* the solid measures or units of weight include grains (gr), ounces (oz), and pounds (lb). One ounce equals 480 gr, and 1 lb equals 16 oz or 7,680 gr. Note that the apothecaries' pound equals 12 oz, but the avoirdupois pound equals 16 oz.

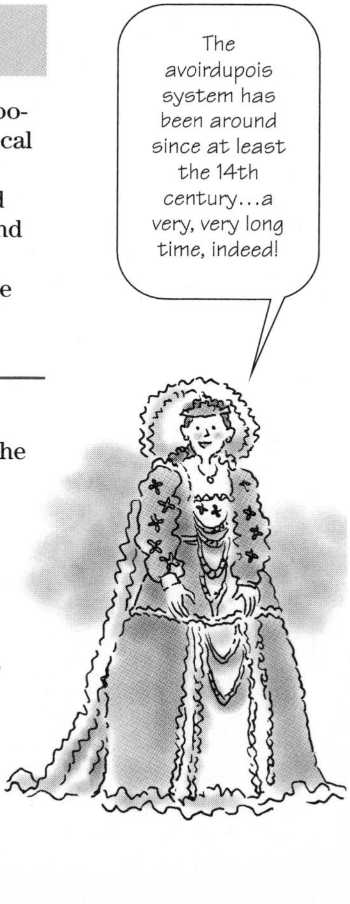

The avoirdupois system has been around since at least the 14th century…a very, very long time, indeed!

Avoirdupois system conversions

The following examples show how to perform conversions in the avoirdupois system:

- How many pounds equal 32 oz? One pound equals 16 oz; therefore, 2 lb equal 32 oz.
- How many ounces equal 7,680 gr? One ounce equals 480 gr; therefore, 16 oz equal 7,680 gr.
- How many grains are in 2 lb? You know that 7,680 gr are in 1 lb; therefore, 15,360 gr are in 2 lb. (See *Measure for measure,* page 109.)

Measure for measure

Here are some approximate liquid and solid equivalents among the household, apothecaries', avoirdupois, and metric systems. Use your facility's protocol for converting measurements from one system to another.

Liquids

Household	*Apothecaries'*	*Metric*
1 drop (gtt)	1 minim (m)	0.06 milliliter (ml)
15 to 16 gtt	15 to 16 m	1 ml
1 teaspoon (tsp)	1 fluidram	5 ml
1 tablespoon (tbs)	½ fluid ounce (oz)	15 ml
2 tbs	1 fluid oz	30 ml
1 cup	8 fluid oz	240 ml
1 pint (pt)	16 fluid oz	480 ml
1 quart (qt)	32 fluid oz	960 ml
1 gallon (gal)	128 fluid oz	3,840 ml

Solids

Avoirdupois	*Apothecaries'*	*Metric*
1 grain (gr)	gr i	0.06 gram (g)
1 gr	gr i	60 milligrams (mg)
15.4 gr	15 gr	1 g
1 oz	480 grains	28.35 g
1 pound (lb)	1.33 lb	454 g
2.2 lb	2.7 lb	1 kilogram (kg)

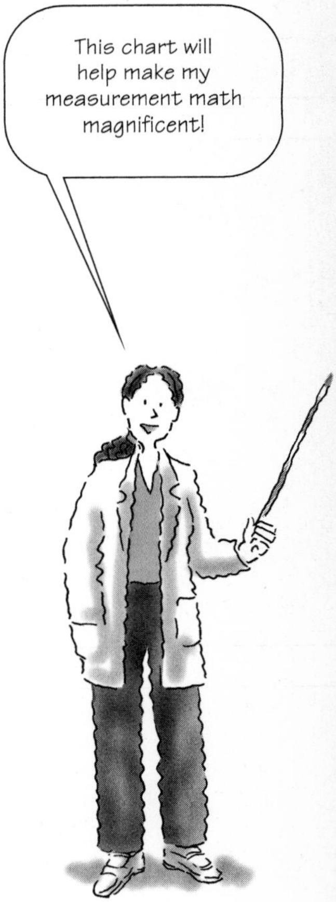

This chart will help make my measurement math magnificent!

Unit system

Some drugs are measured in units, such as United States Pharmacopoeia (USP) units or International Units (IU). The measurement of the unit is unique to each drug that's expressed in units.

U-niquely insulin

The most common drug that's measured in units is insulin, which comes in such measurements as U-100 strength.

With insulin, the U refers to the number of units per milliliter. For example, 1 ml of U-100 insulin contains 100 units.

More units singled out

Some other drugs are also measured in units, for example, the anticoagulant heparin, the topical antibiotic bacitracin, and penicillin G. The hormone calcitonin and the fat-soluble vitamins A, D, and E are measured in IU. Some forms of vitamin A and D are measured in USP units.

All out of proportion

To calculate the dose to be administered when the medication is available in units, use this proportion:

$$\frac{\text{amount of drug in ml or other measure}}{\text{dose required in units}} = \frac{\text{1 ml or other measure}}{\text{drug available in units}}$$

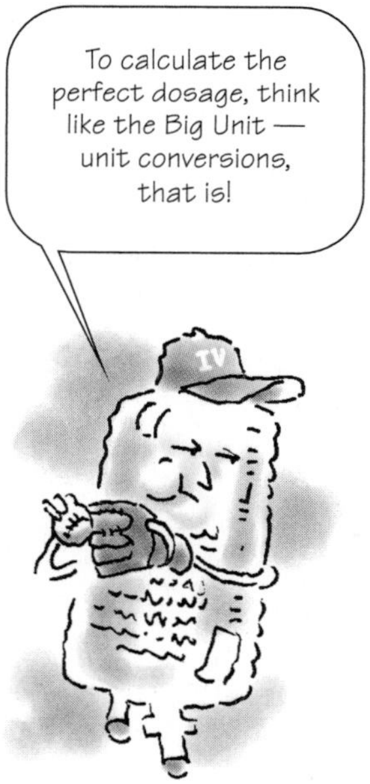

To calculate the perfect dosage, think like the Big Unit — unit conversions, that is!
IV

Unit system conversions

The examples in this section show how to perform conversions in the unit system.

Drip...drip...drip...

A standard heparin drip of 25,000 units in 500 ml of half-normal saline solution is ordered for your patient. The heparin vial that's available has 5,000 units/ml. How many milliliters of heparin should you add to the I.V. fluid? This is how to solve this problem:

- Set up a proportion using X as the unknown quantity:

$$\frac{X}{25{,}000 \text{ units}} = \frac{1 \text{ ml}}{5{,}000 \text{ units}}$$

- Cross-multiply the fractions:

$$X \times 5{,}000 \text{ units} = 1 \text{ ml} \times 25{,}000 \text{ units}$$

- Find X by dividing both sides of the equation by 5,000 units and canceling units that appear in both the numerator and denominator:

$$\frac{X \times \cancel{5{,}000 \text{ units}}}{\cancel{5{,}000 \text{ units}}} = \frac{1 \text{ ml} \times 25{,}000 \cancel{\text{ units}}}{5{,}000 \cancel{\text{ units}}}$$

$$X = 5 \text{ ml}$$

You should add 5 ml of heparin to the I.V. fluid.

Penicillin problem

Your patient needs 500,000 units of penicillin by I.M. injection. The vial of penicillin that's available contains 1,000,000 units/ml. How much of the drug should you draw up? This is how to solve this problem.

- Set up a proportion using *X* as the unknown quantity:

$$\frac{X}{500{,}000 \text{ units}} = \frac{1 \text{ ml}}{1{,}000{,}000 \text{ units}}$$

- Cross-multiply the fractions:

$$X \times 1{,}000{,}000 \text{ units} = 1 \text{ ml} \times 500{,}000 \text{ units}$$

- Find *X* by dividing each side of the equation by 1,000,000 units and canceling units that appear in both the numerator and denominator:

$$\frac{X \times \cancel{1{,}000{,}000 \text{ units}}}{\cancel{1{,}000{,}000 \text{ units}}} = \frac{1 \text{ ml} \times 500{,}000 \cancel{\text{ units}}}{1{,}000{,}000 \cancel{\text{ units}}}$$

$$X = 0.5 \text{ ml}$$

You should inject 0.5 ml of penicillin.

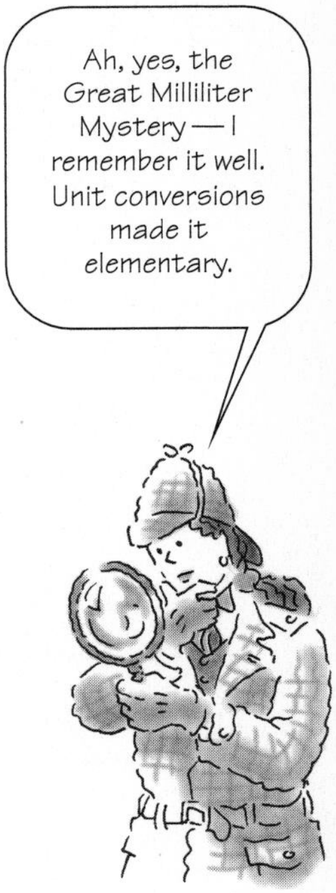

Ah, yes, the Great Milliliter Mystery — I remember it well. Unit conversions made it elementary.

Milliliter mystery

The doctor orders a bolus of 3,000 units of heparin for your patient. The heparin vial that's available contains 1,000 units/ml. How many milliliters should you administer?

- Set up a proportion using *X* as the unknown quantity of heparin:

$$\frac{X}{3{,}000 \text{ units}} = \frac{1 \text{ ml}}{1{,}000 \text{ units}}$$

- Cross-multiply the fractions:

$$X \times 1{,}000 \text{ units} = 1 \text{ ml} \times 3{,}000 \text{ units}$$

- Find *X* by dividing both sides of the equation by 1,000 units and canceling units that appear in both the numerator and denominator:

$$\frac{X \times \cancel{1{,}000 \text{ units}}}{\cancel{1{,}000 \text{ units}}} = \frac{1 \text{ ml} \times 3{,}000 \cancel{\text{ units}}}{1{,}000 \cancel{\text{ units}}}$$

$$X = 3 \text{ ml}$$

You should administer a 3-ml bolus of heparin.

Dosage drill

Test your math skills with this drill.

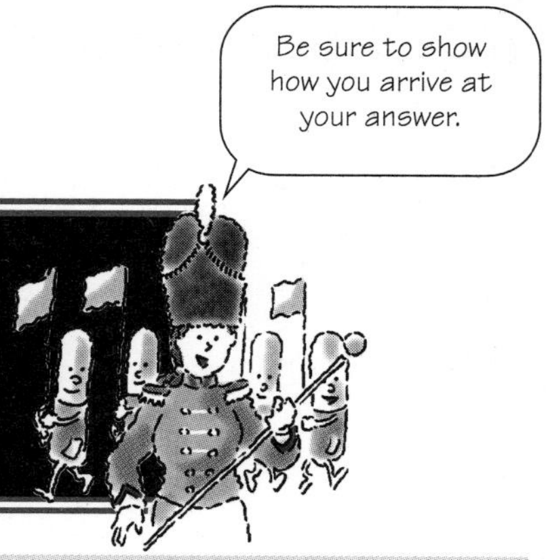
Be sure to show how you arrive at your answer.

Your patient needs a loading dose of streptokinase (Streptase) 250,000 international units. The vial of streptokinase contains 750,000 international units/ml. How much of the drug should you draw up?

Your answer: ______________________

To find the answer, first set up a proportion using *X* as the unknown quantity:

$$\frac{X}{250{,}000 \text{ international units}} = \frac{1 \text{ ml}}{750{,}000 \text{ international units}}$$

Cross-multiply the fractions:

$$X \times 750{,}000 \text{ international units} = 1 \text{ ml} \times 250{,}000 \text{ international units}$$

Find *X* by dividing each side of the equation by 750,000 international units and canceling units that appear in the numerator and denominator:

$$\frac{X \times \cancel{750{,}000 \text{ international units}}}{\cancel{750{,}000 \text{ international units}}} = \frac{1 \text{ ml} \times 250{,}000 \cancel{\text{ international units}}}{750{,}000 \cancel{\text{ international units}}}$$

$$X = 0.3 \text{ ml}$$

You should draw up 0.3 ml of the drug.

Milliequivalent system

Some electrolytes, such as potassium and sodium, are measured in milliequivalents (mEq). Drug manufacturers dispense information about the number of metric units required to provide the prescribed number of milliequivalents. For example, the manufacturer's instructions may indicate that 1 ml equals 4 mEq.

Electrolyte example

Doctors usually order the electrolyte potassium chloride in milliequivalents. Potassium preparations are available for use in I.V. fluids, as oral suspensions or elixirs, and in solid tablet or powder form. Potassium is also available in the combination drug potassium phosphate. The phosphate in this drug is measured in millimoles.

A promising proportion

To calculate the dose to be administered when the medication is available in milliequivalents, use this proportion:

$$\frac{\text{amount of drug in ml or other measure}}{\text{dose required in mEq}} = \frac{\text{1 ml or other measure}}{\text{drug available in mEq}}$$

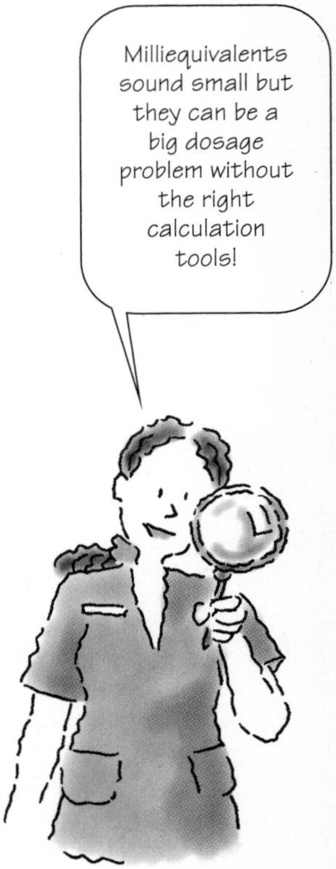

Milliequivalents sound small but they can be a big dosage problem without the right calculation tools!

Milliequivalent system conversions

The problems below show how to do conversions using the milliequivalent system.

Finding the solution solution

The doctor has ordered an I.V. infusion of 40 mEq of potassium chloride in 100 ml of normal saline solution for your patient. The potassium vial that's available contains 10 mEq/ml. How many milliliters of potassium chloride should you add to the normal saline solution? This is how to solve this problem.

- Set up a proportion using X as the unknown quantity:

$$\frac{X}{40\text{ mEq}} = \frac{1\text{ ml}}{10\text{ mEq}}$$

- Cross-multiply the fractions:

$$X \times 10\text{ mEq} = 1\text{ ml} \times 40\text{ mEq}$$

- Find X by dividing each side of the equation by 10 mEq and canceling units that appear in both the numerator and denominator:

$$\frac{X \times \cancel{10\text{ mEq}}}{\cancel{10\text{ mEq}}} = \frac{1\text{ ml} \times 40\ \cancel{\text{mEq}}}{10\ \cancel{\text{mEq}}}$$

$$X = 4\text{ ml}$$

You should dilute 4 ml of potassium chloride in 100 ml of normal saline solution.

Calculate that sodium bicarbonate!

Your patient needs 25 mEq of sodium bicarbonate. The vial from the pharmacy contains 50 mEq in 50 ml. How many milliliters of the solution should you administer? Here's how to solve this problem.

- Set up a proportion using *X* as the unknown quantity:

$$\frac{X}{25\text{ mEq}} = \frac{50\text{ ml}}{50\text{ mEq}}$$

- Cross-multiply the fractions:

$$X \times 50\text{ mEq} = 50\text{ ml} \times 25\text{ mEq}$$

- Find *X* by dividing both sides of the equation by 50 mEq and canceling units that appear in both the numerator and denominator:

$$\frac{X \times \cancel{50\text{ mEq}}}{\cancel{50\text{ mEq}}} = \frac{\cancel{50}\text{ ml} \times 25\ \cancel{\text{mEq}}}{\cancel{50}\ \cancel{\text{mEq}}}$$

$$X = 25\text{ ml}$$

You should administer 25 ml of sodium bicarbonate solution.

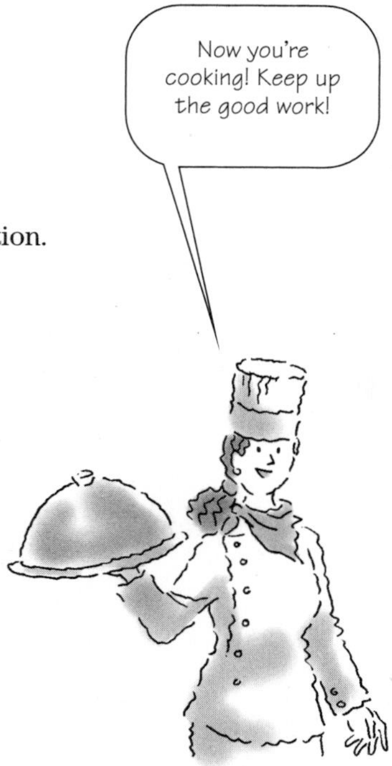

Now you're cooking! Keep up the good work!

Potassium puzzle

The doctor prescribes 30 mEq of potassium chloride oral solution for your patient. The solution contains 60 mEq in every 15 ml. How many milliliters of solution should you give the patient? Here's how to solve this problem.

- Set up a proportion using *X* as the unknown quantity:

$$\frac{X}{30\text{ mEq}} = \frac{15\text{ ml}}{60\text{ mEq}}$$

- Cross-multiply the fractions:

$$X \times 60\text{ mEq} = 15\text{ ml} \times 30\text{ mEq}$$

- Find *X* by dividing both sides of the equation by 60 mEq and canceling units that appear in both the numerator and denominator:

$$\frac{X \times \cancel{60\text{ mEq}}}{\cancel{60\text{ mEq}}} = \frac{15\text{ ml} \times 30\ \cancel{\text{mEq}}}{60\ \cancel{\text{mEq}}}$$

$$X = 7.5\text{ ml}$$

You should administer 7.5 ml of oral potassium chloride solution.

Frequently used conversions

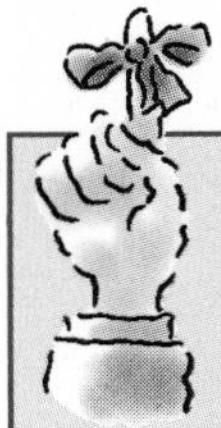

Memory jogger

Remember this jingle when converting inches to centimeters and vice versa: "2.54, that's 1 inch and no more."

In clinical practice, a doctor may write a medication order in one measurement system, but the medication may be available in a different system. For example, he might order gr x of a drug that's available only in milligrams.

To convert medication orders from one system to another, you must know the equivalent measures. If you have trouble remembering the most commonly used equivalents, jot the equivalents on an index card, laminate the card, and tuck it in your pocket for easy reference.

A *conversion* excursion

Two conversions that are commonly used, especially in adult and pediatric intensive care units, are pounds (lb) to kilograms (kg) and inches (″) to centimeters (cm). These conversions are used to determine body weight and body surface.

Making these conversions isn't hard if you remember the general rules:

- Remember that 1 kg equals 2.2 lb. To convert pounds into kilograms, just divide the number of pounds by 2.2. To convert kilograms to pounds, multiply the number of kilograms by 2.2.
- Remember that 1″ equals 2.54 cm. To convert inches to centimeters, just multiply the number of inches by 2.54. To convert centimeters to inches, divide the number of centimeters by 2.54.

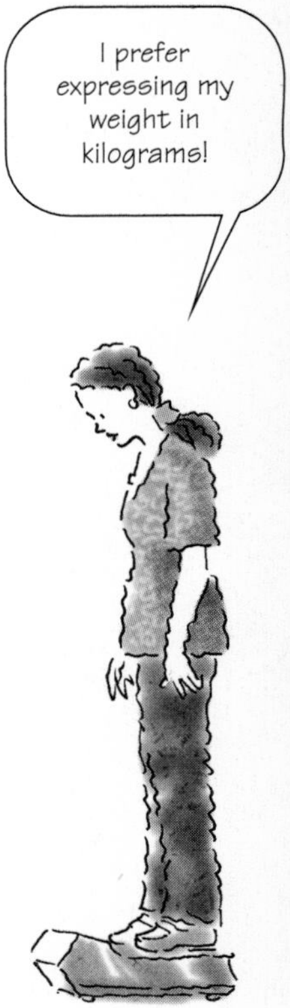
I prefer expressing my weight in kilograms!

Equivalent measure conversions

The following examples show how to do equivalent measure conversions.

You say pounds, I say kilograms

To prepare medications for your hypotensive patient, you must determine her weight in kilograms. You know that she weighs 125 lb, but how much is this in kilograms? Here's how to find out.

- You know that 1 kg equals 2.2 lb. So set up a proportion using X as the unknown weight:

$$\frac{X}{125 \text{ lb}} = \frac{1 \text{ kg}}{2.2 \text{ lb}}$$

- Cross-multiply the fractions:

$$X \times 2.2 \text{ lb} = 1 \text{ kg} \times 125 \text{ lb}$$

- Find X by dividing both sides of the equation by 2.2 lb and canceling units that appear in both the numerator and denominator:

$$\frac{X \times \cancel{2.2\text{ lb}}}{\cancel{2.2\text{ lb}}} = \frac{1\text{ kg} \times 125\ \cancel{\text{lb}}}{2.2\ \cancel{\text{lb}}}$$

$$X = 56.8\text{ kg}$$

Your patient weighs 56.8 kg.

You say milliliters, I say cups

A patient who's on a clear liquid diet must drink 480 ml of water for lunch. How many cups is this equal to? Here's how to find out.

- You know that 1 cup equals 240 ml. So set up a proportion using X as the unknown number:

$$\frac{X}{480\text{ ml}} = \frac{1\text{ cup}}{240\text{ ml}}$$

- Cross-multiply the fractions:

$$X \times 240\text{ ml} = 1\text{ cup} \times 480\text{ ml}$$

- Find X by dividing both sides of the equation by 240 ml and canceling units that appear in both the numerator and denominator:

$$\frac{X \times \cancel{240\text{ ml}}}{\cancel{240\text{ ml}}} = \frac{1\text{ cup} \times 480\ \cancel{\text{ml}}}{240\ \cancel{\text{ml}}}$$

$$X = 2\text{ cups}$$

Your patient must drink 2 cups of water.

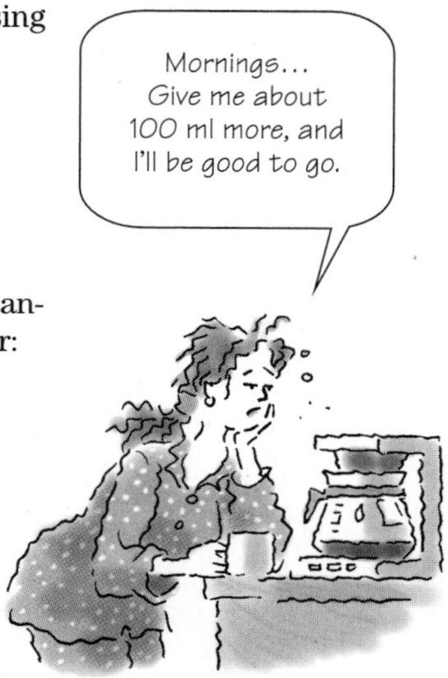
Mornings…
Give me about
100 ml more, and
I'll be good to go.

You say tablespoons, I say milliliters

The doctor orders 30 ml of milk of magnesia for your patient's heartburn. How many tablespoons is this? Here's how to find out.

- You know that 1 tbs contains 15 ml, so set up a proportion using X as the unknown number:

$$\frac{X}{30\text{ ml}} = \frac{1\text{ tbs}}{15\text{ ml}}$$

- Cross-multiply the fractions:

$$X \times 15\text{ ml} = 1\text{ tbs} \times 30\text{ ml}$$

- Find X by dividing both sides of the equation by 15 ml and canceling units that appear in both the numerator and denominator:

$$\frac{X \times \cancel{15\text{ ml}}}{\cancel{15\text{ ml}}} = \frac{1\text{ tbs} \times 30\ \cancel{\text{ml}}}{15\ \cancel{\text{ml}}}$$

$$X = 2\text{ tbs}$$

Your patient needs 2 tbs of milk of magnesia.

Real world problems

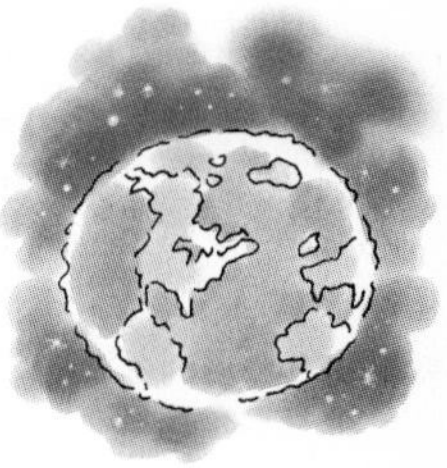

Here are real world examples using alternative measurement systems.

Calcium question

The doctor orders the following I.V. fluid for your patient: 2,000 mg calcium gluconate in 500 ml of dextrose 5% in water (D_5W). The calcium gluconate is available in a vial containing 100 mg calcium gluconate per 1 ml. How many milliliters of calcium gluconate should you add to the D_5W?

- Set up a proportion using X as the unknown quantity.

$$\frac{X}{2{,}000 \text{ mg}} = \frac{1 \text{ ml}}{100 \text{ mg}}$$

- Cross-multiply the fractions:

$$X \times 100 \text{ mg} = 1 \text{ ml} \times 2{,}000 \text{ mg}$$

- Find X by dividing both sides of the equation by 100 mg and canceling units that appear in both the numerator and denominator:

$$\frac{X \times \cancel{100 \text{ mg}}}{\cancel{100 \text{ mg}}} = \frac{1 \text{ ml} \times 2{,}000 \cancel{\text{mg}}}{100 \cancel{\text{mg}}}$$

$$X = 20 \text{ ml}$$

You should add 20 ml of calcium gluconate to the 500 ml of D_5W.

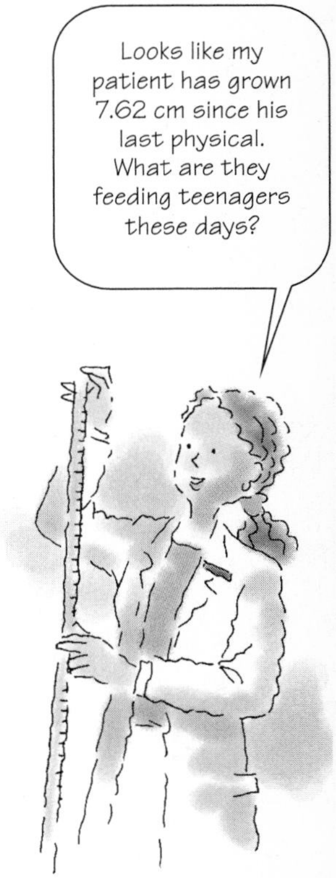

Looks like my patient has grown 7.62 cm since his last physical. What are they feeding teenagers these days?

A tall order

Your patient's height measures 68″. How many centimeters is this?

- Remember that 1″ = 2.54 cm so you can set up a proportion using X for the unknown quantity.

$$\frac{X}{68''} = \frac{2.54 \text{ cm}}{1''}$$

- Cross-multiply the fractions:

$$X \times 1'' = 2.54 \text{ cm} \times 68''$$

- Solve for X by dividing both sides of the equation by 1″ and canceling units that appear in both the numerator and denominator:

$$\frac{X \times \cancel{1''}}{\cancel{1''}} = \frac{2.54 \text{ cm} \times 68\cancel{''}}{1\cancel{''}}$$

$$X = 172.72 \text{ cm}$$

The patient measures 172.72 cm.

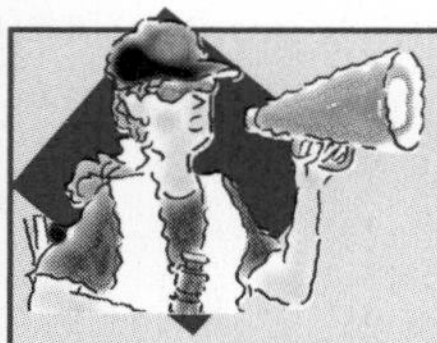

That's a wrap!

Alternative measurement systems review

Keep these important facts in mind when performing calculations with alternative measurement systems.

Apothecaries' system
- Measures liquid volume and solid weight
- Minim – basic unit of liquid volume
- Grain – basic unit of solid weight
- 1 drop = 1 minim = 1 grain
- Traditionally uses Roman numerals

Roman numerals

To convert a Roman numeral to an Arabic numeral:
- if a smaller Roman numeral precedes a larger Roman numeral, subtract the smaller numeral from the larger numeral
- if a smaller Roman numeral follows a larger Roman numeral, add the numerals.

To convert an Arabic numeral to a Roman numeral:
- break the Arabic numeral into its component parts
- translate each part into Roman numerals.

Household system
- Uses droppers, teaspoons, tablespoons, and cups to measure liquid medication doses
- Common household conversions:
  3 tsp = 1 tbs
  8 oz = 1 cup
  4 qt = 1 gal

Avoirdupois system
- Pronounced "av-wah-doo-PWAH"
- Solid measures or units of weight, including grains, ounces, and pounds
- Common avoirdupois conversions:
  1 oz = 480 gr
  1 lb = 16 oz = 7,680 gr

Unit conversions
- Insulin is the most common drug measured in units.
- Divide the units required by the amount of drug available in units.

Milliequivalent conversions
- Measures some electrolytes
- Divide the amount of milliequivalents required by the amount of drug available in milliequivalents.

Commonly used conversions
- Pounds to kilograms: Divide the number of pounds by 2.2.
- Kilograms to pounds: Multiply the number of kilograms by 2.2.
- Inches to centimeters: Multiply the number of inches by 2.54.
- Centimeters to inches: Divide the number of centimeters by 2.54.

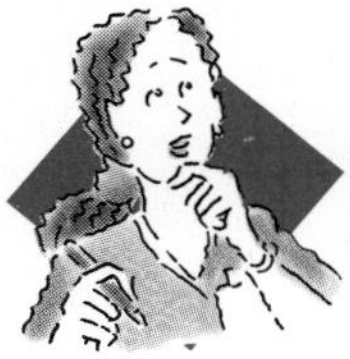

Quick quiz

1. The Arabic numeral 575 in Roman numerals is:
  A. DXXXXXXXV.
  B. DLXXV.
  C. CCCCCLXXV.
  D. DXC.

Answer: B. To convert 575, break it into its component parts (500, 70, and 5); then translate the parts into Roman numerals.

2. The symbol ss represents:
  A. one-half.
  B. the abbreviation for "without."
  C. the dram symbol.
  D. the grain symbol.

Answer: A. The symbol ss represents one-half in Roman numerals.

3. Drugs that are measured in units include:
  A. penicillin G, insulin, and heparin.
  B. co-trimoxazole.
  C. cough medicine.
  D. erythromycin and calcium.

Answer: A. Penicillin G, insulin, and heparin are measured in units.

4. Electrolytes are measured in:
  A. grains.
  B. milligrams.
  C. milliequivalents.
  D. fluidrams.

Answer: C. Most electrolytes, such as potassium chloride, are measured in milliequivalents.

5. When converting pounds to kilograms, you should:
  A multiply by 2.54.
  B. divide by 2.2.
  C. divide by 2.54.
  D. multiply by 2.2.

Answer: B. One kilogram equals 2.2 lb. By dividing pounds by 2.2, you obtain kilograms.

6. Before the metric system was established, doctors and pharmacists used the:

A. apothecaries' system.
B. avoirdupois system.
C. household system.
D. unit system.

Answer: A. Used before the metric system, the apothecaries' system is being phased out today.

7. The doctor prescribes 5,000 units of heparin I.V. for your patient. The heparin vial that's available contains 1,000 units/ml. How many milliliters should you administer?

A. 0.5 ml
B. 0.05 ml
C. 5 ml
D. 50 ml

Answer: C. To solve this problem, set up the proportion.

$$\frac{X}{5{,}000 \text{ units}} = \frac{1 \text{ ml}}{1{,}000 \text{ units}}$$

Cross-multiply the fractions; then divide both sides of the equation by 1,000 units and cancel units that appear in both the numerator and denominator.

$$\frac{X \times \cancel{1{,}000 \text{ units}}}{\cancel{1{,}000 \text{ units}}} = \frac{1 \text{ ml} \times 5{,}000 \cancel{\text{units}}}{1{,}000 \cancel{\text{units}}}$$

$$X = 5 \text{ ml}$$

8. The equivalent of 1 tsp of medication in milliliters is:

A. 15 or 16 ml.
B. 4 or 5 ml.
C. 30 or 32 ml.
D. 10 or 12 ml.

Answer: B. 1 tsp equals 4 or 5 ml.

Scoring

☆☆☆ If you answered all eight items correctly, fantastic! Reward yourself with a minim of ice cream. (Okay, you can have a pint!)

☆☆ If you answered five to seven items correctly, good job! Have a fluidram of champagne. (Enjoy every minim!)

☆ If you answered fewer than five items correctly, keep at it. In the meantime, have a dram of chocolate. (Savor every grain!)

Part III Recording drug administration

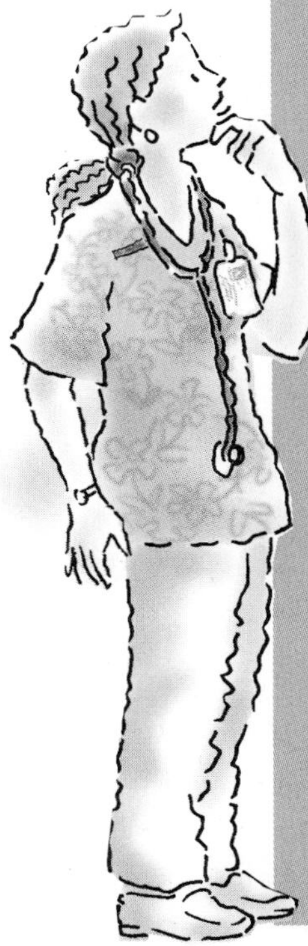

INCREDIBLY EASY MINIGUIDE

Improving patient safety with computerized medication orders

Computerized medication orders prevent medication errors by allowing doctors to enter orders directly into the computer system. This system eliminates transcription errors caused by nurses attempting to decipher illegible handwritten orders.

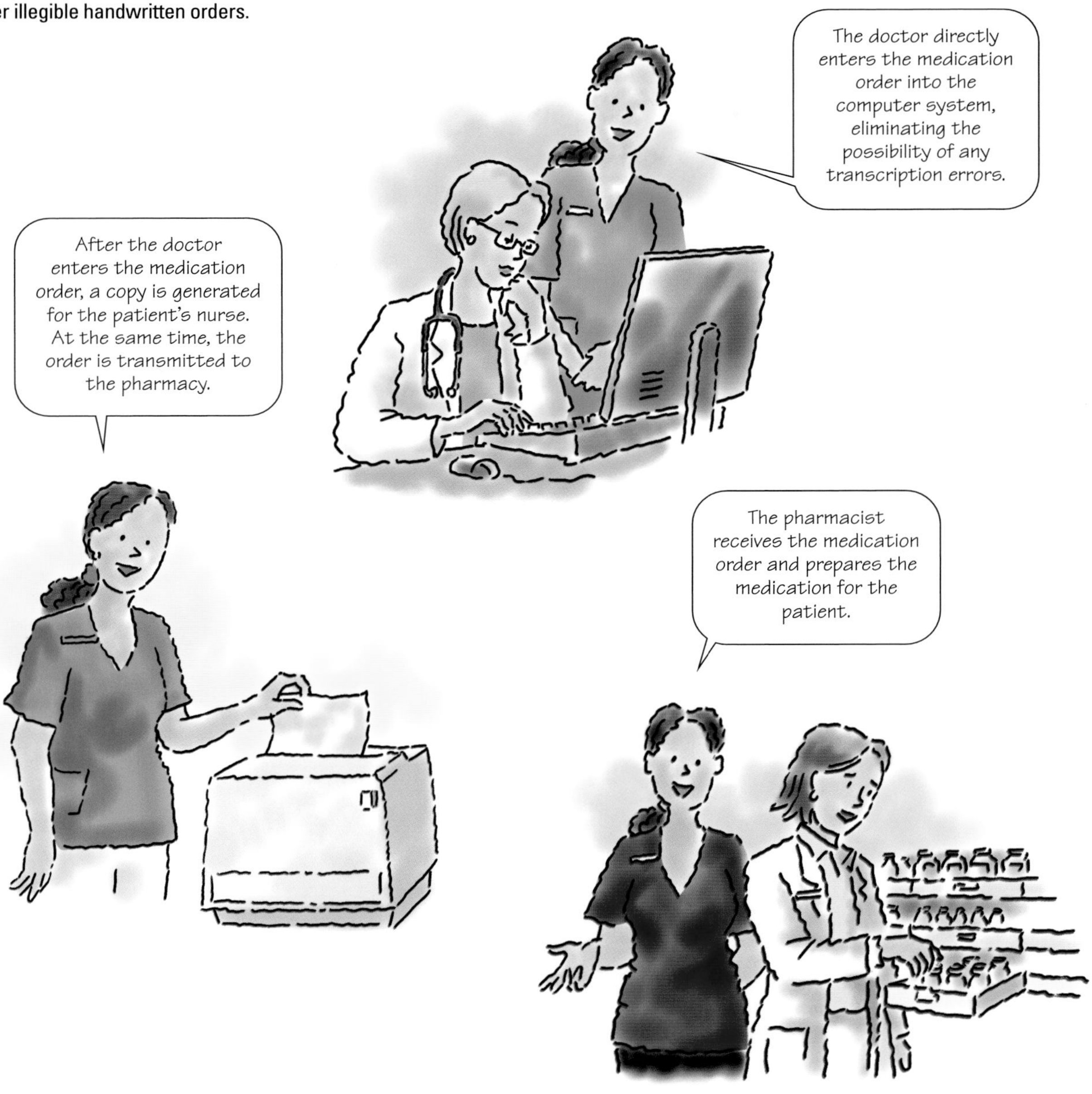

The doctor directly enters the medication order into the computer system, eliminating the possibility of any transcription errors.
After the doctor enters the medication order, a copy is generated for the patient's nurse. At the same time, the order is transmitted to the pharmacy.
The pharmacist receives the medication order and prepares the medication for the patient.

INCREDIBLY EASY MINIGUIDE

Reducing medication administration errors with technology

Automated medication management systems and bar code technology have both contributed to a reduction in medication administration errors.

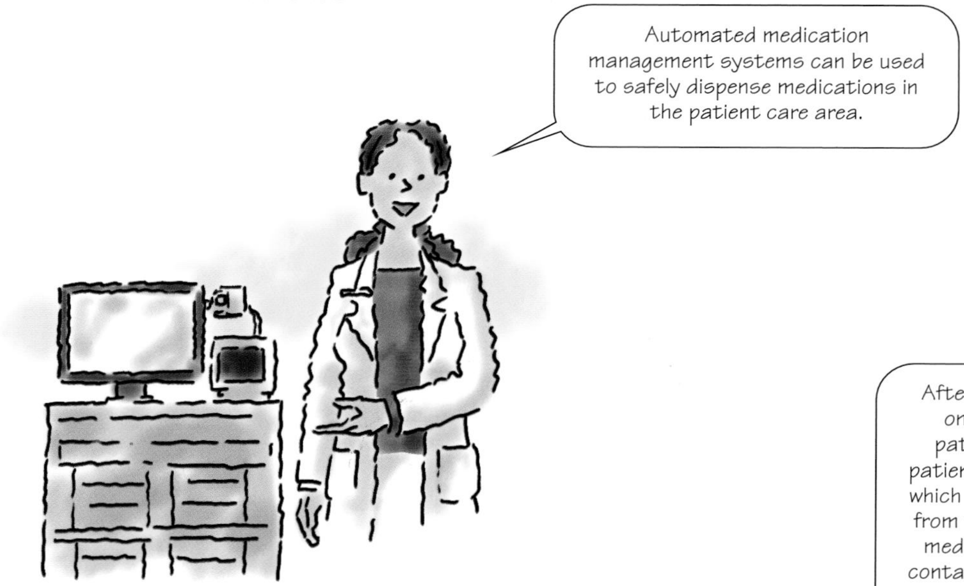
Automated medication management systems can be used to safely dispense medications in the patient care area.

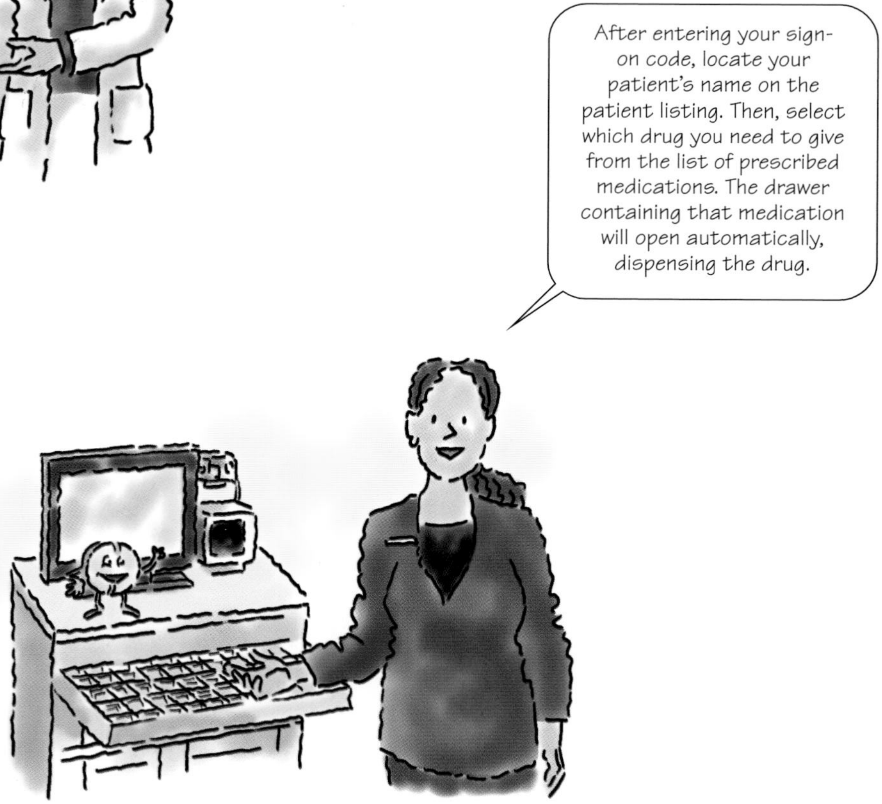
After entering your sign-on code, locate your patient's name on the patient listing. Then, select which drug you need to give from the list of prescribed medications. The drawer containing that medication will open automatically, dispensing the drug.

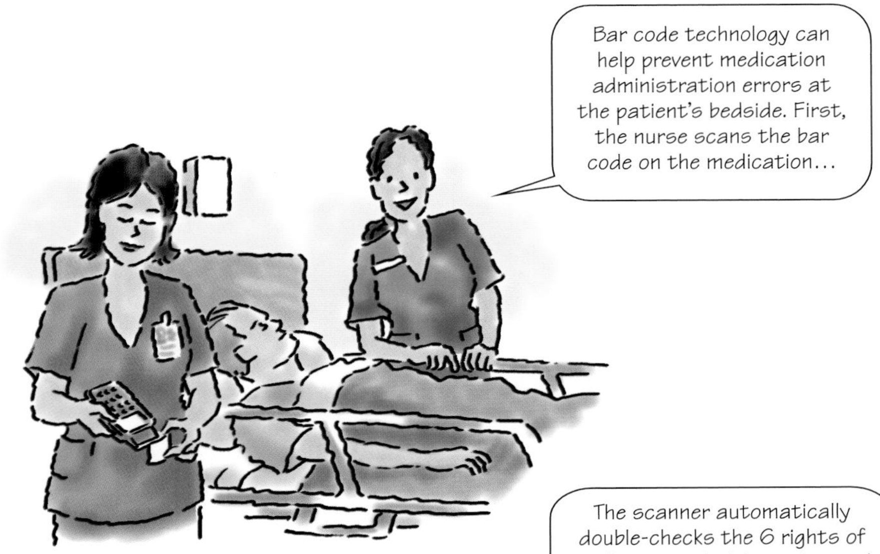
Bar code technology can help prevent medication administration errors at the patient's bedside. First, the nurse scans the bar code on the medication...

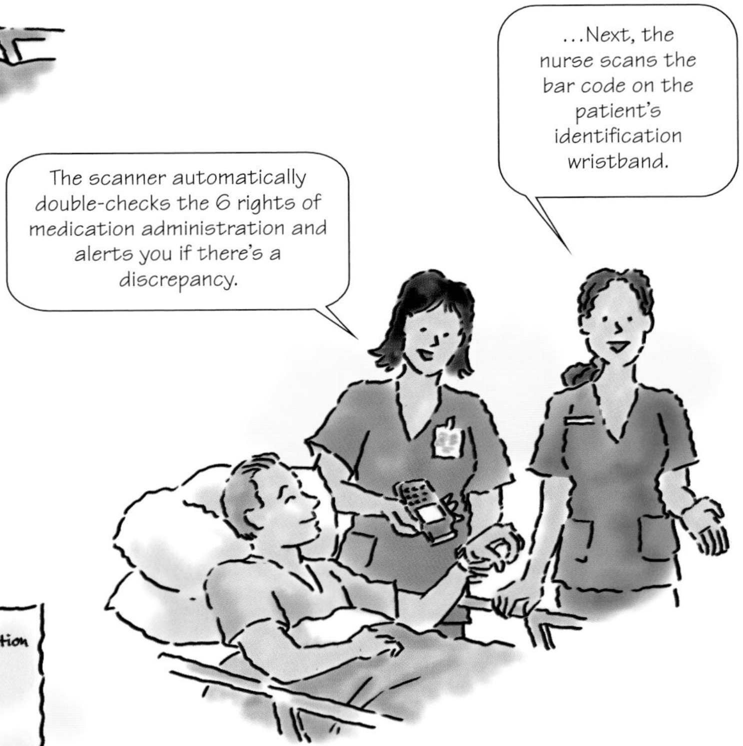
...Next, the nurse scans the bar code on the patient's identification wristband.
The scanner automatically double-checks the 6 rights of medication administration and alerts you if there's a discrepancy.

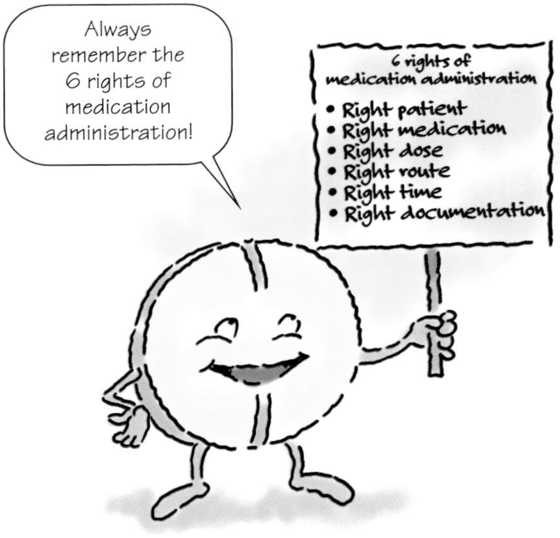
Always remember the 6 rights of medication administration!
6 rights of medication administration
• Right patient
• Right medication
• Right dose
• Right route
• Right time
• Right documentation

INCREDIBLY EASY MINIGUIDE

Preventing medication errors without technology

Technology has greatly reduced medication errors. However, when technology isn't available, remember the basics.

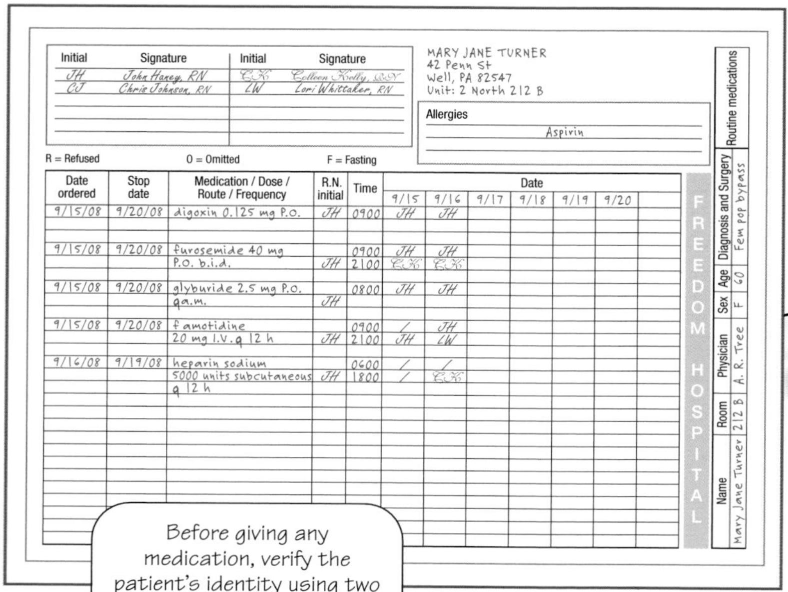

Initial	Signature	Initial	Signature
JH	John Haney, RN	CK	Colleen Kelly, RN
CJ	Chris Johnson, RN	LW	Lori Whittaker, RN

MARY JANE TURNER
42 Penn St
Well, PA 82547
Unit: 2 North 212 B

Allergies: Aspirin

R = Refused 0 = Omitted F = Fasting

Date ordered	Stop date	Medication / Dose / Route / Frequency	R.N. initial	Time	9/15	9/16	9/17	9/18	9/19	9/20
9/15/08	9/20/08	digoxin 0.125 mg P.O.	JH	0900	JH	JH				
9/15/08	9/20/08	furosemide 40 mg		0900	JH	JH				
		P.O. b.i.d.	JH	2100	CK	CK				
9/15/08	9/20/08	glyburide 2.5 mg P.O.		0800	JH	JH				
		qa.m.	JH							
9/15/08	9/20/08	famotidine		0900	/	JH				
		20 mg I.V. q 12 h	JH	2100	JH	LW				
9/16/08	9/19/08	heparin sodium		0600	/	/				
		5000 units subcutaneous	JH	1800	/	CK				
		q 12 h								

FREEDOM HOSPITAL

Name	Room	Physician	Sex	Age	Diagnosis and Surgery	Routine medications
Mary Jane Turner	212 B	A. R. Tree	F	60	Fem pop bypass	

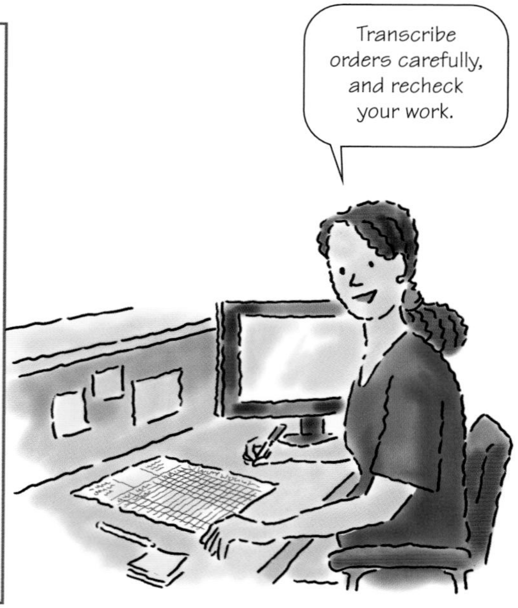
Transcribe orders carefully, and recheck your work.

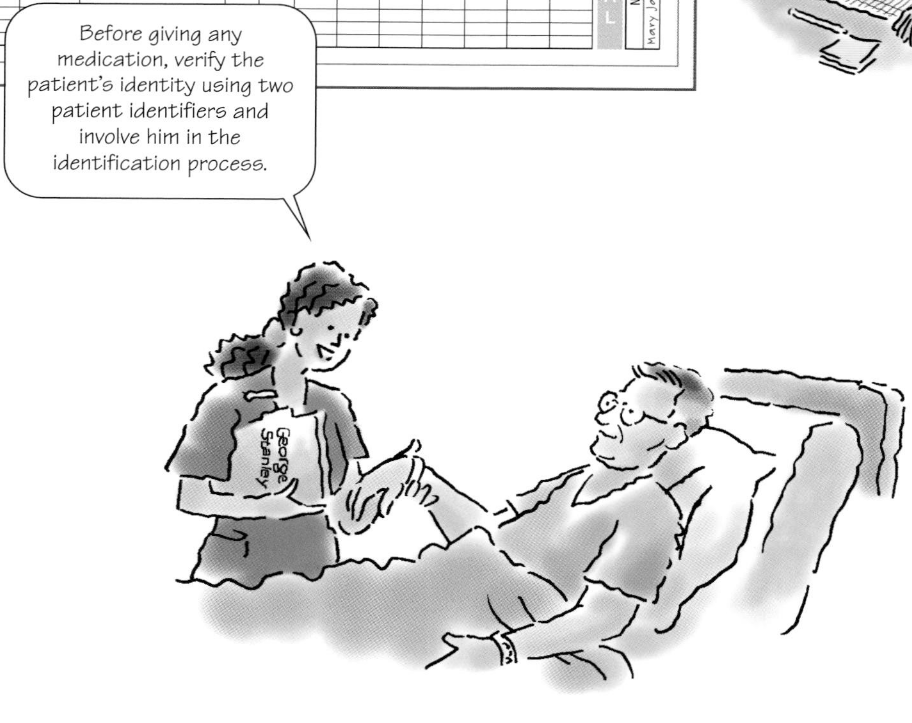
Before giving any medication, verify the patient's identity using two patient identifiers and involve him in the identification process.
George Stanley

7

Drug orders

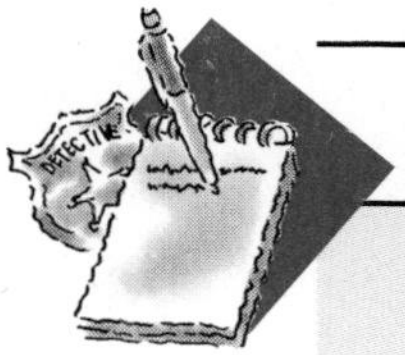

Just the facts

In this chapter, you'll learn:

- what a drug order consists of
- how to interpret drug orders using standard abbreviations
- how to use military time
- what to do about unclear drug orders.

A look at drug orders

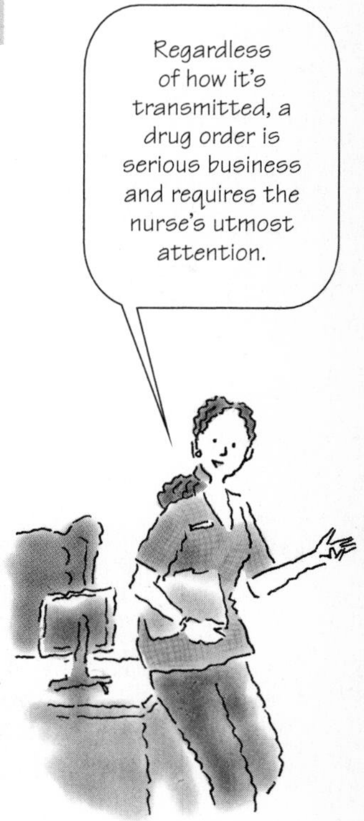

Regardless of how it's transmitted, a drug order is serious business and requires the nurse's utmost attention.

Administering drugs is one of your most critical nursing responsibilities. It's also the area with the smallest margin for error. How can you prevent drug errors? The best way is by knowing how to read and correctly interpret drug orders. To do this, you need to understand what a drug order is and how it's used.

Direct handoff

In an outpatient setting, a doctor or other health care professional who's licensed to prescribe drugs typically writes an order on a prescription form and gives it directly to the patient.

Keyboard, form, or fax

The routine for prescribing drugs is different in inpatient facilities. There, a doctor generates a drug order in one of these ways:

- by entering the order into a computer system that transmits it to the pharmacy and to the nurses' station
- by writing the order on the drug order sheet in the patient's chart
- by faxing the order to a pharmacy (which saves time by preventing an order from staying in a patient's chart or computer until the chart or computer is checked, although the patient's confidentiality may be breached by this method).

What's in a drug order?

If a drug order sheet is used, the order sheet is located in the patient's chart. It must include all patient information, so it's usually stamped with the patient's admission data plate. When writing the order, the doctor includes:

- date and time of the order
- name of the drug, either generic or trade
- dosage form in metric, apothecaries', or household measurement
- abbreviation for the route of administration, such as P.O., I.M., I.V., P.R., or S.L.
- administration schedule written as times per day or as number of hours between doses
- restrictions or specifications related to the order
- doctor's signature, or name and code number in a computerized system (one signature, or name and code number, is sufficient after a group of orders)
- doctor's registration number for controlled drugs, if applicable.

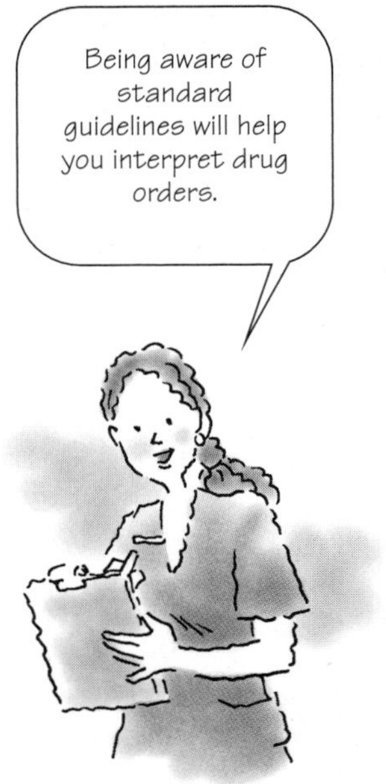
Being aware of standard guidelines will help you interpret drug orders.

Following orders

Standard guidelines exist for writing drug orders. Being aware of these guidelines will help you interpret drug orders:

- The generic name of a drug is written entirely in lowercase letters.
- The trade or brand name of a drug begins with a capital letter.
- Drug names shouldn't be abbreviated to avoid errors.
- Information is written down following a standard sequence: drug name first, then dose, administration route, and lastly time and frequency of administration.

A brief look at abbreviating

Standard abbreviations are used to describe drug measurements, dosages, routes and times of administration, and related terms. The Joint Commission requires every health care facility to develop a list of approved abbreviations for staff use. (See *Standard abbreviations.*)

However, The Joint Commission has also developed a "Do not use" list of abbreviations known for causing medication errors. See chapter 9, "Preventing Drug Errors," for more information on this list.

Remember that abbreviations can be easily misinterpreted, especially if they're written carelessly or quickly. If an abbreviation seems unusual or doesn't make sense to you, contact the doctor for clarification. Then clearly write the correct term in your revision and transcription.

Standard abbreviations

Standard abbreviations are handy for quick and accurate transcription of medication orders and documentation of drug administration. However, some abbreviations used commonly in the past have been identified as possible patient safety risks; these are labeled as "Do not use!"

Abbreviation	Meaning	Use or do not use
Drug and solution measurements		
cc	cubic centimeter	Do not use!
fl dr	fluid dram	✔
fl oz	fluid ounce	✔
g	gram	✔
gal	gallon	✔
gr	grain	✔
gtt	drop	✔
kg	kilogram	✔
L	liter	✔
mcg	microgram	✔
ml	milliliter	✔
Drug dosage forms		
cap	capsule	✔
DS	double strength	✔
elix	elixir	✔
LA	long-acting	✔
liq	liquid	✔
SA	sustained action	✔
SR	sustained release	✔
Sol	solution	✔
Susp tab	suspension tablet	✔
Routes of drug administration		
A.D.	right ear	Do not use!
A.S.	left ear	Do not use!
A.U.	each ear	Do not use!
I.M.	intramuscular	✔
I.V.	intravenous	✔
NG tube	nasogastric tube	✔
O.D.	right eye	Do not use!

(continued)

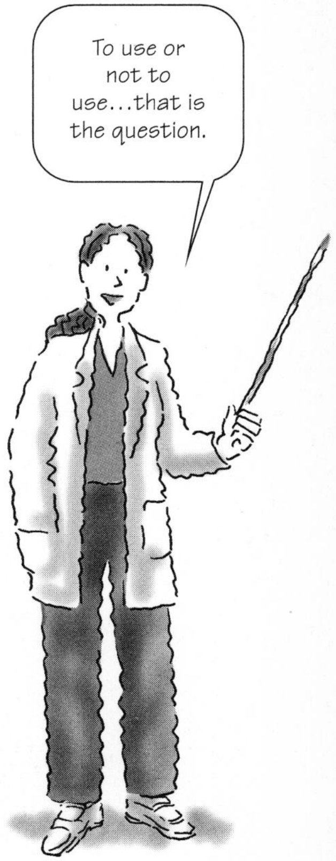

To use or not to use…that is the question.

Standard abbreviations *(continued)*

Abbreviation	Meaning	Use or do not use
***Routes of drug administration** (continued)*		
O.S.	left eye	Do not use!
O.U.	each eye	Do not use!
P.O. or p.o.	by mouth	✔
P.R.	rectally	✔
P.V.	vaginally	✔
S.C.	subcutaneously	Do not use!
S.L.	sublingually	✔
Times of drug administration		
a.c.	before meals	✔
b.i.d.	twice a day	✔
h.s.	at bedtime	Do not use!
p.c.	after meals	✔
p.r.n.	as needed	✔
q.a.m.	every morning	✔
q.d.	every day	Do not use!
q.o.d.	every other day	Do not use!
q4h	every 4 hours	✔
stat	immediately	✔
Miscellaneous abbreviations		
AMA	against medical advice	✔
ASAP	as soon as possible	✔
BP	blood pressure	✔
BPM	breaths (or beats) per minute	✔
$\bar{c}$	with	✔
D/C or dc	discontinue	Do not use!
KVO	keep vein open	✔
MR	may repeat	✔
NKA	no known allergies	✔
NPO	nothing by mouth	✔
P	pulse	✔
R	respiration	✔
<	less than	Do not use!
>	greater than	Do not use!
$\bar{s}$	without	✔

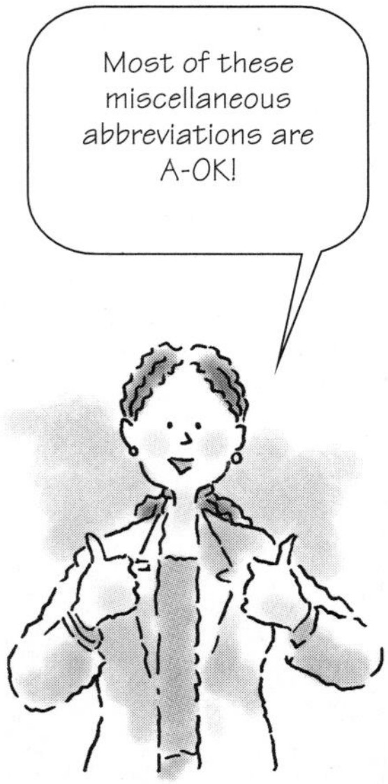
Most of these miscellaneous abbreviations are A-OK!

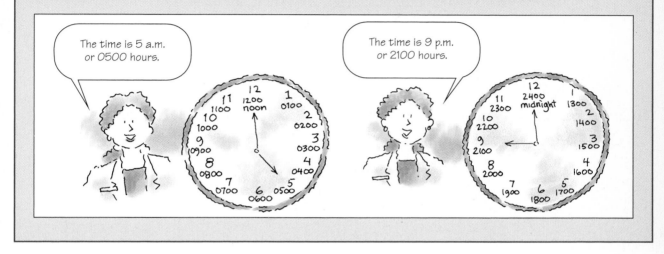

Military time

Study the two clocks below to better understand military time. The clock on the left represents the hours from 1 a.m. (0100 hours) to noon (1200 hours). The clock on the right represents the hours from 1 p.m. (1300 hours) to midnight (2400 hours).

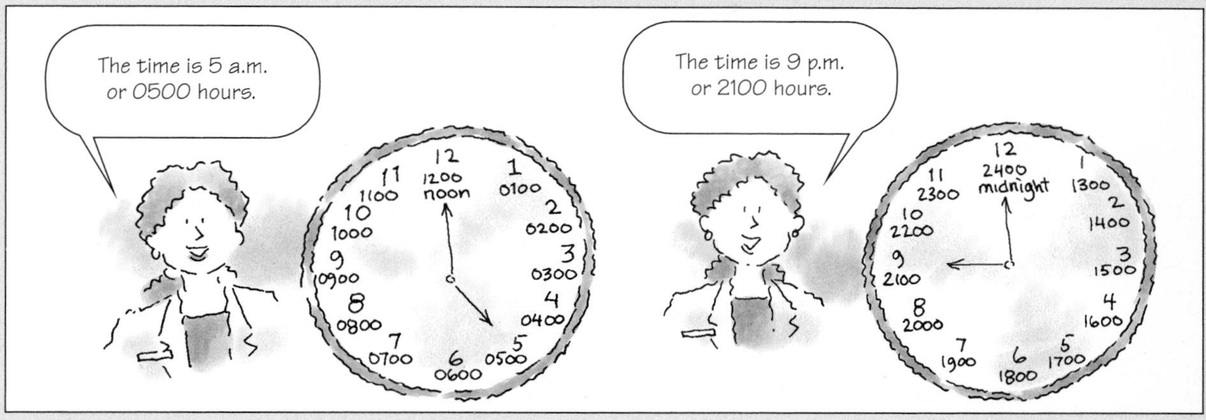
The time is 5 a.m. or 0500 hours.
12 1200 noon
1 0100
2 0200
3 0300
4 0400
5 0500
6 0600
7 0700
8 0800
9 0900
10 1000
11 1100
The time is 9 p.m. or 2100 hours.
12 2400 midnight
1 1300
2 1400
3 1500
4 1600
5 1700
6 1800
7 1900
8 2000
9 2100
10 2200
11 2300

Marching in time (military time, that is)

Some doctors and health care facilities require pharmacologic orders and medication administration records to be written and transcribed in military time. For example, an order might read *Lasix 40 mg I.V. b.i.d. at 0900 and 2100 hours.* (See *Military time.*)

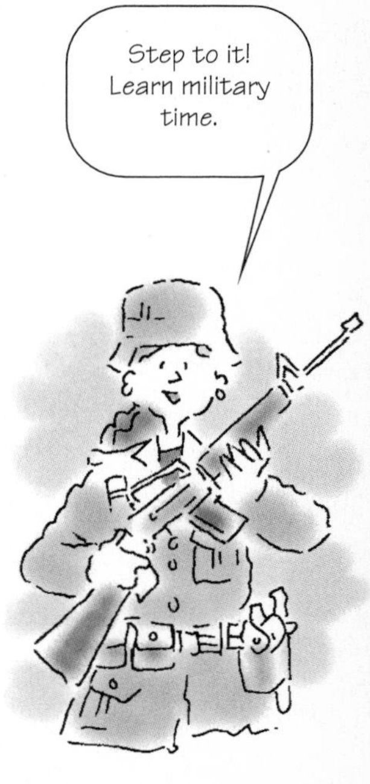
Step to it! Learn military time.

Simply confusing or confusingly simple?

Military time might seem confusing at first, but it's actually simple to use. This method of time is based on a 24-hour system. Here's how it works:

- To write single-digit times from 1:00 a.m. to 9:59 a.m., put a zero before the times and remove the colon. For example, 1:00 a.m. is written 0100 hours.
- To write double-digit times from 10:00 a.m. to 12:59 p.m., just remove the colon. For example, 11:00 a.m. becomes 1100 hours.
- The minutes after the hour remain the same. For example, 4:45 a.m. becomes 0445 hours.
- To write times from 1:00 p.m. to 12 midnight, simply add 1200 to the hour and remove the colon. For example, 1:00 p.m. becomes 1300 hours (1:00 + 12:00); 3:30 p.m. becomes 1530 hours (3:30 + 12:00); and 12:00 a.m (midnight) becomes 2400 hours (12:00 + 12:00).

- To write the minutes between 12:01 a.m. and 12:59 a.m., start over with zero. For example, 12:33 a.m. becomes 0033 hours.

Dealing with drug orders

After you determine that a drug order contains all the necessary information, you can begin to interpret it. Read on to find guidelines for dealing with illegible handwriting, timing drug administration, renewing drug orders, and discontinued drug orders. (See *Say it in English.*)

Hospital hieroglyphics

If any required information is missing or if the doctor's handwriting is illegible, check with the doctor and clarify the order before signing the transcription. Also ask the doctor for clarification if nonstandard abbreviations are used.

When the order is clear, sign it and send a copy to the pharmacy where the drug will be dispensed according to your facility's policy.

Calibrating the clinical clock

Although the drug order sheet tells you when to give a drug, the actual administration time depends on three things:

- your facility's policy (for drugs that are given a specific number of times per day)
- the nature of the drug
- the drug's onset and duration of action.

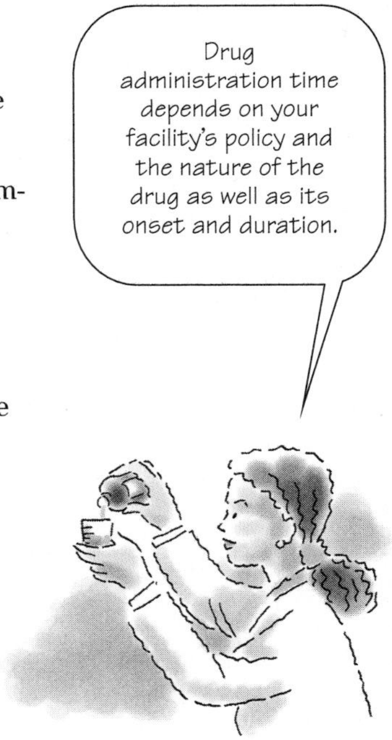
Drug administration time depends on your facility's policy and the nature of the drug as well as its onset and duration.

Be sure to administer drugs within a half-hour of the times specified on the drug order sheet. After giving a drug, record the actual time of administration on the medication administration record.

Reevaluate, renew, reorder

Health care facilities also have policies for how often drug orders must be renewed. For example, opioids may need to be reordered every 24, 48, or 72 hours. This requirement allows health care professionals to reevaluate the patient's need for the drug and to adjust the dosage or frequency of administration, if necessary.

Remember that I.V. fluids — such as normal saline solution, dextrose and water, and total parenteral nutrition solutions — are considered drugs. Check all I.V. fluid orders carefully. Most health care facilities provide guidelines for the renewal of I.V. fluids as well as for other drugs.

Say it in English

The following examples illustrate how to read and interpret a wide range of drug orders.

Drug order	Interpretation
Colace 100 mg P.O. b.i.d. p.c.	Give 100 mg of Colace by mouth twice per day after meals.
Vistaril 25 mg I.M. q3h p.r.n. anxiety	Give 25 mg of Vistaril intramuscularly every 3 hours as needed for anxiety.
Increase Duramorph to 6 mg I.V. q8h	Increase Duramorph to 6 mg intravenously every 8 hours.
folic acid 1 mg P.O. daily	Give 1 mg of folic acid by mouth daily.
Minipress 4 mg P.O. q6h, hold for sys BP less than 120	Give 4 mg of Minipress by mouth every 6 hours; withhold the drug if the systolic blood pressure falls below 120 mm Hg.
nifedipine 30 mg S.L. q4h	Give 30 mg of nifedipine sublingually every 4 hours.
Begin aspirin 325 mg P.O. daily	Begin giving 325 mg of aspirin by mouth daily.
Persantine 75 mg P.O. t.i.d.	Give 75 mg of Persantine by mouth three times per day.
aspirin grains v P.O. t.i.d.	Give 5 grains of aspirin by mouth three times per day.
Vasotec 2.5 mg P.O. daily	Give 2.5 mg of Vasotec by mouth daily.
1,000 ml D_5W $\bar{c}$ KCl 20 mEq I.V. at 100 ml/hr	Give 1,000 ml of dextrose 5% in water with 20 milliequivalents of potassium chloride intravenously at a rate of 100 milliliters per hour.
Discontinue penicillin I.V., start penicillin G 800,000 units P.O. q6h	Discontinue intravenous penicillin; start 800,000 units of penicillin G by mouth every 6 hours.
diphenhydramine 25–50 mg P.O. at bedtime p.r.n. insomnia	Give 25 to 50 mg of diphenhydramine by mouth at bedtime as needed for insomnia.

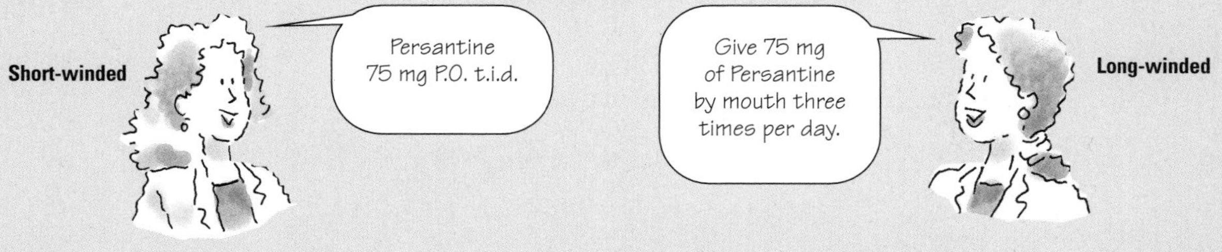
Short-winded
Persantine 75 mg P.O. t.i.d.
Give 75 mg of Persantine by mouth three times per day.
Long-winded

Stop! That's an order.

If the doctor decides to discontinue a drug before the original order runs out, he must write a new order. These orders must also be precise.

For example, if an order reads *discontinue K* and the patient is receiving vitamin K and potassium chloride, you'll need to contact the doctor to clarify which medication he wants to discontinue.

Handling ambiguous drug orders

All too often, drug orders are unclear because of nonstandard abbreviations, illegible handwriting, incorrect dosages, or missing information. It helps if handwritten orders are neat, with drugs spelled correctly. (See *Don't struggle with difficult orders*.)

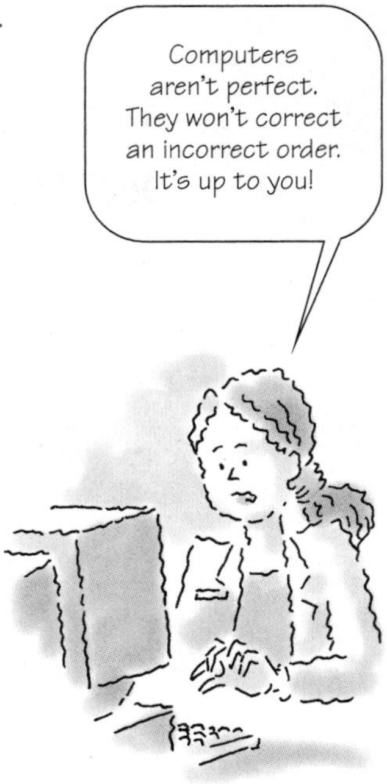

Computers aren't perfect. They won't correct an incorrect order. It's up to you!

Rule #1: Bad input equals bad output.

Even if the doctor enters drug orders into the computer system, your interpretation skills are still extremely important. Although computers solve the problem of illegible handwriting, they can't correct human error. A computer will accept the wrong drug, the wrong dose, the wrong route, and the wrong frequency. Remember, some safeguards are programmed into computer systems to minimize errors, but it's still up to you to verify the orders.

Rule #2: Advocate appropriate administration.

Your responsibility in interpreting orders includes making sure that the ordered drug is an appropriate treatment. Your role as patient advocate comes into play in this situation. To make sure the drug you're asked to administer is appropriate:

- Think critically; don't be timid about asking for clarification and justification.
- Know the action of each drug you give, the purpose for which it's given, and its possible adverse effects.
- Know your patient. Drugs should be used with caution in very young or very old patients as well as those who are pregnant or who have known kidney or liver disease, a compromised immune system, or diabetes.

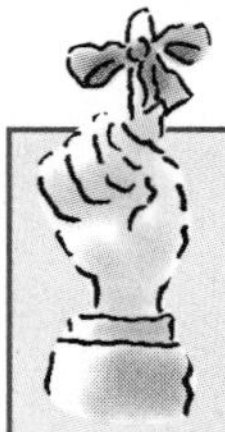

Memory jogger

Repetition is key!

Use repetition to remember your responsibilities when it comes to drug administration. As you prepare to administer each drug, think of the actions you must take. To remember the steps in sequence, think of the phrase "**U**ntil **C**lear, **A**sk **M**any **T**imes":

Understand the drug and how it works.

Clarify the drug order as needed.

Administer the drug.

Monitor the patient for therapeutic response to the drug and for adverse effects.

Teach the patient about the drug as needed.

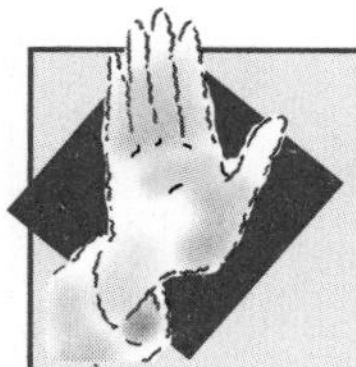

Before you give that drug!

Don't struggle with difficult orders

The combination of poor handwriting and inappropriate abbreviations on a drug order can lead to confusion and medication errors. Ask the doctor to clarify an order that's difficult to understand or one that seems wrong.

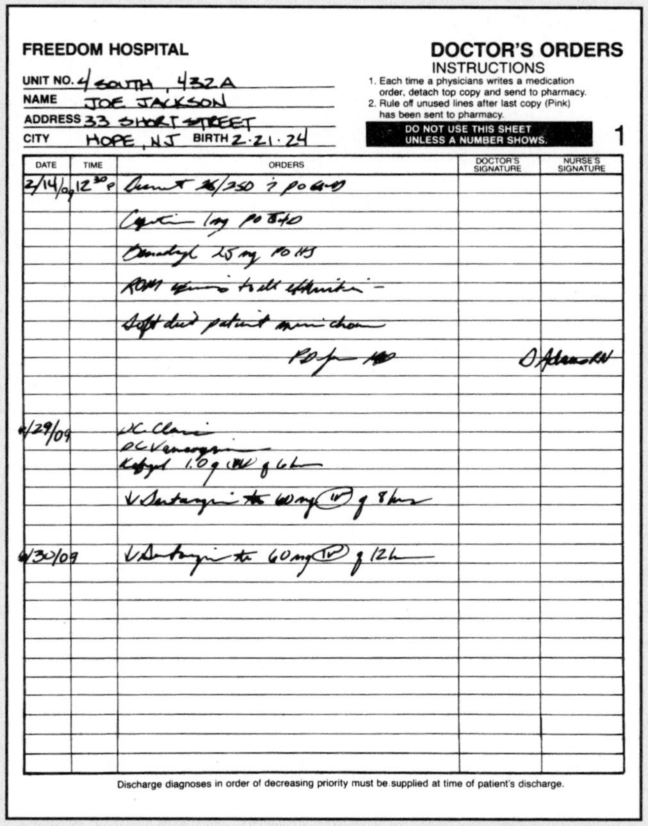

FREEDOM HOSPITAL

UNIT NO. 4 SOUTH, 432A
NAME JOE JACKSON
ADDRESS 33 SHORT STREET
CITY HOPE, NJ BIRTH 2·21·24

DOCTOR'S ORDERS
INSTRUCTIONS
1. Each time a physicians writes a medication order, detach top copy and send to pharmacy.
2. Rule off unused lines after last copy (Pink) has been sent to pharmacy.

DO NOT USE THIS SHEET UNLESS A NUMBER SHOWS. 1

DATE	TIME	ORDERS	DOCTOR'S SIGNATURE	NURSE'S SIGNATURE

Discharge diagnoses in order of decreasing priority must be supplied at time of patient's discharge.

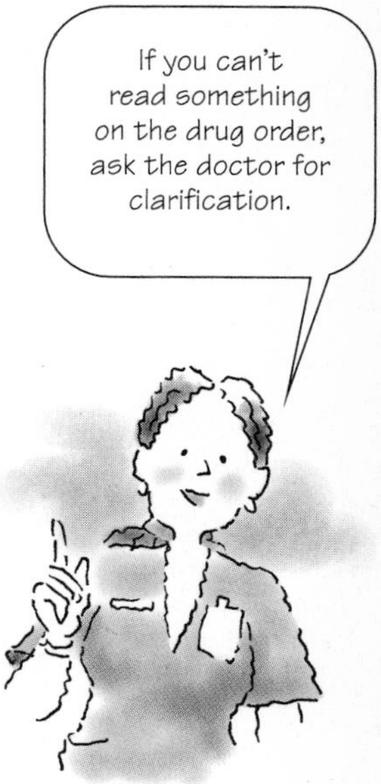

If you can't read something on the drug order, ask the doctor for clarification.

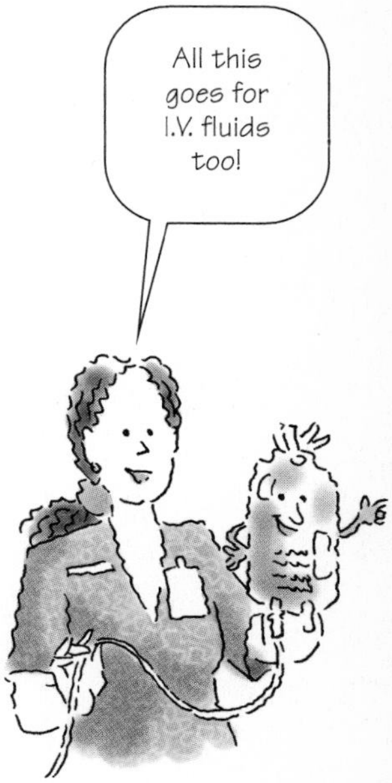

All this goes for I.V. fluids too!

- If a drug order seems questionable, use all available resources to check it. For example, ask the doctor, the pharmacist, and your colleagues and refer to a drug handbook.
- Always check the six "rights" before giving a drug. (See *Right on target*, page 132.)
- Check and recheck all your drug calculations.
- Never administer a drug that's improperly labeled or missing a label or that you personally didn't draw from a vial.
- Never use open or unmarked I.V. solution bags.

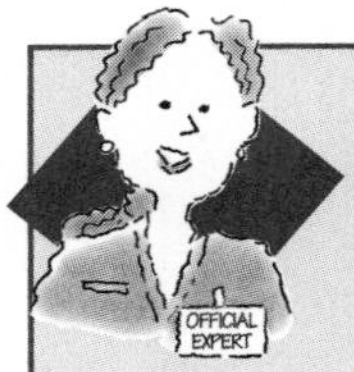

Advice from the experts

Right on target

No matter how careful you are when administering drugs, occasional errors can still occur. The pharmacy may even send the wrong drug. To avoid errors and keep your patient safe, never administer a drug without first checking off the "six rights" at your patient's bedside.

- Right drug
- Right dose
- Right route
- Right time
- Right patient
- Right documentation

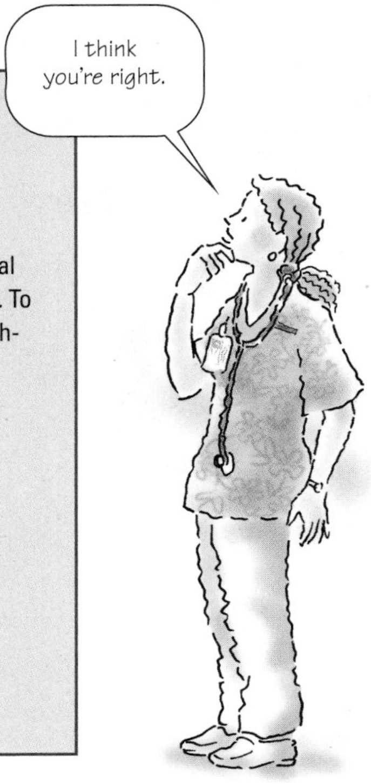

Real world problems

The following are examples of poorly written drug orders that need to be clarified by the doctor who wrote them. See if you can find the errors.

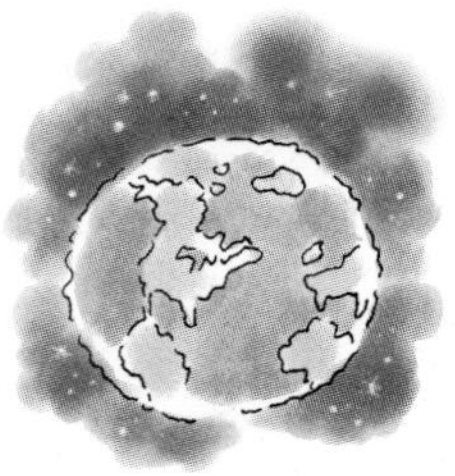

What?

K 40 mEq I.V. daily — It's unclear what drug is being ordered. Is it vitamin K or potassium chloride (KCl)? If it's KCl, remember that this electrolyte must be diluted in a large volume of I.V. fluid before administration.

How?

Digoxin 0.25 mg daily — The administration route is missing. Digoxin may be given orally as a pill or elixir or may be given I.V.

When?

Nifedipine 10 mg P.O. — The frequency of administration is missing. Nifedipine can be given in a single dose for hypertension, or it can be given on another schedule as a maintenance drug. In the latter case, it's usually given orally.

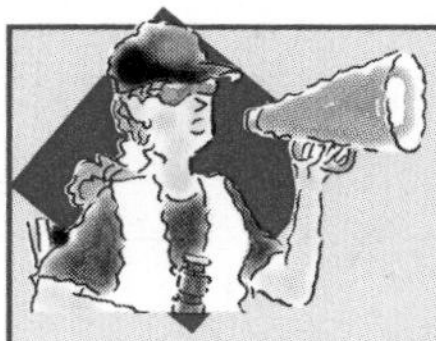

That's a wrap!

Drug orders review

Here's a quick review of important points about drug orders.

Reading and transcribing drug orders

Make sure the drug order includes all of the following information:

- drug name
- dose
- administration route
- time and frequency of administration.

Using military time

- To write single-digit times from 1:00 a.m. to 12:59 p.m., put a zero before the time and remove the colon. (Example: 4:00 a.m. is 0400 hours)
- To write double-digit times from 1:00 a.m. to 12:59 p.m., just remove the colon. (Example: 12:00 p.m. [noon] is 1200 hours)
- To write times from 1:00 p.m. to 12 a.m. (midnight), add 1200 to the hour and remove the colon. (Example: 9:00 p.m. is 2100 hours)
- Minutes after the hour remain the same. (Example: 10:36 p.m. is 2236 hours)

Administering drugs

- Give within 30 minutes of the specified time.
- Record the actual administration time.
- If the drug is discontinued, make sure the doctor writes a new order.
- With each order, ensure that the appropriate drug is being administered.

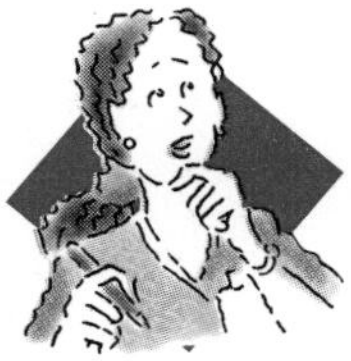

Quick quiz

1. Drug abbreviations should be:
A. written in lowercase letters.
B. written in capital letters.
C. written with the first letter in capitals.
D. avoided.

Answer: D. Drug abbreviations should generally be avoided to prevent errors.

2. The correct abbreviation for "after meals" is:
A. P.O.
B. P.R.
C. p.c.
D. a.c.

Answer: C. P.O. stands for "by mouth," P.R. stands for "by rectum," and a.c. stands for "before meals."

3. Which abbreviation is unacceptable according to The Joint Commission's "Do not use" list?

A. p.r.n.
B. p.o.
C. mcg
D. S.C.

Answer: D. The abbreviation S.C. should be avoided. Instead, write out *subcutaneously.*

4. The order *morphine 4 mg I.M. q4h p.r.n. pain, hold for respiratory rate less than 12 BPM* means:

A. Give morphine 4 mg intramuscularly four times per day for pain; hold for respiratory rate less than 12 breaths per minute.
B. Give morphine 4 mg intramuscularly every 4 hours for pain; hold for respiratory rate greater than 12 breaths per minute.
C. Give morphine 4 mg intramuscularly every 4 hours as needed for pain; hold for respiratory rate less than 12 breaths per minute.
D. Give morphine 4 mg intramuscularly every 6 hours for pain; hold for respiratory rate greater than 12 breaths per minute.

Answer: C. "Every 4 hours" is abbreviated q4h and the abbreviation p.r.n. means "as needed."

5. "Give Dilantin 150 mg by mouth twice per day at 0900 hours and 2100 hours; draw Dilantin levels every other day" can be written on a drug order as:

A. Dilantin 150 mg P.O. b.i.d. at 9:00 a.m. and 9:00 p.m., draw Dilantin levels every other day.
B. Dilantin 150 mg P.O. t.i.d. at 9:00 a.m. and 9:00 p.m., draw Dilantin levels q.d.
C. Dilantin 150 mp I.V. b.i.d. at 9:00 a.m. and 9:00 p.m., draw Dilantin levels q.o.d.
D. Dilantin 150 mg P.R. b.i.d. at 0900 and 2100, draw Dilantin levels q.o.d.

Answer: A. In option B, t.i.d. means "three times per day," and q.d., meaning daily, shouldn't be used. In option C, mp isn't a standard abbreviation, I.V. means "intravenously," and "q.o.d" shouldn't be used. In option D, "P.R." means "per rectum" and "q.o.d." shouldn't be used.

Scoring

☆☆☆ If you answered all five items correctly, wow! You're error-free!

☆☆ If you answered four items correctly, you're almost there! You can spot an incorrect order and read hospital hieroglyphics.

☆ If you answered fewer than four items correctly, keep going! You're acquiring the art of the drug order.

8

Administration records

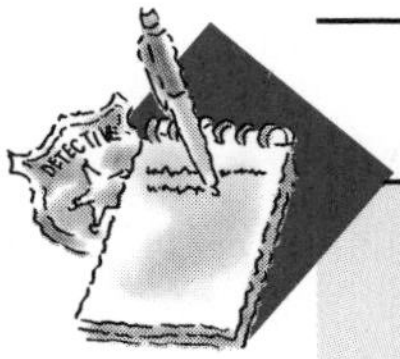

Just the facts

In this chapter, you'll learn:

- what types of medication administration record systems are used
- how to document patient information on the administration record
- how to record drug information on the administration record
- how to document administration of controlled substances.

A look at administration records

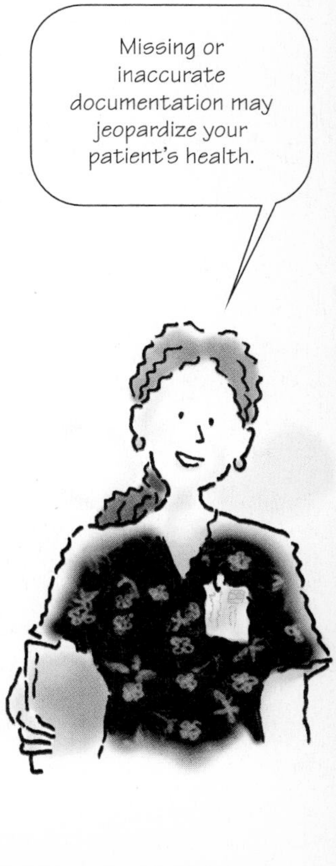
Missing or inaccurate documentation may jeopardize your patient's health.

Maintaining accurate medication administration records is a vital nursing responsibility, both for legal reasons and for patient safety. The liability risk of the health care provider may increase if medication administration isn't properly documented. Missing or inaccurate documentation can lead to drug errors that may jeopardize your patient's health.

Record-keeping systems

Two main types of medication administration record systems are used today: the medication administration record (MAR) and computer charting.

The MAR

The MAR is an 8½″ × 11″ form that goes into the patient's chart. It also may be kept in the medication room on the medication cart in a three-ring binder or may be attached to the patient's chart or clipboard while the patient is hospitalized. On discharge, the MAR is placed in the patient's chart with the other MARs already used for that patient.

Computer charting

Another system, computer charting, is being used increasingly by more health care facilities. Information is entered into a computer that automatically generates a list of administration times for all scheduled medications. Computer systems cut the risk of drug errors caused by illegible handwriting. (See *Record keeping in the computer age.*)

Record keeping in the computer age

As health care facilities purchase or develop computer systems, manufacturers offer increased choices among medication monitoring programs.

From simple...

Computerized record systems range from simple to sophisticated. In the simplest systems, the computer is used as a word processor or typewriter.

...to sophisticated

In more sophisticated systems, doctors can order drugs from the pharmacy by typing the drug's name, or they can select specific drugs by searching through various listings, such as pharmacologic categories, pharmacokinetic categories, and disease-related uses.

The computer indicates whether the pharmacy has the drug. The order then goes into the pharmacy's computer for filling. The order also generates a copy of the patient's record, on which the nurse can document medication administration. In some cases, the nurse can document medication administration right on the computer.

Benefits bit by bit

Computer systems offer the following advantages:

- When drug orders are changed, the pharmacy receives immediate notification, so drugs arrive on the unit faster.
- The pharmacy's computer can immediately confirm or deny a drug's availability.
- Nurses can document on medication administration records quickly and easily.
- Nurses can see at a glance which drugs have been administered and which still must be given.
- Errors from misinterpreted handwriting are eliminated.
- Records can be stored electronically in addition to, or instead of, paper copies.

Now we're cooking with gas! Changing orders by computer means instant notification — and less delay.

Different forms, same info

The medication administration record below illustrates the kind of information required on all types of medication administration forms. Although different facilities may use different forms, virtually all require the patient information, date, drug information, time of administration, and the nurse's initials after administering the drug.

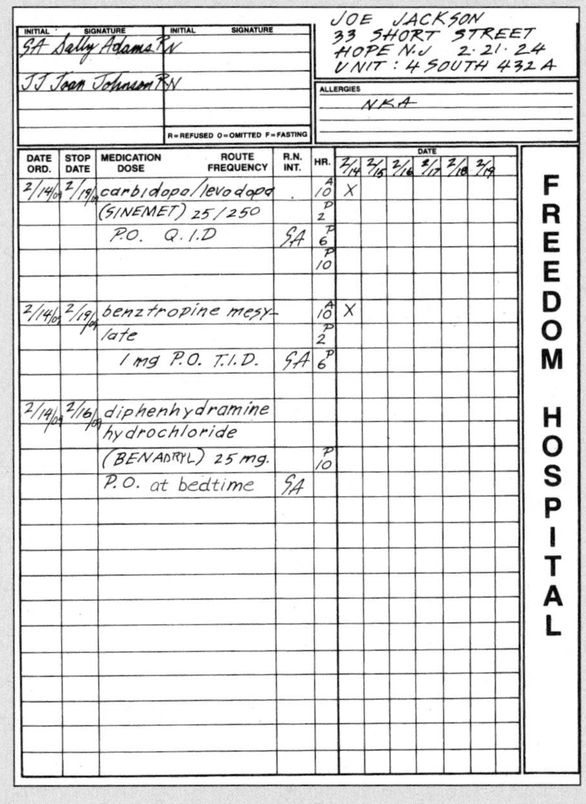

INITIAL	SIGNATURE	INITIAL	SIGNATURE
SA	Sally Adams RN		
JJ	Joan Johnson RN		

R = REFUSED O = OMITTED F = FASTING

JOE JACKSON
33 SHORT STREET
HOPE N.J 2·21·24
UNIT : 4 SOUTH 432 A

ALLERGIES
NKA

DATE ORD.	STOP DATE	MEDICATION DOSE ROUTE FREQUENCY	R.N. INT.	HR.	DATE 2/14	2/15	2/16	2/17	2/18	2/19	
2/14/09	2/19/09	carbidopa/levodopa		A 10	X						
		(SINEMET) 25/250		P 2							
		P.O. Q.I.D	SA	P 6							
				P 10							
2/14/09	2/19/09	benztropine mesy-		A 10	X						
		late		P 2							
		1 mg P.O. T.I.D.	SA	P 6							
2/14/09	2/16/09	diphenhydramine									
		hydrochloride									
		(BENADRYL) 25 mg.		P 10							
		P.O. at bedtime	SA								

FREEDOM HOSPITAL

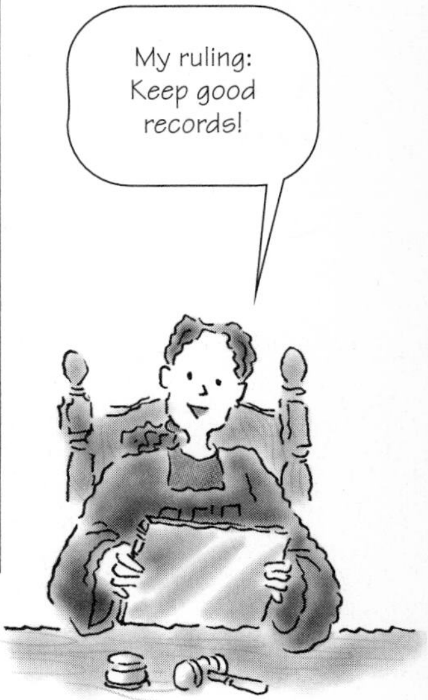
My ruling: Keep good records!

See you in court

No matter what type of medication charting system your facility uses, you must still record certain standard information. Standardization allows medication administration records to be used as legal documents if it ever becomes necessary to prove that a drug dose was given. (See *Different forms, same info*.)

Documentation

In general, documentation reflects the tasks, assessments, and procedures nurses perform. Documenting on the administration record indicates that you've carried out the doctor's order.

Does that say subcutaneous or subcuticular?

Before transcribing the doctor's orders, make sure that they're complete, clear, and correct. If you detect a problem, contact the doctor before sending the order to the pharmacy. If you detect a problem after the order goes to the pharmacy, contact both the doctor and the pharmacy.

Is that 1 mg I.V. over 10 minutes or 10 mg over 1 minute?

Information recorded on an MAR must be written legibly in ink. Most facilities require the use of blue or black ink to allow for clear reproduction of the record. All handwritten or computerized administration records must contain patient information, drug information, and signatures. *Remember:* Transcribing drug orders requires close attention because even a small discrepancy can cause a major drug error.

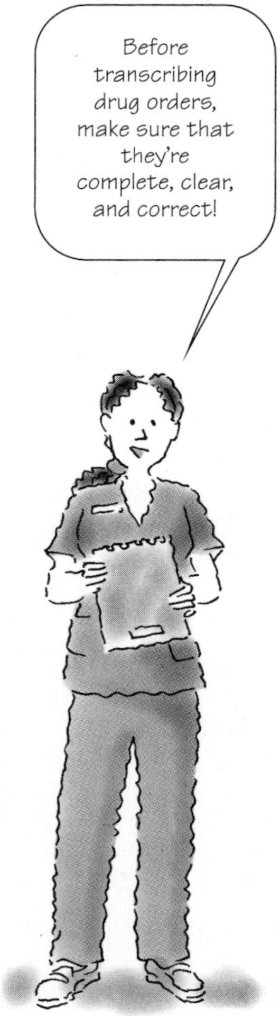
Before transcribing drug orders, make sure that they're complete, clear, and correct!

Recording patient information

If your facility uses a computerized system, you don't need to transcribe patient information onto the administration record. It's already there because the admissions office enters the patient information into the system, and the pharmacy adds information, such as the patient's height, weight, and allergies. In some systems, however, nurses may also enter this information.

If you use an MAR, stamp the form with the patient's admission data plate. If this isn't available, copy the information from the patient's identification bracelet.

Identification, please

Record the patient's full name, hospital identification number, unit number, bed assignment, and allergies, even those that aren't drug related. If the patient doesn't have any known allergies, write "NKA."

If the name of his insurance carrier is written on his identification bracelet, record this, too. *Transcribe the information exactly as it appears on the bracelet.*

Recording drug information

Next, transcribe from the doctor's order complete information about every drug the patient is taking. Include dates and drug names, dosages, strengths, dosage forms, administration routes, and administration times.

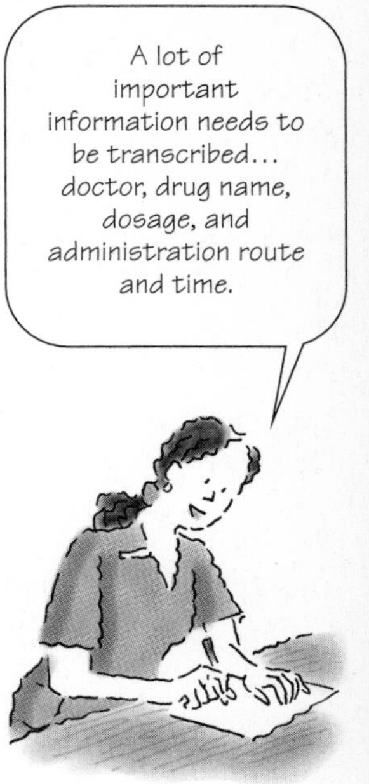

A lot of important information needs to be transcribed… doctor, drug name, dosage, and administration route and time.

It's a date!

You must always record these dates on the administration record: the date the prescription was written; the date the drug should begin, if this is different from the original order date; and the date the drug should be discontinued.

At some facilities, the time and date the drug should begin are recorded together. This serves as a reference for the time to discontinue a drug when a limited period is indicated. Many facilities also have a standard length of time a drug may be given before it's automatically discontinued.

Full name, please

Record the drug's full generic name. If the doctor ordered the drug using a proprietary (trade or brand) name, record this name as well. Don't use abbreviations, chemical symbols, research names, or special facility names. Doing so can cause medication errors or delay therapy.

Working on your strength

When recording drug strength, be sure to write the amount of the drug to be administered.

As a matter of form…

Also record the drug dosage form that the doctor ordered. Then decide whether the form is appropriate, considering the patient's special needs.

For example, if sustained-action theophylline tablets are ordered for a patient with a nasogastric tube, he won't be able to take the tablets orally. You'll have to crush them before administering them through the tube.

However, crushing sustained-action tablets destroys the drug's integrity and alters its therapeutic action. So, you'll need to contact the doctor and discuss an alternative drug dosage form.

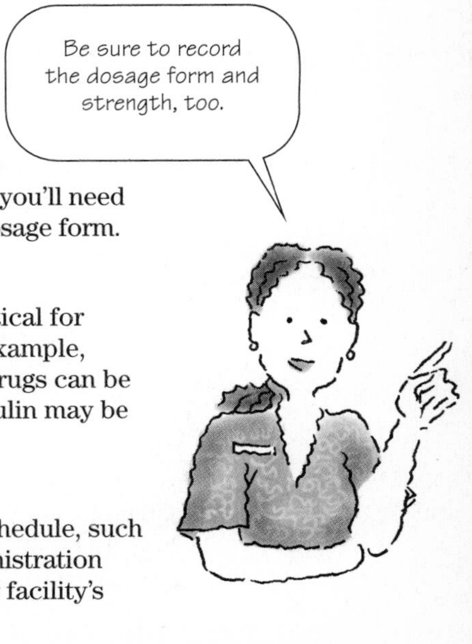

Be sure to record the dosage form and strength, too.

Tracking the route

Recording the route of administration is especially critical for drugs that may be given by two different routes. For example, acetaminophen can be given orally or rectally. Other drugs can be given by only one correct route; for example, NPH insulin may be given subcutaneously but not I.V.

Schedule scheme

The doctor's order should include an administration schedule, such as *t.i.d.* or *q6h.* Transcribe the schedule onto the administration record; then convert it into actual times based on your facility's policy and the drug's availability, characteristics, onset, and duration of action.

For example, t.i.d. may mean 9 a.m., 1 p.m., and 5 p.m. in one facility and 10 a.m., 2 p.m., and 6 p.m. in another. Similarly, b.i.d. may be 10 a.m. and 6 p.m. or 10 a.m. and 10 p.m.

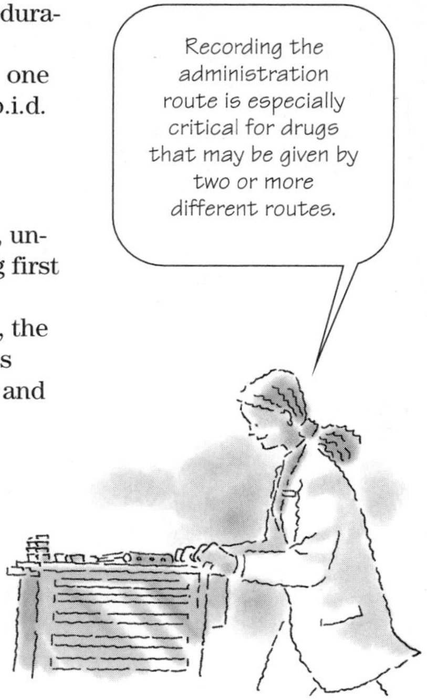

Working around the clock

Remember that time notations are based on a 24-hour clock, unless otherwise specified. This means that the hour appearing first on a 24-hour clock should appear first in the time notation.

In other words, if an administration schedule is 2-10-2-10, the first 2 represents 2 a.m., or 0200 hours; the first 10 represents 10 a.m., or 1000 hours; the second 2 is 2 p.m., or 1400 hours; and the second 10 is 10 p.m., or 2200 hours.

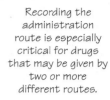

Under special circumstances

Some facilities have separate administration records or specially designated areas of the regular administration record for transcribing single orders or special drug orders. Special orders include drugs given p.r.n., large-volume parenteral drugs, and dermatologic and ophthalmic medications dispensed in bottles or tubes.

Other facilities put single orders or special drugs on the regular administration record. If this is the case where you work, be careful to distinguish these drugs from those that are regularly scheduled. All facilities have special forms for recording controlled substances. (See *Controlling controlled substances*.)

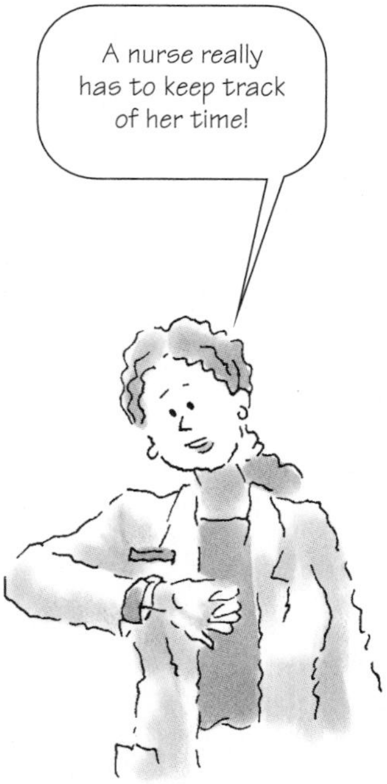

A nurse really has to keep track of her time!

Don't forget to sign

Remember that every time you transcribe orders onto the administration record, you must sign it. First initial the record after transcribing from the doctor's order sheet. Many facilities also require the nurse to perform a chart check and initial the doctor's order sheet on a line after the last order. This indicates that all orders have been transcribed correctly onto the administration record. If someone other than the nurse transcribes the order, a nurse must co-sign the order sheet and the administration record.

After you give that drug, document!

Immediately after giving a drug, document the time of administration to prevent you from mistakenly giving the drug again. For scheduled drugs, you'll usually initial the appropriate time slot for the date that the drug is administered.

Scheduled drugs are considered on time if they're given within a half-hour of the ordered time. For unscheduled drugs, such as

Controlling controlled substances

Federal and state laws regulate the dispensation, administration, and documentation of controlled substances. When these substances are issued to a unit, they're accompanied by a perpetual inventory record, commonly called a *controlled inventory record.*

A paper trail

If the doctor orders a controlled substance for your patient, document its administration on the administration record and the perpetual inventory record. When you remove a dose from the locked storage site, note this information on the perpetual inventory record:

- date and time the dose is removed
- amount of the drug remaining in the locked storage site
- patient's full name
- doctor's name
- drug dose
- your signature.

If you have to discard any of the dose, have another nurse verify the amount discarded and ask her to sign the form, too.

Paperless trail

Most facilities now have computerized drug dispensing systems such as a Pyxis on every unit. These systems may dispense controlled substances as well as other medications. Your username and password serve as your signature to access and withdraw medications. You'll still need another nurse to witness any part of a controlled substance that you discard — the system will usually display a prompt screen for her to enter her username and password to serve as her signature.

Computerized drug dispensing systems provide you with access to medications that are commonly needed in the patient care area. So, when a new drug is ordered, you can obtain it from the computerized drug dispensing system instead of waiting for the pharmacy to deliver it. A safety feature allows the pharmacist to review and approve the medication before you can select and administer the medication from the system.

Computerized drug dispensing systems also have software that promotes patient safety by utilizing readable bar-codes for restocking and choosing medications, providing automated refilling systems, giving medication safety alerts, and linking to satellite pharmacies after hours so drugs can be verified and distributed.

single doses and p.r.n. drugs, record the exact time of administration in the appropriate slot.

If the dose you administer varies in any way from the strength or amount ordered, note this in a special area on the administration record or, if there isn't an administration record, in the progress notes. For example, you would document whether the patient refused to take a drug, consumed only part of a drug, or vomited shortly after taking a drug.

Document detours

If you administer a drug by a different route from that which the doctor originally ordered, indicate that change, along with the reason and authorization for the change. Also document if a special administration technique, such as a Z-track I.M. injection, was used.

Citing the site

When administering a drug by a parenteral route, record the injection site to facilitate site rotation. Most administration forms include a numbered list of recognized sites, allowing you to record the site by its number. However, if necessary, describe anatomical landmarks used to locate the specific site.

When the timing's off

If you don't give a drug on time or if you miss a dose, document the reason on either the administration record or the patient's progress notes. Facility policy may require you to initial and circle the particular time missed on the administration record to draw attention to it.

Initiate initialing

You need to sign the administration record after giving a drug. Put your initials in the appropriate space on the form. Make sure that they're legible and always sign them the same way. If another nurse on your unit has the same initials or name, use your middle initial to avoid confusion.

In addition, write your full name, title, and initials in the signature section of the administration record. This information must appear on every record you initial when administering drugs.

Real world problems

Here are some examples of administration record problems you may encounter in the real world.

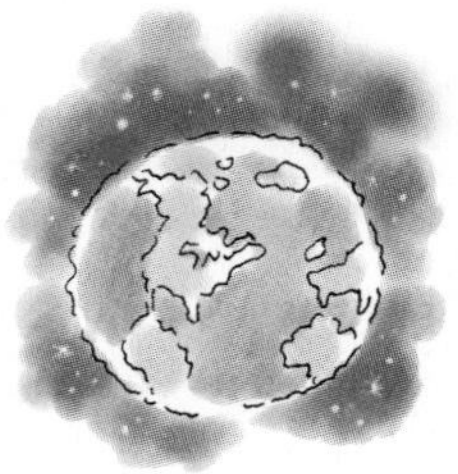

The old NPO holdup

Your patient receives oral potassium chloride supplements. You're due to give a dose but the patient was made NPO for a test, so you withheld the dose. How do you record this?

In most facilities still using written charts, you record a withheld dose by placing your initials in the appropriate time slot on the MAR, and then circling them. You can dictate the reason you withheld the dose (in this case, the patient was made NPO) in the progress notes.

In control

Your patient needs a dose of morphine sulfate, a controlled substance. You only need 2 mg of the 4-mg prefilled syringe available. On the record, how do you indicate that the extra morphine was appropriately discarded?

First, ask another nurse to watch as you appropriately discard the extra medication. Then, have her sign the controlled inventory record (or follow your facility's policy) to verify this process.

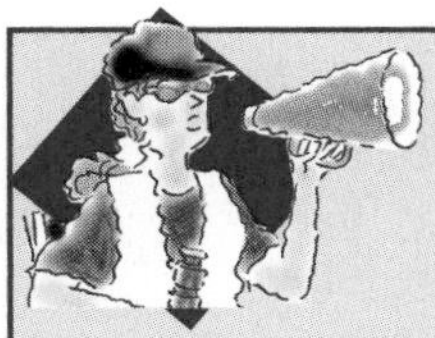

That's a wrap!

Administration records review

Keep these important points about administration records in mind.

Drug administration record systems

- MAR
  - Uses a form to record medication administration
- Computer charting
  - Medication administration information entered into a computer
  - Automatic, computer-generated list of scheduled medications and their administration times
  - Used increasingly over other systems

Documenting drug administration

- Write legibly in blue or black ink.
- Record allergy information if it isn't already documented, using "NKA" if no allergies are known.
- Transcribe from the doctor's order complete information about each drug (dates and drug names, dosages, strengths, dosage forms, administration routes, and administration times).
- If parenteral, record the injection site.
- Immediately document the times of all administrations.
- If unscheduled, record the exact time the drug was given.
- If given late or not at all, document the reason.
- Always sign any documentation on the administration record.

Recording controlled-substance administration

- Include date and time dose is removed from locked storage area.
- Include amount of drug remaining in locked storage area.
- Record the patient's full name.
- Document the doctor's full name.
- Enter the drug dose given.
- Include your full signature (if a form is used; the nurse's password serves as a signature if a computer is used).
- If any part of the drug was discarded, obtain the signature of another nurse who verified the amount discarded (or have her enter her password as verification if using a computer).

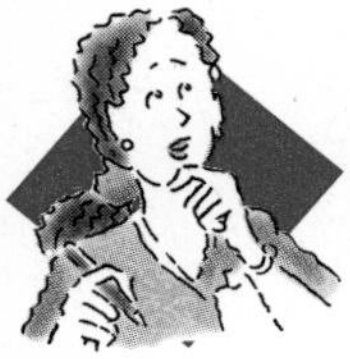

Quick quiz

1. You may be required to circle and initial the time slot of a medication if:

A. you missed the dose or gave it late.
B. the administration time has changed.
C. another nurse forgot to administer a drug.
D. the medication has been discontinued.

Answer: A. Circling and initialing the time slot signals to the next nurse that the dose was missed or late. The nurse then refers to the single-order or p.r.n. section of the MAR to find the actual administration time. That way, she doesn't mistakenly administer the next dose too soon.

2. The abbreviation NKA stands for:

A. no known adverse reactions.
B. no known administration.
C. no known alteration.
D. no known allergies.

Answer: D. Allergy information should always be recorded. If there are no known allergies, document NKA.

3. To avoid confusion, nurses with the same initials should sign the administration record with:

A. their identification numbers.
B. pens with different colors of ink.
C. their middle initials.
D. their birth dates.

Answer: C. Middle initials should be used. In addition, be sure to write legibly and always sign the same way.

4. Immediately after you administer a drug, you should:

A. document its effectiveness.
B. document the time of administration.
C. order the next dose of the drug from the pharmacy.
D. take the patient's vital signs.

Answer: B. Documenting the time of administration immediately after you give the drug prevents you from mistakenly giving the drug again.

Scoring

☆☆☆ If you answered all four items correctly, amazing! You've been voted best nurse at the Administration Academy Awards!

☆☆ If you answered three items correctly, fantastic! Here's your Oscar for best supporting nurse!

☆ If you answered fewer than three items correctly, keep your chin up! You're still a record setter!

9

Preventing drug errors

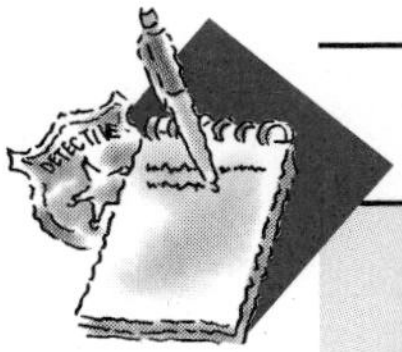

Just the facts

In this chapter, you'll learn:

- the types and causes of common drug errors
- how to prevent drug errors
- how to report drug errors.

A look at drug errors

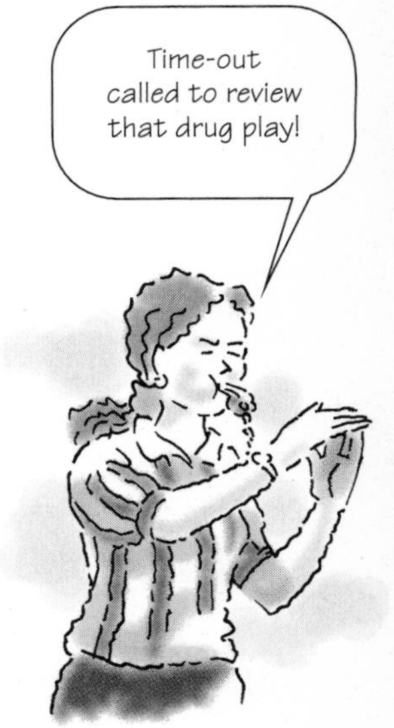

Time-out called to review that drug play!

Drug errors cause thousands of injuries and deaths in health care settings every year. In fact, in U.S. hospitals alone, they're responsible for about 15,000 deaths annually. Because only about 1 out of every 10 drug errors is reported, no one knows exactly how many errors actually occur. Despite such discouraging statistics, finding better ways to safeguard patients against these kinds of errors has become a national health care priority.

Are you legal?

Depending on where you practice nursing, several different health care professionals, including doctors, nurse practitioners, dentists, podiatrists, and optometrists, may be legally permitted to prescribe, dispense, and administer medications. Usually, however, doctors prescribe medications, pharmacists prepare and dispense the drugs, and nurses administer them to patients.

An integral team player

As a nurse, you're almost always on the front line when it comes to medication administration. That means you also bear a major share of the responsibility in protecting patients from all types of drug errors.

Doing your part

Many kinds of drug errors can occur in everyday nursing practice. Consequently, each institution has its own set of guidelines for how and when to properly administer drugs to patients, and each nurse is responsible for knowing what those guidelines are. Besides faithfully following your facility's administration policies, you can

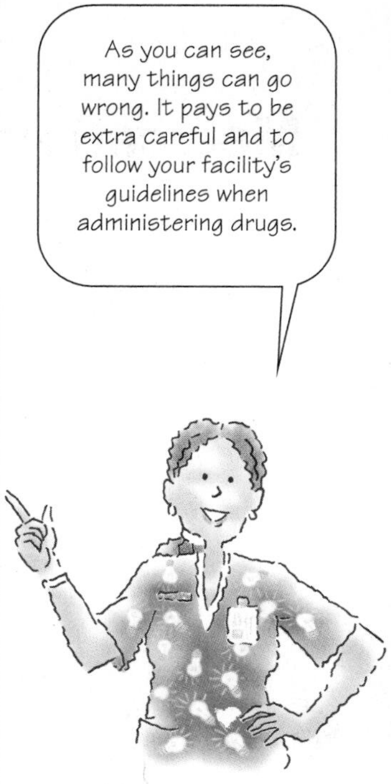

As you can see, many things can go wrong. It pays to be extra careful and to follow your facility's guidelines when administering drugs.

Common drug errors

Certain situations or activities can place nurses at high risk for making a drug error. Some of the most common types and causes of errors are highlighted here.

Types of errors

- Giving the wrong drug
- Giving the wrong dose
- Using the wrong diluent
- Preparing the wrong concentration
- Missing a dose or failing to give an ordered drug
- Giving the drug at the wrong time
- Administering a drug to which the patient is allergic
- Infusing the drug too rapidly
- Giving the drug to the wrong patient
- Administering the drug by the wrong route

Causes

- Insufficient knowledge
- Chaotic work environment
- Use of floor stock medications
- Failure to follow facility policies and procedures
- Incorrect preparation or administration techniques
- Use of I.V. solutions that aren't premixed
- Failure to verify drug and dosage instructions
- Following oral, not written, orders
- Inadequate staffing
- Typographical errors
- Use of acronyms or erroneous abbreviations
- Math errors
- Poor handwriting
- Failure to check dosages for high-risk drugs or pediatric medications
- Inadequate drug information
- Preparation of the drug in a clinical area instead of the pharmacy
- Unlabeled syringes

help prevent drug errors by studying and avoiding the common slip-ups that allow them to happen. (See *Common drug errors*.)

Medication errors in practice

In addition to dosage calculation errors (which account for roughly 7% of all reported drug errors), common errors include mistakes with drug or patient names, missed allergy alerts, errors compounded by two or more practitioners, errors involving routes of administration, misinterpreted abbreviations, misinterpreted drug orders, preparation errors, reconciliation errors, and errors caused by stress.

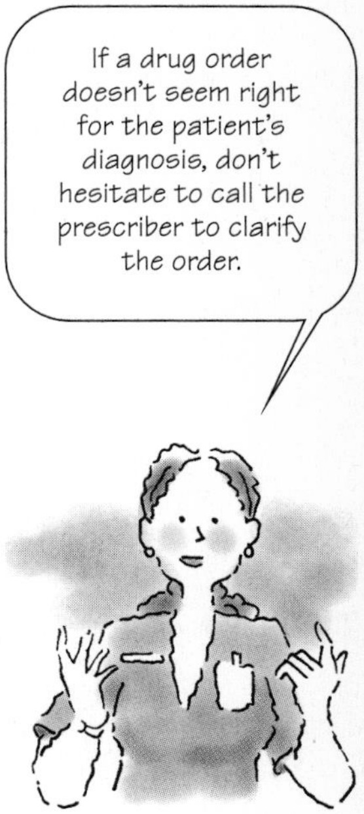
If a drug order doesn't seem right for the patient's diagnosis, don't hesitate to call the prescriber to clarify the order.

Drug name errors

Drugs with similar-sounding names are easy to confuse. Even different-sounding names can look similar when written out rapidly by hand on a medication order. Remember, if the patient's drug

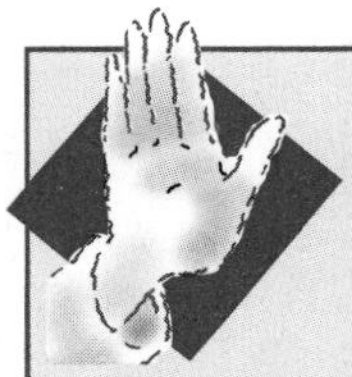

Before you give that drug

Look-alike and sound-alike drug names

The drug names listed here resemble each other in terms of spelling or sound. Always double-check the medication order carefully before administering one of them to your patient. If you have any doubt about the appropriateness of the drug, consult the prescriber, the pharmacist, or a drug reference:

- amantadine and rimantadine
- amiodarone and amiloride
- amoxicillin and amoxapine
- benztropine and bromocriptine
- Celebrex and Celexa
- Celebrex and Cerebyx
- cimetidine and simethicone
- codeine and Cardene
- dexamethasone and desoximetasone
- digoxin and doxepin
- epinephrine and ephedrine
- epinephrine and norepinephrine
- flunisolide and fluocinonide
- hydromorphone and morphine
- hydroxyzine and hydralazine
- imipramine and desipramine
- Imuran and Inderal
- insulin glargine and insulin glulisine
- levothyroxine and liothyronine
- metformin and metronidazole
- naloxone and naltrexone
- nifedipine and nicardipine
- nitroglycerin and nitroprusside
- oxycontin and oxycodone
- pentobarbital and phenobarbital
- propylthiouracil and Purinethol
- Ritalin and Rifadin
- sitagliptin and sumatriptan
- sulfisoxazole and sulfasalazine
- vinblastine and vincristine
- Xanax and Zantac
- Zyrtec and Zyprexa.

order doesn't seem right for his diagnosis, call the prescriber to clarify the order. (See *Look-alike and sound-alike drug names*, page 147.)

Morphing the name

For example, an order for morphine can be easily confused with one for hydromorphone. Both drugs are available in 4-mg prefilled syringes, and both cause respiratory depression. However, morphine has a greater effect on a patient's respiratory status. If you administer morphine when the prescriber really ordered hydromorphone, the patient could develop respiratory depression or even respiratory arrest.

Posting prevention

To prevent errors, consider posting a notice prominently on your unit where opioids are kept, to warn the staff about this common mix-up. Or try attaching a fluorescent or brightly colored sticker with the words "NOT MORPHINE" to each hydromorphone syringe.

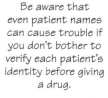

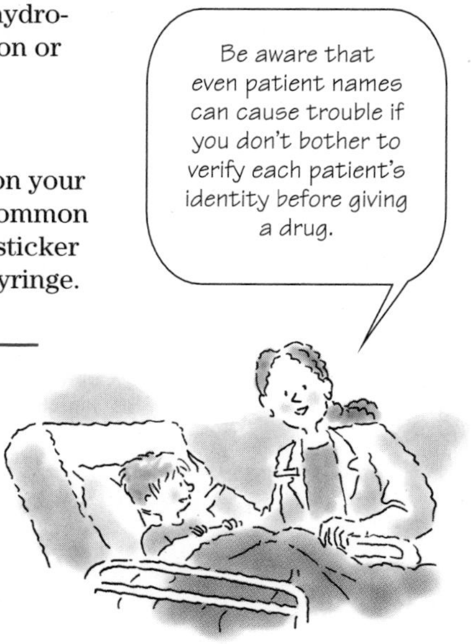

Patient name errors

Drug names aren't the only names subject to confusion. Sometimes, patient names can cause trouble as well, especially when nurses don't verify each patient's identity before administering medications. Caring for two patients with the same or similar first or last name can further complicate matters. Consider the following scenario.

A tale of two Bobs

Five-year-old Robert Brewer is hospitalized with measles. Robert Brinson, also age 5, is admitted to the same pediatric unit after a severe asthma attack. The boys are assigned to adjacent rooms. Each has a nonproductive cough.

The nurse caring for Robert Brewer enters his room to give him an expectorant. As the nurse is about to administer the drug, the child's mother informs her that someone else came into the room a few minutes ago to give Robert a medication that he inhaled by mask. The nurse quickly determines that another nurse mistakenly gave Robert Brinson's medication (acetylcysteine—a mucolytic) to Robert Brewer.

Fortunately, no harmful adverse effects developed. However, if the other nurse had checked the patient's identity more carefully, this error would never have occurred.

Check and double-check

Always verify the patient's identity using two patient identifiers. The two identifiers may be included in the same location, such as the hospital identification bracelet. Acceptable identifiers include the patient's first and last names, his assigned identification number (such as the medical record number), and his birth date. Involve the patient in the identification process by asking him his full name.

Raising the bar with bar coding

Bar-code medication administration technology is one way to help prevent medication errors before they reach the patient. With this technology, a bar code is placed on each medication the patient is to receive. Each medication bar code contains the National Drug Code, which includes the drug's name, its dose, and packaging information. Another bar code is placed on the patient's hospital identification bracelet.

Before administering a medication, the nurse scans the medication bar code and the patient's bar code using an optical scanner. Scanning both bar codes in this manner helps ensure administration of the right medication to the right patient at the right time by alerting the nurse about any discrepancies.

Bar codes in action

Two examples of how bar-code medication technology prevented medication errors are illustrated here.

A nurse attempting to administer furosemide (Lasix) 40 mg I.V. to a patient scanned the product at the patient's bedside and received a warning message that read "No order in the system." She didn't administer the medication and immediately reviewed the patient's chart. After reviewing the chart, she realized that the medication wasn't intended for that patient.

In another incident, a nurse scanned the bar code on the patient's identification bracelet and then scanned the bar code on the patient's levofloxacin (Levaquin) container. The nurse received a warning message that read "Dose early." The nurse didn't administer the medication until 2 hours later, when the medication was due to be administered.

Preventing drug errors through teaching

Drug errors aren't limited to hospital settings. Patients sometimes make drug errors when taking their medications at home. To prevent such errors, take the time to educate your patient thoroughly about each medication he'll be taking. Be sure to cover these points:

- drug's name (generic and trade name)
- drug's purpose
- correct dosage and how to calculate it (such as breaking scored tablets or mixing liquids when necessary)
- how to take the drug
- when to take the drug
- what to do if a dose is missed
- how to monitor the drug's effectiveness (for example, checking blood glucose levels when taking an antidiabetic drug)
- potential drug interactions (including the need to avoid certain over-the-counter and herbal drugs)
- required dietary changes (including the use of alcohol)
- possible adverse effects and what to do if they occur
- proper storage, handling, and disposal of the drug or supplies (such as syringes)
- required follow-up.

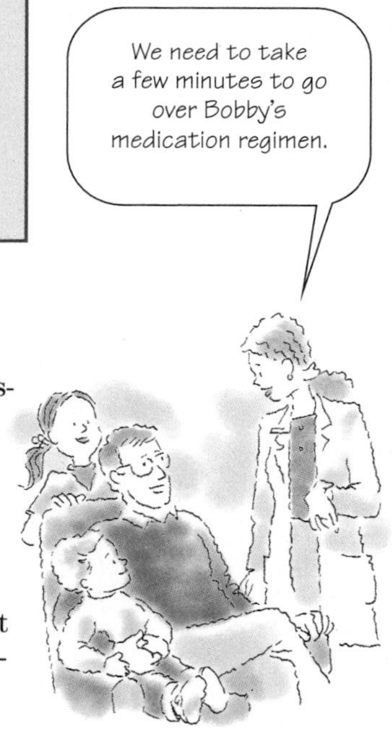

We need to take a few minutes to go over Bobby's medication regimen.

Teach the patient (or parents if the patient is a child) to offer his identification bracelet for inspection when anyone—including the nurse, doctor, nurse practitioner, anesthetist, or respiratory therapist—enters his room to administer a medication. Also urge patients to tell you or another nurse whenever an identification bracelet falls off, is removed, or becomes misplaced. Then, replace it or substitute a new one immediately. (See *Raising the bar with bar coding*, page 149.)

Patients can also be taught what their medications look like, how they're given, and at what times they should take them. That way, they know what they should be receiving while in the hospital and are prepared to safely use the drug after discharge. (See *Preventing drug errors through teaching*.)

Missed allergy alerts

After you've verified your patient's identity, check to see if he's wearing allergy identification, such as MedicAlert jewelry. All allergy identification tags or jewelry should have the name of the specific allergen conspicuously written or embossed on them.

This same allergy information should be recorded on the front of the patient's chart and on his medication record. Always double-check the information against the chart. Regardless of whether the patient is wearing allergy identification, take the time to ask the patient directly about drug allergies — even if he's in distress.

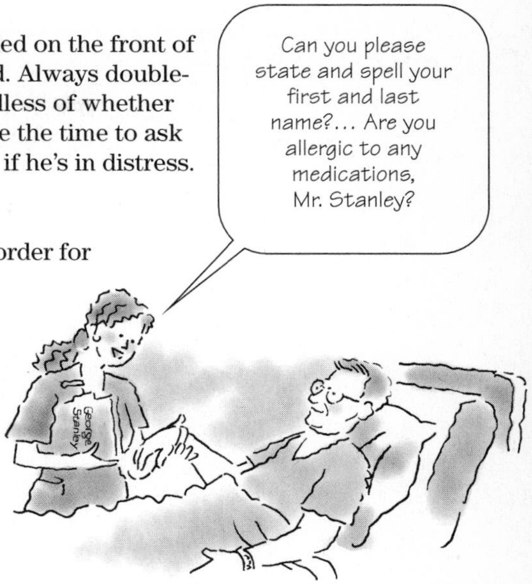

Can you please state and spell your first and last name?... Are you allergic to any medications, Mr. Stanley?
George Stanley

A distressing situation

Consider this example. The doctor issues a stat order for lorazepam (Ativan) for a distressed patient. By the time the nurse arrives with the drug, the patient has grown more visibly distressed. Unnerved by the patient's demeanor, the nurse quickly administers the drug — without verifying the patient's identity and checking the patient's allergy bracelet or medication administration record first, and without documenting the order. The patient has an immediate allergic reaction.

Because the patient's allergy bracelet clearly stated his known allergy, and this same information was clearly indicated on his chart and medication administration record, this error was fully preventable.

Resisting temptation

Any time you're in a tense situation with a patient who needs or wants medication fast, resist the temptation to act first and document later. Skipping this crucial step can easily lead to a medication error.

Not just talking peanuts

Certain medications should never be given to patients allergic to peanuts, soy, or sulfa compounds. Keep these tips in mind to help prevent allergic reactions in these patients:

- A patient who's severely allergic to peanuts or soy may have an anaphylactic reaction (a severe, life-threatening reaction) to ipratropium (Atrovent) aerosol given by metered-dose inhaler. Ask the patient (or parents) whether he's allergic to peanuts or soy before giving this drug. If you find that he has such an allergy, you'll need to use the nasal spray or inhalation solution (nebulizer) form of the drug. Because neither form contains soy lecithin (an emulsifier used in the metered-dose formula), it's safe for patients allergic to peanuts or soy.
- Patients allergic to sulfa drugs shouldn't receive sulfonylurea antidiabetic agents, such as chlorpropamide (Diabinese), glyburide (Micronase), and glipizide (Glucotrol).

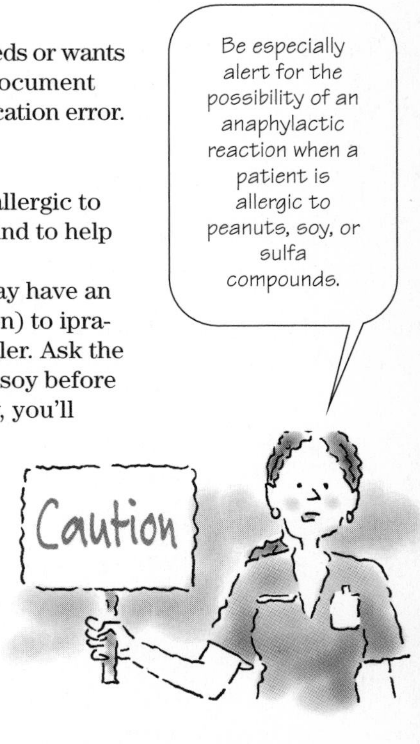

Compound errors

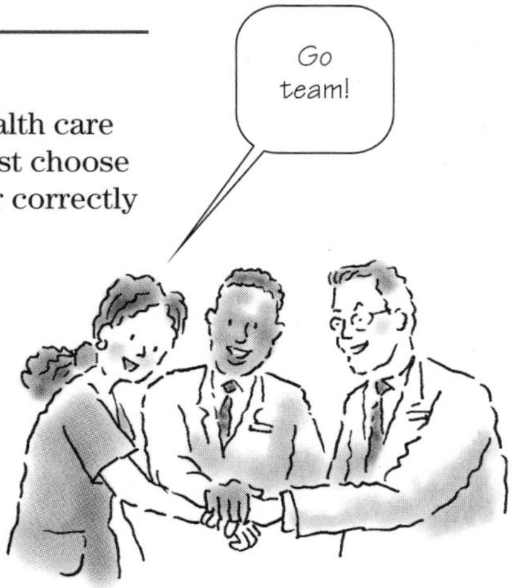

For a drug to be given correctly, each member of the health care team must fulfill an appropriate role: The prescriber must choose the right medication for the patient, then write the order correctly and legibly or enter it into the computer correctly. The pharmacist must interpret the order, determine whether it's complete, and prepare the drug using precise measurements. Finally, the nurse must evaluate whether the medication is appropriate for the patient, then administer it correctly according to facility guidelines.

Never break the chain

A breakdown along this chain of events can easily lead to a medication error, an error that's further compounded because of the number of people who could have prevented it. That's why it's vital for all health care providers to work together as a team, supporting and helping each other to promote the best patient care. In some cases, working as a team may be as simple as asking for further clarification or as complicated as double-checking another practitioner's action and calling him to task.

Calling all pharmacists

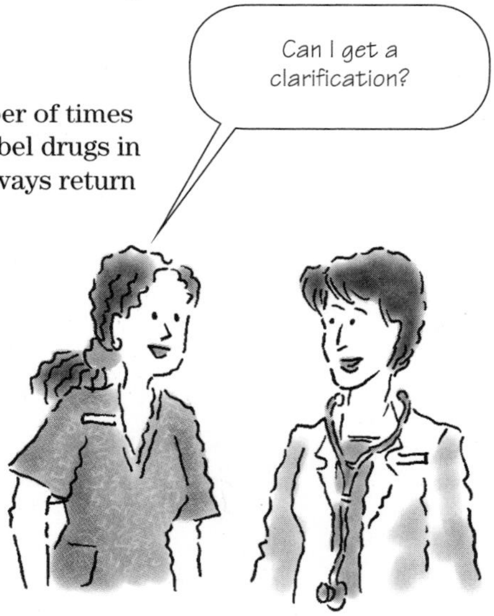

For instance, the pharmacist can help clarify the number of times a drug must be given each day. He can also help you label drugs in the most appropriate way. Or, he can remind you to always return unused or discontinued medications to the pharmacy.

I can see clearly now

As a nurse, you're responsible for clarifying a prescriber's order that doesn't seem clear or correct. You must also correctly handle and store multidose vials obtained from the pharmacist, and administer only those drugs that you've personally prepared. Never give a drug with an ambiguous label or no label at all. Here's an example of what could happen if you do.

A shocking mistake

The nurse places an unlabeled syringe on a tray near a patient in the operating room. The nurse gets called away unexpectedly and the doctor administers the medication. The doctor thought the syringe contained bupivacaine (Marcaine), but instead it contained

30 ml of epinephrine 1:1,000, which the nurse had drawn up into the syringe. The patient developed ventricular fibrillation, was immediately defibrillated, and then needed to be transferred to the intensive care unit, where he later recovered.

Obviously, this was a compound medication error. The nurse should have labeled the syringe clearly, and the doctor should never have given an unlabeled drug to the patient.

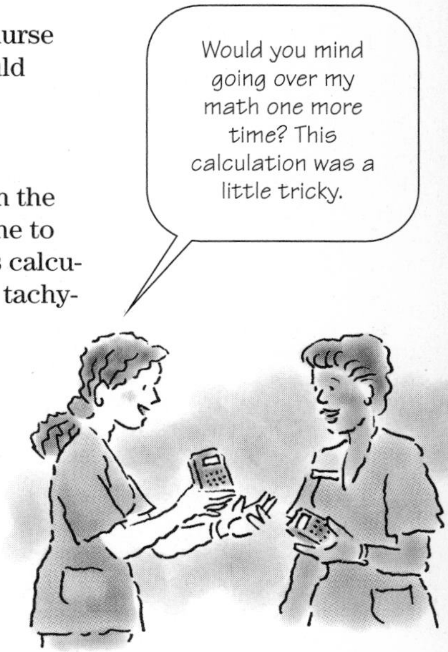

Would you mind going over my math one more time? This calculation was a little tricky.

Liters vs. grams

In another example of a compound error, a nurse working in the neonatal intensive care unit prepares a dose of aminophylline to administer to an infant. No one bothers to check the nurse's calculations. Shortly after receiving the drug, the infant develops tachycardia and other signs of theophylline toxicity and later dies. The nurse thought that the order read *7.4 ml of aminophylline*. Instead, it read *7.4 mg.*

This tragedy might have been avoided if the doctor had written a clearer order, if the nurse had clarified the order before administering it, if the pharmacist had prepared and dispensed the drug, or if another nurse had double-checked the dosage calculation. To avoid this type of problem, many facilities require pharmacists to prepare and dispense all nonemergency parenteral doses whenever commercial unit doses aren't available.

Take necessary precautions to breathe easier

Here's another example: A nurse mistakenly leaves a container of 5% acetic acid (used to clean tracheostomy tubing) near nebulization equipment in the room of a 10-month-old infant. A respiratory therapist mistakes the liquid for normal saline solution and uses it to dilute albuterol for the child's nebulizer treatment. During the treatment, the child experiences bronchospasm, hypercapneic dyspnea, tachypnea, and tachycardia.

Leaving dangerous chemicals near patient-care areas is extremely risky, especially when container labels don't warn of toxicity. To prevent such problems, always read the label on every drug you prepare, and never administer a drug or solution that isn't labeled or that's labeled poorly.

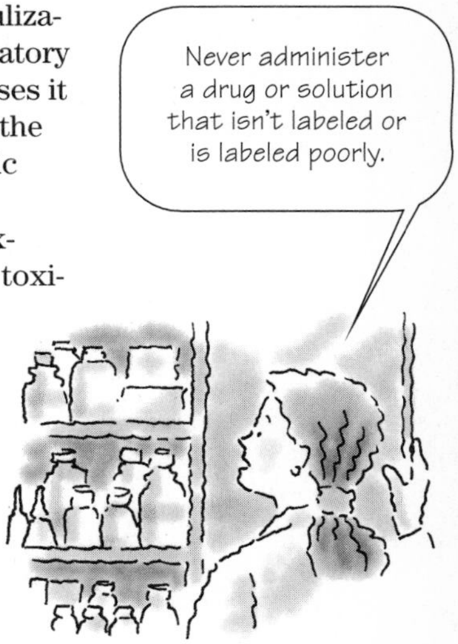

Route errors

Many drug errors stem, at least in part, from problems involving the route of administration. The risk of error increases when a patient has several lines running for different purposes, as illustrated in the following scenario.

Crossing the line

A nurse prepares a dose of digoxin elixir for a patient with a central I.V. line and a jejunostomy tube in place. She mistakenly administers the oral drug into the central I.V. line. Fortunately, the patient suffers no adverse effects.

To help prevent similar mix-ups in the route of administration, prepare all oral medications in a syringe that has a tip small enough to fit an abdominal tube but too large to fit a central line. Some facilities even use designated tubing for enteral feedings, so that it can't be inadvertently connected to an I.V. line.

Clearing the air

Here's another error that could have been avoided: To clear air bubbles from a 9-year-old patient's insulin infusion, the nurse disconnects the tubing and raises the pump rate to 200 ml/hour, flushing the bubbles through quickly. She then reconnects the tubing and restarts the infusion, but she forgets to reset the drip rate back to 2 units/hour. The child receives 50 units of insulin before the nurse detects the error.

To prevent this kind of mistake, never increase the drip rate to clear bubbles from a line. Instead, remove the tubing from the pump, disconnect it from the patient, and use the flow-control clamp to establish gravity flow of the I.V. fluid to purge the air from the line.

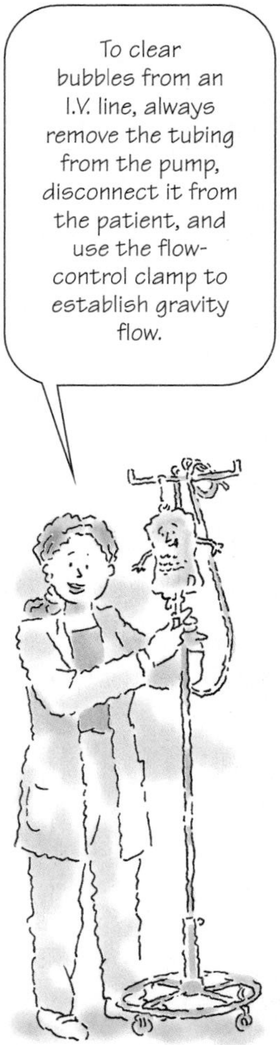
To clear bubbles from an I.V. line, always remove the tubing from the pump, disconnect it from the patient, and use the flow-control clamp to establish gravity flow.

Misinterpreted abbreviations

Some commonly used abbreviations are known to contribute significantly to drug errors. For example, in a doctor's order reading *levothyroxine (Synthroid) 50 µg PO daily*, the *µg* (meaning micrograms) may be easily misinterpreted to mean *milligrams*. The patient could mistakenly receive 50 mg of levothyroxine, or 1,000 times the ordered dose.

The Joint Commission guidelines

To prevent such devastating errors, every facility should make a "Do not use" list readily available for all health care workers. This list identifies abbreviations that should *never* be used in any form, under any circumstances. In fact, The Joint Commission has compiled a list of dangerous abbreviations that should be avoided in all clinical documentation, including doctor's orders, patient charts, progress notes, consultation reports, operative reports, educational materials, and protocols and pathways. (See *The Joint Commission's "Do not use" list*, pages 156 and 157.)

Shorthand for shortsighted

Abbreviating or using a shorthand version of a drug name is equally risky, as shown in this example: Epoetin alfa (Epogen), a synthetic form of erythropoietin that's commonly abbreviated as EPO, is

Incredibly Easy miniguide

Anatomy of a medication label

Before you can safely administer a medication, you must check the doctor's order against the medication you have on hand. To do so, you must have a good understanding of the anatomy of the medication label.

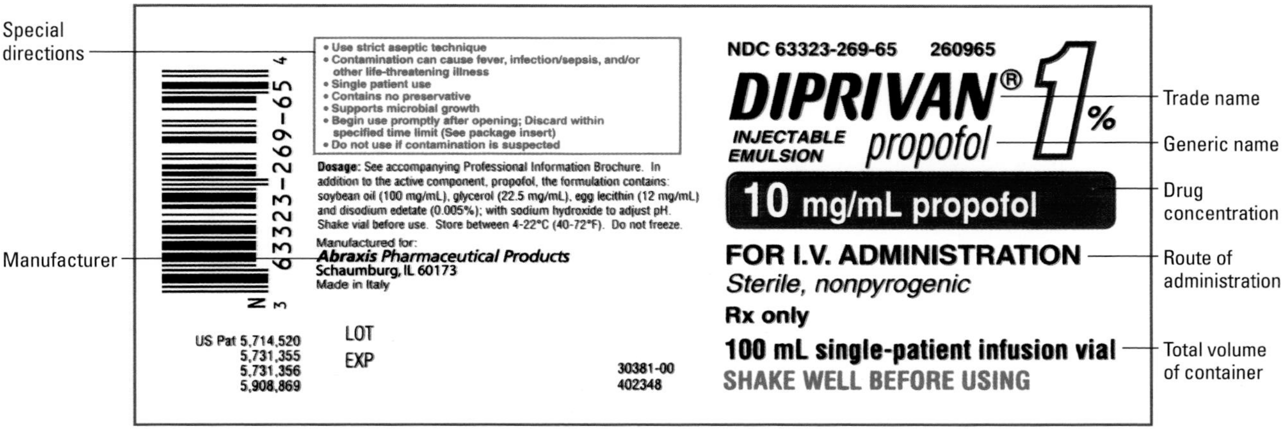

Special directions
Manufacturer
Trade name
Generic name
Drug concentration
Route of administration
Total volume of container
• Use strict aseptic technique
• Contamination can cause fever, infection/sepsis, and/or other life-threatening illness
• Single patient use
• Contains no preservative
• Supports microbial growth
• Begin use promptly after opening; Discard within specified time limit (See package insert)
• Do not use if contamination is suspected
Dosage: See accompanying Professional Information Brochure. In addition to the active component, propofol, the formulation contains: soybean oil (100 mg/mL), glycerol (22.5 mg/mL), egg lecithin (12 mg/mL) and disodium edetate (0.005%); with sodium hydroxide to adjust pH. Shake vial before use. Store between 4-22°C (40-72°F). Do not freeze.
Manufactured for:
Abraxis Pharmaceutical Products
Schaumburg, IL 60173
Made in Italy
N 3 63323-269-65 4
US Pat 5,714,520
5,731,355
5,731,356
5,908,869
LOT
EXP
30381-00
402348
NDC 63323-269-65 260965
DIPRIVAN® 1%
INJECTABLE EMULSION propofol
10 mg/mL propofol
FOR I.V. ADMINISTRATION
Sterile, nonpyrogenic
Rx only
100 mL single-patient infusion vial
SHAKE WELL BEFORE USING

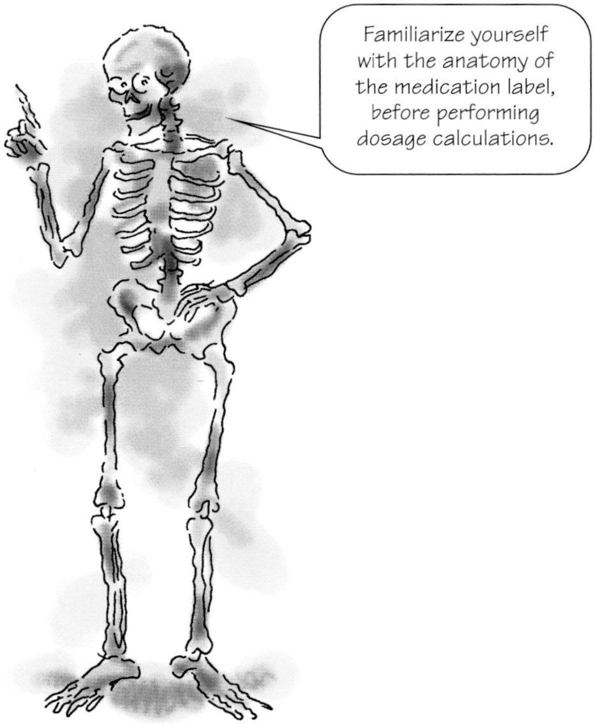

Familiarize yourself with the anatomy of the medication label, before performing dosage calculations.

Incredibly Easy miniguide

Improving patient safety using infusion devices

Electronic infusion pumps help facilitate I.V. fluid and medication administration. They allow easy control of the infusion rate by programming it into the machine. They also keep track of the amount of fluid infused and signal when mechanical problems occur or the fluid container is empty. Some infusion pumps even calculate medication dosages for you.

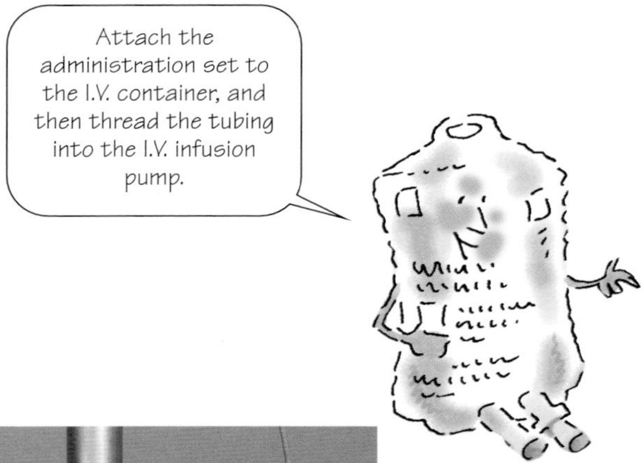
Attach the administration set to the I.V. container, and then thread the tubing into the I.V. infusion pump.

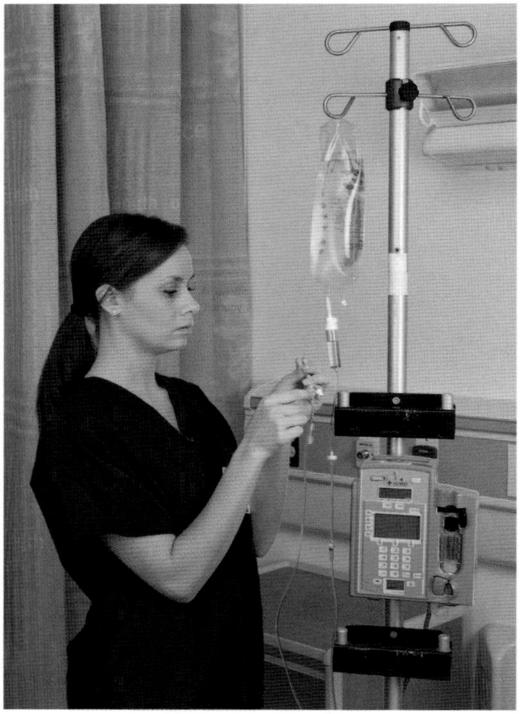

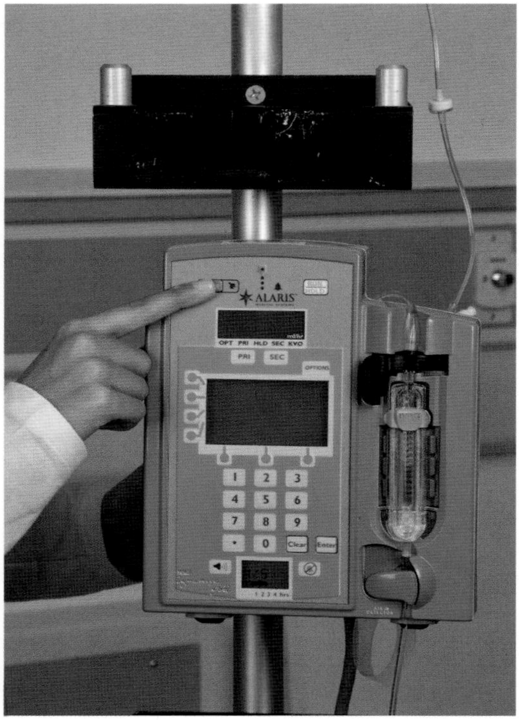

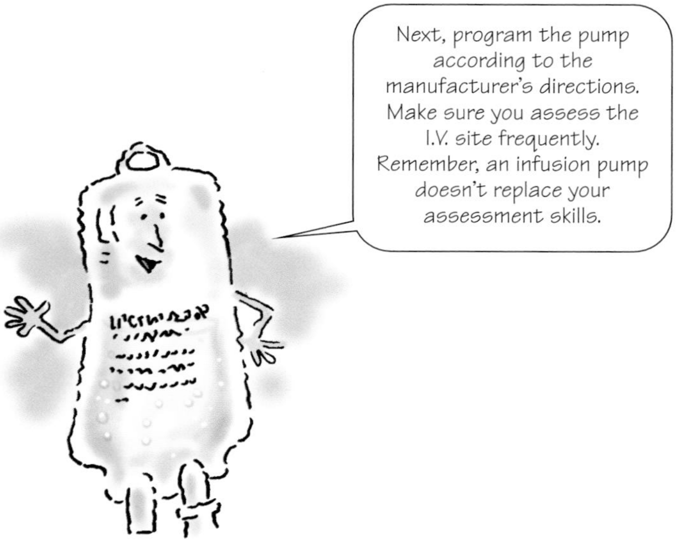
Next, program the pump according to the manufacturer's directions. Make sure you assess the I.V. site frequently. Remember, an infusion pump doesn't replace your assessment skills.

A patient-controlled analgesia system is another device that helps promote patient safety. The device allows the patient to self-administer analgesic doses while providing optimal opioid dosing and maintaining a constant serum drug level.

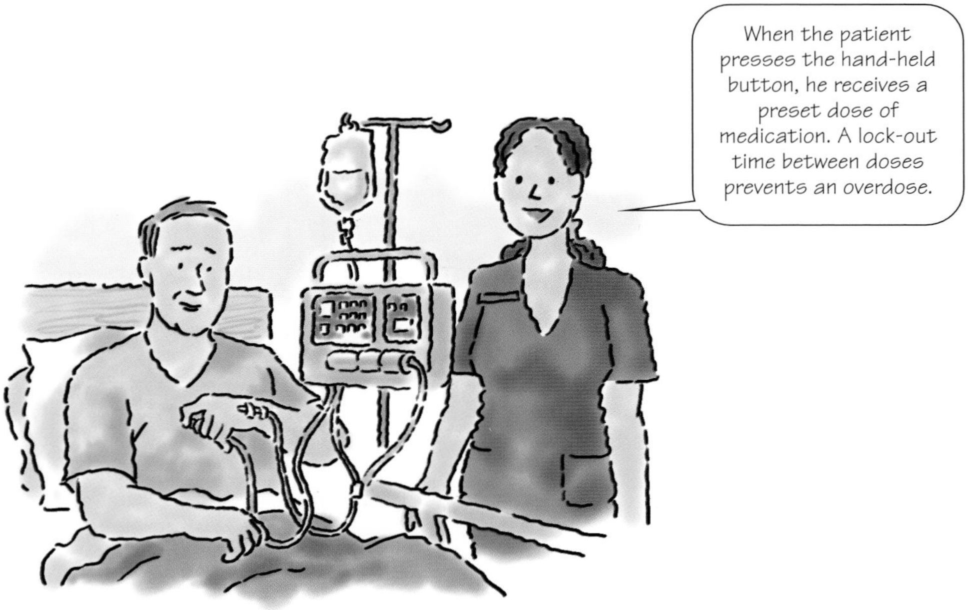

When the patient presses the hand-held button, he receives a preset dose of medication. A lock-out time between doses prevents an overdose.

INCREDIBLY EASY MINIGUIDE

Administering medications safely through the enteral route

Patients sometimes require enteral feeding tubes for nutrition and medication administration. Before administering medications through a feeding tube, make sure the medication can be given safely by that route.

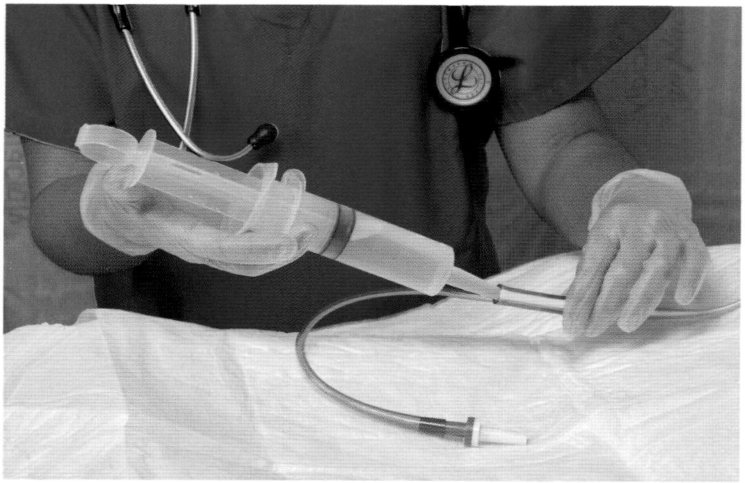

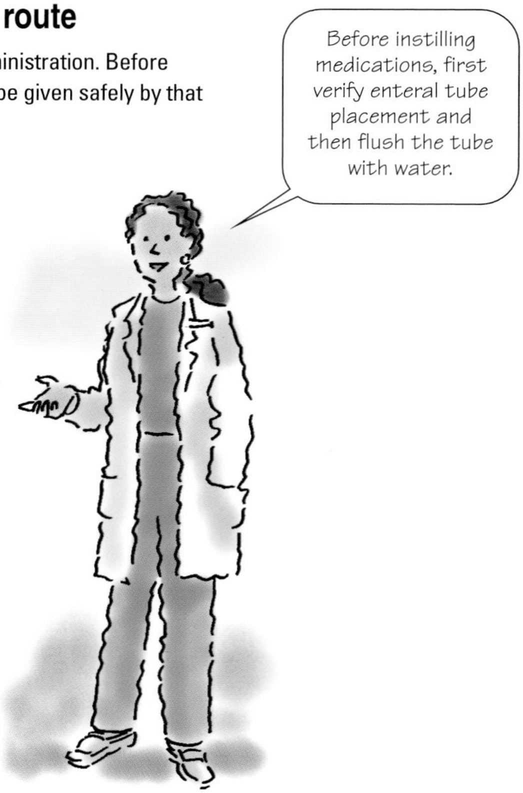

Before instilling medications, first verify enteral tube placement and then flush the tube with water.

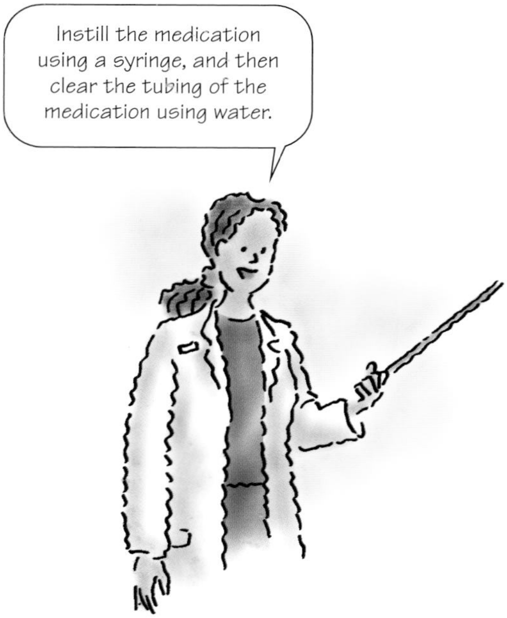

Instill the medication using a syringe, and then clear the tubing of the medication using water.

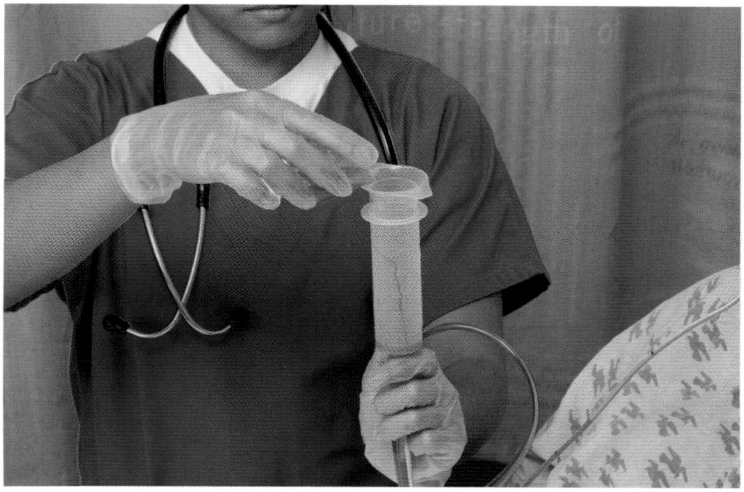

occasionally used by anemic cancer patients to stimulate red blood cell production. In one case, a doctor wrote, "May take own supply of EPO" on the discharge orders of a patient whose cancer was in remission. However, the patient wasn't anemic.

Sensing that something was wrong with ordering epoetin alfa for a patient who isn't anemic, the pharmacist interviewed the patient, who confirmed that he was taking "EPO," or evening primrose oil, to lower his cholesterol level. Fortunately, the pharmacist became aware of his misinterpretation of the abbreviation before an error could occur in this situation.

To avoid this type of error, ask prescribers to spell out all drug names.

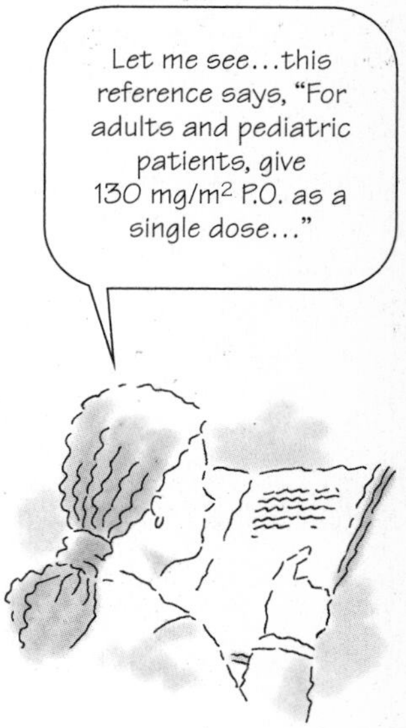
Let me see...this reference says, "For adults and pediatric patients, give 130 mg/m^2 P.O. as a single dose..."

Misinterpreted orders

As a rule of thumb, if you're unfamiliar with a drug that a doctor prescribes, always consult a drug reference before administering the medication to the patient. Also, ask the prescriber to clarify vague or ambiguous terms. Don't assume that you'll get it right on your own.

Guessing is always wrong

Here's an example. A patient was supposed to receive one dose of the antineoplastic drug lomustine (Ceena) to treat brain cancer. (Lomustine is typically given as a single oral dose once every 6 weeks.) The doctor's order read, "Administer at night." Because the evening shift nurse misinterpreted the order to mean "every night" when the doctor meant "at bedtime," the patient received three daily doses of a drug he should have only received once, developed severe thrombocytopenia and leukopenia, then died.

Remember to clarify confusing orders with the prescriber, and to read each order carefully. Also remember to look up in a drug reference any drugs you're unfamiliar with—doing so may prevent an error and save a life.

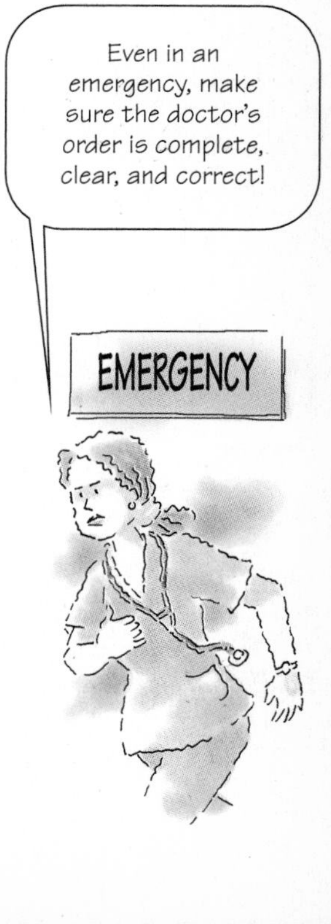
Even in an emergency, make sure the doctor's order is complete, clear, and correct!
EMERGENCY

Did I hear you right?

In rare cases, you may need to follow a doctor's verbal order to administer a drug. These situations typically involve emergencies, such as resuscitation of a patient, when there's no time to write out an order. If you find yourself in this type of situation, be sure to listen closely to the instruction, repeating it back to the doctor as necessary to ensure you've heard him correctly, before administering the drug. Then promptly document the order and the details of the incident in the patient's chart. Make sure that the doctor reviews and signs all orders as necessary as soon as the patient has stabilized.

The Joint Commission's "Do not use" list

All health care facilities accredited by The Joint Commission are required to maintain a "Do not use" list—a list of abbreviations that should never be used in any form (upper or lower case, with or without periods) in clinical documentation because they're confusing and subject to misinterpretation.

Official "Do not use" list

These abbreviations must appear on a "Do not use" list and should be avoided in *all* orders and medication-related documentation that is handwritten (including free-text computer entry) or on preprinted forms.

Abbreviation	Potential problem	Preferred term
U (for unit)	Mistaken as 0 (zero), 4 (four), or cc	Write *unit.*
IU (for international unit)	Mistaken as I.V. (intravenous) or 10 (ten)	Write *international unit.*
Q.D., QD, q.d., qd (daily) Q.O.D., QOD, q.o.d., qod (every other day)	Mistaken for each other (the period after the *Q* may be mistaken for an *I,* and the *O* may be mistaken for an *I*)	Write *daily* and *every other day.*
Trailing zero (as in *X.0 mg*), *absence of leading zero (as in *.X mg*)	Inaccuracies with numbers or values due to missed decimal point	Write *X mg* and *0.X mg.*
MS, MSO_4, $MgSO_4$	Confused for one another (can mean morphine sulfate or magnesium sulfate)	Write *morphine sulfate* or *magnesium sulfate.*

***Exception:** A "trailing zero" may be used only where required to demonstrate the level of precision of the value being reported, such as for laboratory results, imaging studies that report size of lesions, or catheter/tube sizes. It may not be used in medication orders or other medication-related documentation.

It's extremely important to know your facility's policy on accepting and documenting verbal orders. Be aware that many facilities have started phasing out verbal orders and telephone orders because of the prevalence of computers at nurse's stations and throughout key departments on every floor, allowing medical orders to be entered and retrieved quickly from virtually any location.

Preparation errors

Sometimes the incorrect selection of a drug compound or solution strength when preparing a medication can be harmful, even fatal, to the patient. With practice, nurses can develop a sharp eye for

Additional abbreviations

These abbreviations, acronyms, and symbols may represent a risk to patient safety. They are not part of the official "Do not use" list but are reviewed annually for possible inclusion.

Do not use	Potential problem	Use instead
> (greater than) < (less than)	Misinterpreted as the number "7" (seven) or the letter "L" Confused for one another	Write *greater than.* Write *less than.*
Abbreviations for drug names	Misinterpreted due to similar abbreviations for multiple drugs	Write drug names in full.
Apothecary units	Unfamiliar to many practitioners Confused with metric units	Use metric units.
@	Mistaken for the number "2" (two)	Write *at.*
cc	Mistaken for U (units) when poorly written	Write *ml* or *milliliters.*
μg	Mistaken for mg (milligrams), resulting in one thousand-fold overdose	Write *mcg* or *micrograms.*

this type of error, as illustrated in the following situations. In both cases, the alert nurses noticed that antineoplastics prepared in the pharmacy appeared suspiciously different and took the appropriate action.

The sleuthing Holmes...

The first case involves a 6-year-old child who was to receive 12 mg of methotrexate intrathecally. The pharmacist handling the order mistakenly selected a 1-g vial of methotrexate instead of a 20-mg vial and reconstituted the drug with 10 ml of normal saline solution. The preparation containing 100 mg/ml was incorrectly labeled as containing 2 mg/ml, and 6 ml of the solution was drawn into a syringe. Although the syringe label indicated 12 mg of methotrexate, the syringe actually contained 600 mg of the drug.

The nurse who received the syringe observed that the drug's color didn't appear correct, and she returned it to the pharmacy for verification. The pharmacist retrieved the vial he had used to prepare the dose and withdrew the remaining solution into another syringe. He compared the solutions in both syringes and, noting that they matched, concluded that the color change was due to a change in the manufacturer's formula. No one noticed the vial's 1-g label.

The child received the 600-mg dose and experienced seizures 45 minutes later. A pharmacist responding to the emergency detected the error. The child received an appropriate antidote and soon recovered.

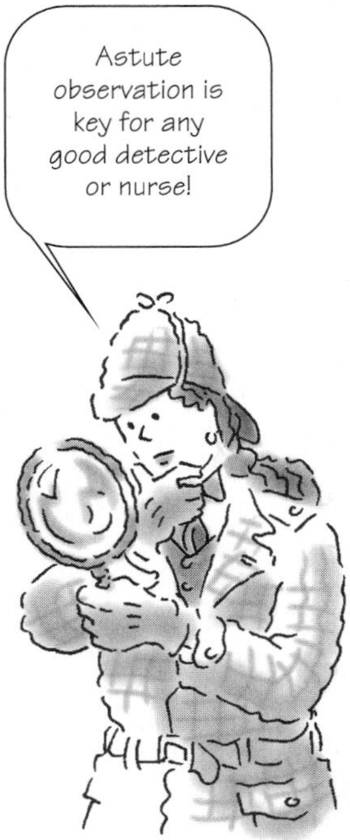

Astute observation is key for any good detective or nurse!

...and Dr. Watson

In a similar case, a 20-year-old patient with leukemia was supposed to receive mitomycin (Mitozytrex) instead of mitoxantrone (Novantrone). These drugs are both antineoplastic antibiotics; however, mitoxantrone is a dark blue liquid.

Upon receiving the medication from the pharmacy, the nurse noticed the unusual bluish tint of what was labeled mitomycin and immediately questioned the pharmacist. The pharmacist assured her that the color difference was due to a change in manufacturer, so she administered the drug. Upon further investigation, however, it was discovered that the pharmacist had mislabeled a solution of mitoxantrone as mitomycin. Fortunately, the patient suffered no harmful effects.

It's elementary!

If a familiar drug seems to have an unfamiliar appearance, investigate the cause. If the pharmacist cites a manufacturing change, ask him to double-check whether he's received verification from the manufacturer. Always document the appearance discrepancy, your actions, and the pharmacist's response in the patient record.

Reconciliation errors

Medication errors can occur when communication about medications isn't clear as patients move from one health care setting to another. Therefore, it's important to obtain, maintain, and communicate an accurate list of the patient's medications whenever new medications are ordered or medication dosages are changed.

List and compare

Whenever a patient is admitted to your facility, create a list of all his current medications. Involve the patient and his family to make sure that the list is accurate and complete. Then use this list to compare the medications he was receiving at home to those ordered in your facility, and reconcile any discrepancies.

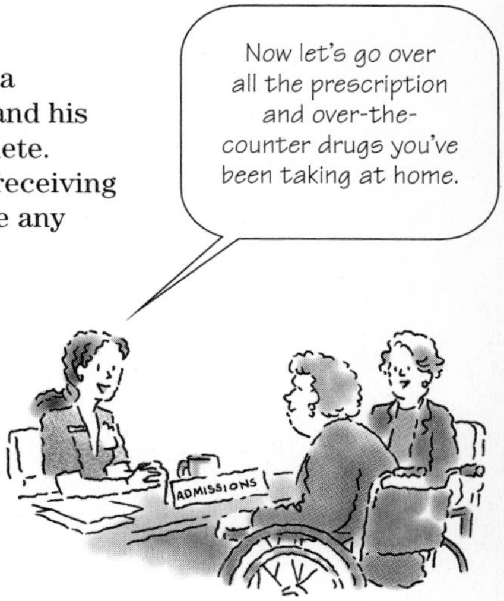

Now let's go over all the prescription and over-the-counter drugs you've been taking at home.
ADMISSIONS

The big hand-off

If the patient is transferred to other areas within your facility, communicate the current list of medications to the next care team and document that communication took place in the patient's medical record. Likewise, if the patient is transferred to another health care facility, provide a complete reconciled list to the receiving facility and document in the patient's medical record that communication took place.

Can I have that to go?

When a patient is discharged home, give the complete reconciled list of medications to the patient and his family. Take time to explain the list so they understand the medications and any possible adverse reactions. The reconciled list should also be sent to the patient's primary doctor or next known health care provider.

A day of reckoning

Here's an example of what can go wrong when a patient's medication list isn't reconciled. When a 56-year-old man was admitted to the cardiac intensive care unit with acute myocardial infarction, he was prescribed nitroglycerin, morphine, metoprolol, aspirin, oxygen, and betaxolol (to treat his glaucoma). Within 2 days, the patient's condition improved and he was transferred to the cardiac step-down unit, where his medication regimen included nitroglycerin, morphine, metoprolol, aspirin, and oxygen, as needed. The following morning, the patient asked the nurse why he hadn't received his eye drops. Had the medication list been reconciled on admission to the step-down unit, this error would have been prevented.

Stress-related errors

No one will argue that nursing is sometimes a difficult, stressful occupation, even under the best circumstances. Clearly, nurses carry a great deal of responsibility in drug administration, ensuring that the right patient gets the right drug, in the right concentration, at the right time, and by the right route.

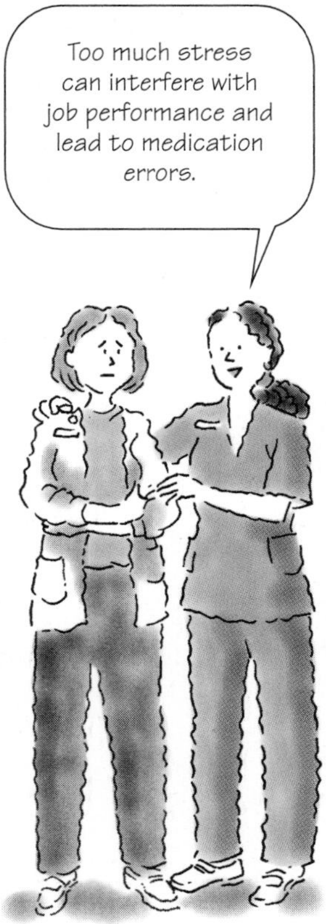

Too much stress can interfere with job performance and lead to medication errors.

Recognizing stressors

Too much stress — whether personal, job-related, or environmental — can cause or contribute to drug errors. Avoiding stress, or at least learning to recognize and minimize it, will help lower your risk of making errors and maximize the therapeutic effects of your patients' drug regimen.

Added stress from error

Committing a serious medication error can cause enormous stress that might cloud your judgment. If you're administering a medication and realize that you've made a mistake, seek help immediately instead of trying to remedy the situation yourself, as in the following situation.

A nurse-anesthetist just gave the sedative midazolam to the wrong patient. Discovering her error, she reaches for what she thinks is a vial of the antidote, flumazenil (Romazicon), then withdraws 2.5 ml of the drug and administers it to the patient. When the patient fails to respond, the nurse-anesthetist realizes that she must have inadvertently reached for a vial of ondansetron (Zofran), an antiemetic. She quickly calls for another practitioner, who assists with proper I.V. administration of flumazenil. The patient recovers unharmed.

Assuring quality and preventing errors

Each facility has its own method of tracking errors in drug administration. Unfortunately, many errors aren't documented because the administering nurses are afraid to report them or don't recognize the event as an error. What they fail to realize, however, is that tracking and documenting errors allows the performance improvement (quality assurance) team to recommend ways to prevent future episodes, thereby benefiting both nurses and patients.

Stepping up to the challenge

On a more personal level, you can take several steps to help decrease your risk of making drug errors. Perhaps the easiest way is to strictly adhere to your facility's policies, suggested safety precautions, and performance improvement recommendations.

Other measures you can take include being especially careful when transcribing orders from the doctor's order sheet to the administration record, being aware of your right to refuse administering potentially dangerous drugs, and maintaining a calm, professional demeanor.

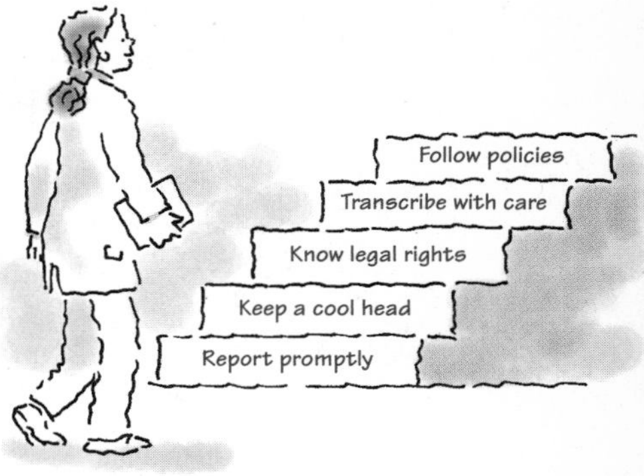
Follow policies
Transcribe with care
Know legal rights
Keep a cool head
Report promptly

Overcoming your fear

Keep in mind that, despite the best intentions and circumstances, mistakes are bound to happen. You may very well find yourself in a situation where you caused or contributed to a medication error. If this occurs, you'll need to swallow your fear and take the proper measures and report the incident promptly.

Transcribe carefully

Taking the time to carefully document drug orders is one of the easiest ways to prevent errors. To avoid transcription errors, follow these guidelines:

- Transcribe all orders from the doctor's order sheet to the administration record in a quiet area, where you can concentrate without interruption.
- Before signing the order sheet and initialing the administration record, carefully check both forms to make sure that you've copied the orders accurately.
- Follow your facility's policy for reviewing orders. Some require nurses to check all patient charts for new orders several times each shift. Others require checking all orders written within the past 24 hours. (In many cases, this responsibility falls on the night shift.)

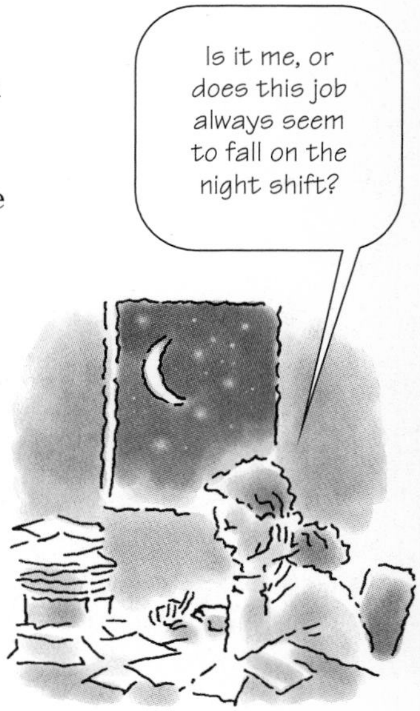
Is it me, or does this job always seem to fall on the night shift?

Know your rights

On rare occasions, you may be asked to administer a drug that you know you'd feel uncomfortable giving. Be aware that you can legally refuse to administer a drug under these circumstances:

- if you think the dosage prescribed is too high
- if you think the drug might interact dangerously with other drugs the patient is taking, including alcohol
- if you think the patient's physical condition contraindicates use of the drug.

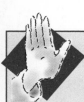

The right way to just say "No"

When you refuse to carry out a drug order, follow these steps:

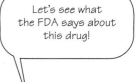

1. Notify your immediate supervisor so she can make alternative arrangements (such as assign a new nurse or clarify the order).
2. Notify the prescribing doctor if your supervisor hasn't already done so.
3. Document that the drug wasn't given and explain why (if your facility requires you to do so).

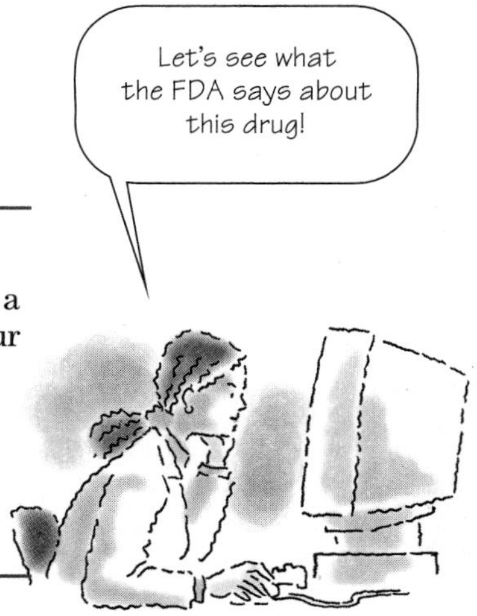

Let's see what the FDA says about this drug!

Keep a cool head

Many drug errors occur because nurses are in a hurry, are under a great deal of stress, or are unfamiliar with a drug. Try to take your time, and do what you can to avoid distractions and stress. Remember that many drugs are derivatives of other drugs, so they have similar names. If a drug is new to you, use available resources, such as drug references and online medical services, to find out all you can about it. (See *Conquering confusion.*)

Report drug errors promptly

Whenever you're involved in a drug error—regardless of whether you or someone else caused the mistake—you need to report it immediately and meticulously document what occurred.

Before you give that drug

Conquering confusion

Before giving a drug, remind yourself of these essential tactics.

Remember the six rights.
Check that you're giving the right *drug,* at the right *dose,* by the right *route,* at the right *time,* and to the right *patient* and that you include the right *documentation.*

Double-check the math.
You can never be too safe. Go over your math at least twice to make sure your calculations are correct, or have a coworker check your calculations.

Look at the label.
Examine drug labels closely—many of them look alike.

Notice the name.
Pay attention! Many drugs have similar-sounding or similar-looking names.

The right response

If you make an error, follow these steps:

1. Notify the doctor immediately.

2. Consult the pharmacist. He can provide information about drug interactions, solutions to dose-related problems (such as what to do about an overdose or an omitted dose), and an antidote (if needed).

3. Follow your facility's policy for documenting drug errors. You may have to complete an incident report for legal purposes. If so, clearly document what happened, without defending your actions or placing blame. Record the names and functions of everyone involved and what actions they took to protect the patient after the error was discovered.

4. Consider reporting the error to the United States Pharmacopeia (USP). Their Web site provides a confidential and anonymous way to report actual or potential drug errors. The USP can then use this information to help improve patient safety through the development of educational programs to prevent future errors of the same nature. (For information and a link to the reporting form, you can access the USP Web site at *www.usp.org/hqi/patientSafety/mer/*.)

Real world problem

Here's a complex scenario involving some of the medication errors discussed in this chapter. See if you can unravel what went wrong.

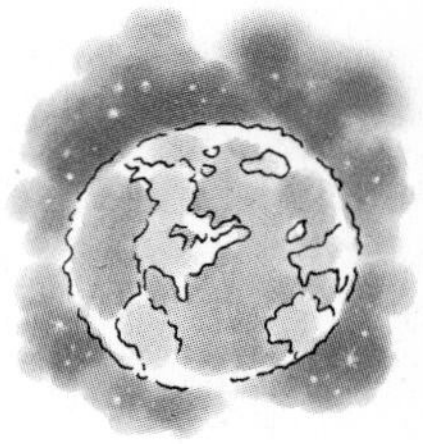

All the wrong moves

The nurse pages the doctor to ask if he'll order an antiemetic for a patient who's complaining of nausea. The doctor calls the nurse back from the hospital cafeteria, giving a verbal order for the antiemetic prochlorperazine. The nurse documents the order on a patient chart; however, it's the wrong patient's chart. She then receives a call to report to the emergency department and asks another nurse to administer the drug before leaving the unit.

The second nurse reads the chart with the order for prochlorperazine and administers the drug to the wrong patient. Fortunately, the patient was not harmed after taking the prochlorperazine; however, the patient who should have received it continued to suffer from nausea until he was administered his dose of the medication.

No hits, no runs...and how many errors?

This situation shows how carelessness and failure to follow proper procedures can lead to various errors, in this case involving two patients: one who received a drug that he shouldn't have, and one who failed to receive a drug that he needed.

Starting from the beginning of the scenario, the verbal order should never have been accepted from the doctor, because this clearly wasn't an emergency. Having the doctor write the order on the patient's chart or enter it into the computer system could have prevented the medication error.

This case also involved a transcription error; no matter how busy the nurse was, she needed to take the time to make sure that she was documenting on the correct patient's chart. It also demonstrates a compound error because of the number of practitioners involved, each of whom could have taken an extra step to reduce the likelihood of error.

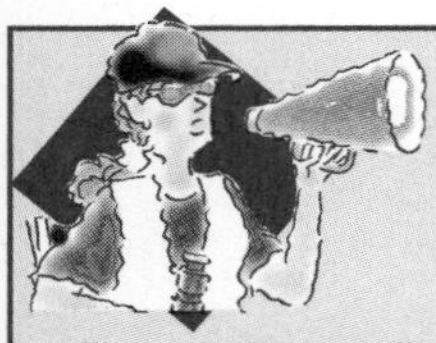

That's a wrap!

Preventing drug errors review

These bullets outline important points about preventing drug errors.

Common drug errors
- Dosage calculation errors
- Drug name errors
- Patient name errors
- Missed allergy alerts
- Compound errors
- Route errors
- Misinterpreted abbreviations
- Misinterpreted orders
- Preparation errors
- Reconciliation errors
- Stress-related errors

Avoiding transcription errors
- Transcribe orders in a quiet area.
- Carefully check your work before signing.
- Follow your facility's policy for reviewing orders.

Refusing to carry out an order
- Notify your supervisor.
- Notify the prescribing doctor.
- Document according to your facility's policy.

The six "rights" of drug administration
- Right drug
- Right dose
- Right route
- Right time
- Right patient
- Right documentation

In case of error
- Notify the doctor.
- Consult the pharmacist.
- Assess the patient throughout.
- Follow your facility's drug error documentation policy.
- If you desire, report the error on the USP Web site.

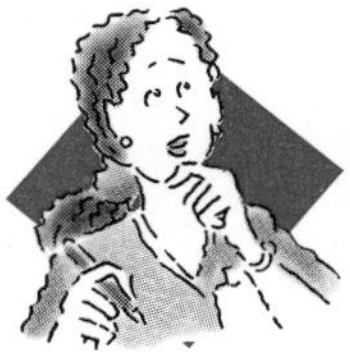

Quick quiz

1. Remembering the six rights of drug administration will help:
- A. save time.
- B. increase drug awareness.
- C. ensure compliance with the drug regimen.
- D. prevent drug errors.

Answer: D. The six rights (right drug, dose, patient, time, route, and documentation) help prevent drug errors, thereby promoting patient safety.

2. The nurse is preparing to administer a dose of chlorpropamide (Diabinese) to a patient with type 2 diabetes. She checks for allergy identification and notices that the patient is wearing an allergy alert bracelet that indicates he's allergic to sulfa drugs. Which action should the nurse take?
- A. Administer the drug as ordered.
- B. Notify the nursing supervisor immediately.
- C. Withhold administering the drug and notify the doctor.
- D. Confirm that the dosage is correct, then administer the drug.

Answer: C. Patients who are allergic to sulfa drugs shouldn't receive sulfonylurea antidiabetic drugs, such as chlorpropamide, because of the possibility of an allergic reaction. The nurse should withhold the drug and notify the doctor, who can order an alternative treatment.

3. The nurse must administer a bolus dose of dextrose 10% in water ($D_{10}W$) to a patient. Another nurse drew the solution into a syringe and left it at the patient's bedside, but forgot to label the syringe. What action should the nurse take?
- A. Administer the medication in the unlabeled syringe.
- B. Verbally confirm the contents of the syringe with the other nurse before administering it.
- C. Discard the unlabeled syringe.
- D. Call the pharmacist.

Answer: C. By discarding this unlabeled syringe, the nurse eliminates the risk of giving the wrong drug or solution to the patient. Never administer unlabeled syringes or solutions. If you do, there's no way to be certain that you're giving the right drug. Even if the other nurse confirms the syringe's contents, it's possible that the syringe became mixed up with another one at the bedside. It's best to be safe — draw up and label a new syringe with $D_{10}W$ to administer to the patient.

4. The USP is interested in nurses reporting drug errors to:
   A. prevent future errors.
   B. place blame on the nurse.
   C. use the information in future lawsuits.
   D. discredit noncompliant health care facilities.

Answer: A. Currently, it's difficult to assess fully the incidence of drug errors and how and why they occur. Many nurses fear that reporting their errors will allow them to be blamed, disciplined, or worse. However, by reporting actual or potential errors directly to the USP, which assures confidentiality and anonymity, nurses can help to identify the types and causes of errors, track their incidence, and initiate educational programs to prevent future occurrences.

Scoring

☆☆☆ If you answered all four items correctly, fantastic! You haven't misinterpreted a thing.

☆☆ If you answered three items correctly, wonderful! You're avoiding mistakes and calculating your responses well.

☆ If you answered fewer than three items correctly, keep on trying! Dwelling on your errors will only compound the problem.

Part IV Oral, topical, and rectal drugs

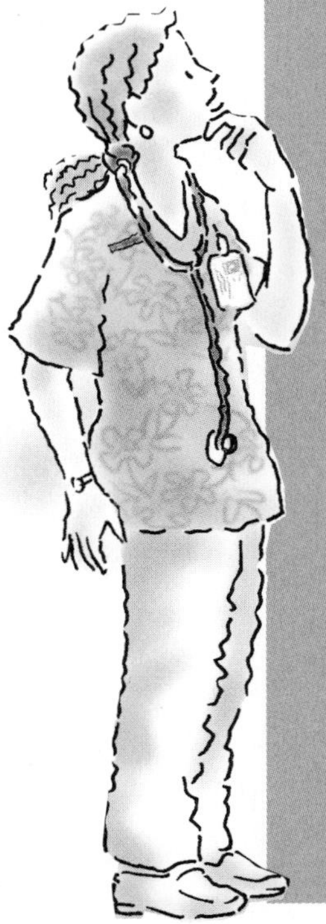

10

Calculating oral drug dosages

Just the facts

In this chapter, you'll learn:

- how to read drug labels to obtain accurate information for calculations
- how to administer drugs safely
- the correct way to calculate oral dosages of tablets, capsules, and liquids
- how to calculate dosages using different measurement systems.

A look at oral drugs

Drugs that are administered orally are usually in tablet, capsule, or liquid form. Most oral drugs are available in a limited number of strengths or concentrations. Therefore, your ability to calculate prescribed dosages for various drug forms and strengths is an important skill.

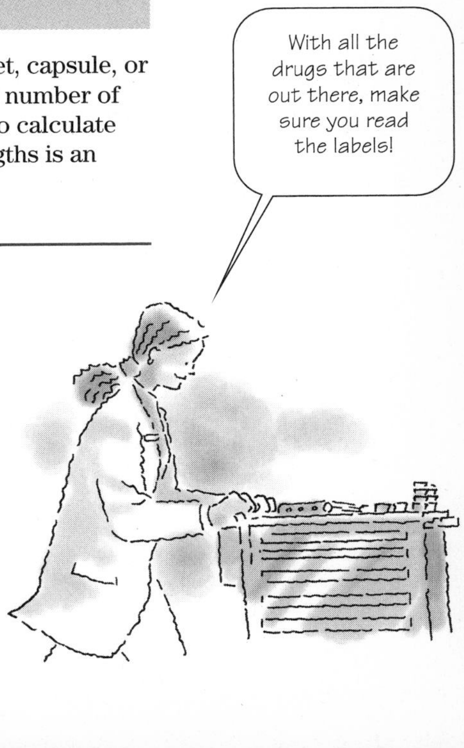

With all the drugs that are out there, make sure you read the labels!

Reading oral drug labels

Before you can administer an oral drug safely, you must make sure that it's the correct drug and the correct dosage. Your first step is to read the label carefully, noting the drug's name, dose strength, and expiration date.

Drug name

When reading a drug label, check the generic name first. If the drug has two names, the generic name typically appears in lowercase print, sometimes in

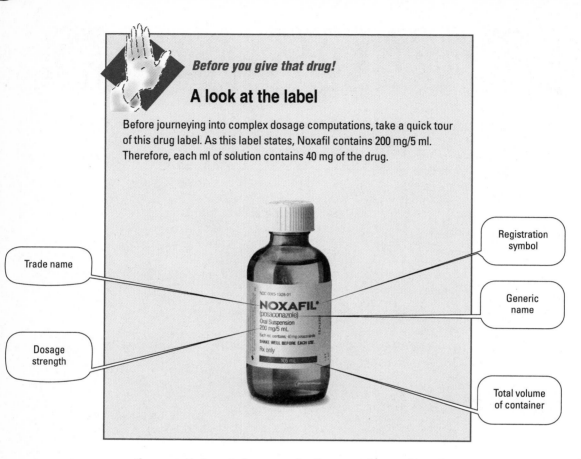

Before you give that drug!

A look at the label

Before journeying into complex dosage computations, take a quick tour of this drug label. As this label states, Noxafil contains 200 mg/5 ml. Therefore, each ml of solution contains 40 mg of the drug.

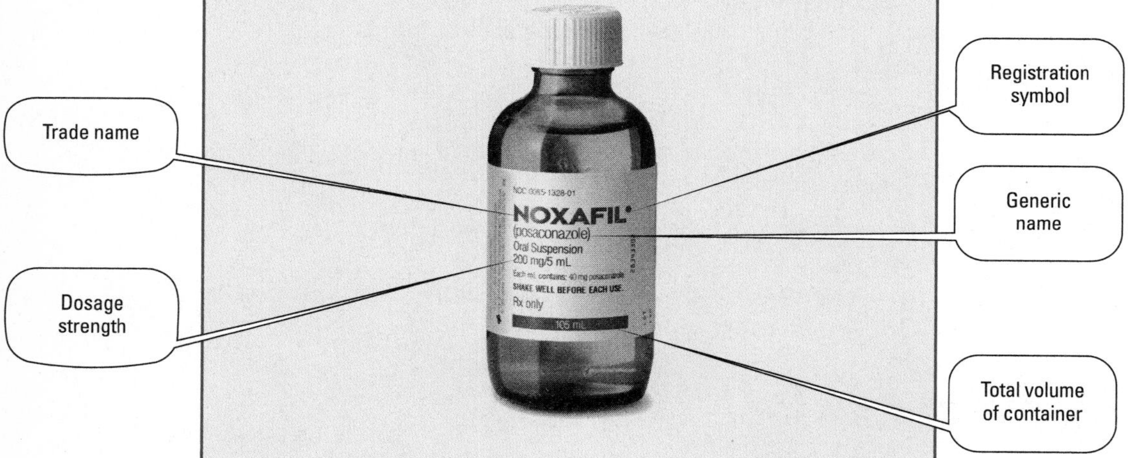

parentheses and almost always under the manufacturer's trade name. The generic name is the accepted nonproprietary name, which is a simplified form of the drug's chemical name.

Next, note the drug's trade name, also called the *brand* or *proprietary* name. This name, given by the manufacturer, typically appears prominently on the label—usually above or before the generic name with the first letter capitalized, followed by the registration symbol. (See *A look at the label.*)

Two in one

Some oral medications contain two drugs. The labels for these combination drugs list both generic names and their doses. These drugs are ordered by the trade name and the number of capsules or tablets or the volume of elixir to be given — for example, atovaquone and proguanil is ordered as *Malarone 1 adult-strength tablet P.O. daily with food.*

The name game

A drug may have several trade names, but it has only one generic name. For example, the generic drug diazepam goes by the trade names Valium and Diastat. The generic drug ibuprofen goes by the trade names Advil, Motrin, and Profen.

However, some drugs are so widely used and so well known by their generic names that the manufacturer never gives them a trade name. One example is *atropine sulfate.*

Worth a second glance

Whether a generic or trade name is used, be extra careful when reading the label to avoid errors.

Meeting the standard

The initials *U.S.P.* or *N.F.* may appear after the drug name. They stand for two legally recognized standards for drugs: *United States Pharmacopeia* and *National Formulary.* These initials mean that a drug has met standards of purity, potency, and storage, which are enforced by the Food and Drug Administration.

Dose strength

After checking the drug name, look for the dose strength on the label. Pay close attention: the labels and containers for different concentrations of the same drug may look exactly alike except for the listing of the drug's concentration. (See *Look-alike labels: Oral solutions*, page 172.)

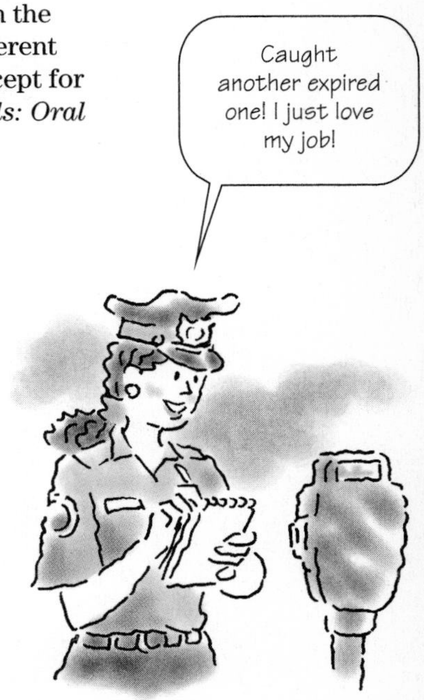

Caught another expired one! I just love my job!

Expiration date

Lastly, check the expiration date. This vital information is commonly overlooked. Expired drugs may be chemically unstable or may no longer provide the correct dose. If a drug has expired, return it to the pharmacy so that it can be disposed of properly and the patient can be reimbursed.

Before you give that drug!

Look-alike labels: Oral solutions

The simulated oral solution labels below are examples of look-alikes that you may encounter. Reading labels carefully can help you avoid medication errors.

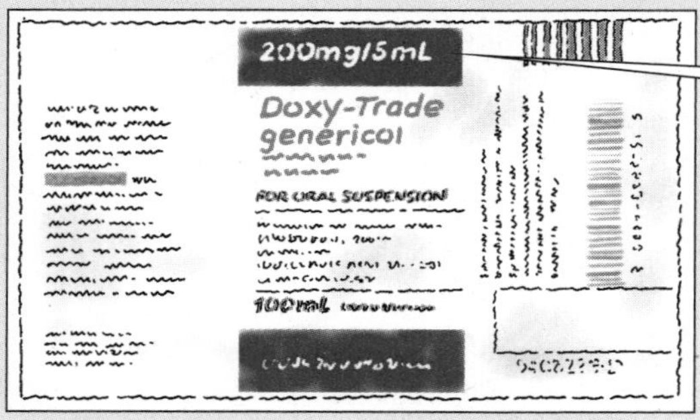

The dose strength of this drug is 200 mg/5 ml.

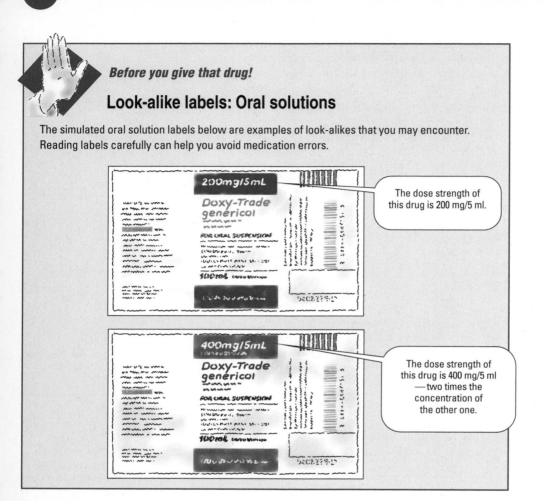

The dose strength of this drug is 400 mg/5 ml —two times the concentration of the other one.

Administering oral drugs safely

The first rule in assuring the safest possible administration of drugs is to check the "six rights" of medication administration—right drug, right route, right dose, right time, right patient, and right documentation. Another important rule is to triple-check drug labels and drug orders. Safe drug administration requires you to compare the doctor's order as transcribed on the medication administration record against the drug label three times. (See *Say it three times: Check orders and labels.*)

Before you give that drug!

Say it three times: Check orders and labels

The secret of drug safety is to check, check, and check again. Before giving a drug, carefully compare the drug's label with each part of the medication administration record, holding the label next to the administration record to ensure accuracy. The example below walks you through the steps for administering *furosemide (Lasix) 40 mg P.O.*

Check drug names.

- Read the drug's generic name on the administration record and compare it to the generic name on the label. They both should say *furosemide.*
- Read the trade name on the administration record and compare it to the trade name on the label. They both should say *Lasix.*

Check the dosage, route, and record.

- Read the dosage on the administration record and compare it to the dose on the label. They both should say *40 mg.*
- Read the route specified on the administration record and note the dose form on the label. The record should say *P.O.,* and the label should say *oral tablet.*
- Note any special considerations on the administration record, such as "known drug allergies," "aspiration precautions (head of bed elevated to 45 degrees for all P.O. intake)," "Patient is HOH (hard of hearing)," or "Patient is blind."

Check orders and labels three times.

Follow this routine three times before giving the drug. Do it the first time when you obtain the drug from the patient's supply. Do it the second time before placing the drug in the medication cup or other administration device. Lastly, do it the third time before removing the drug from the unit-dose package at the patient's bedside.

Proceed with caution

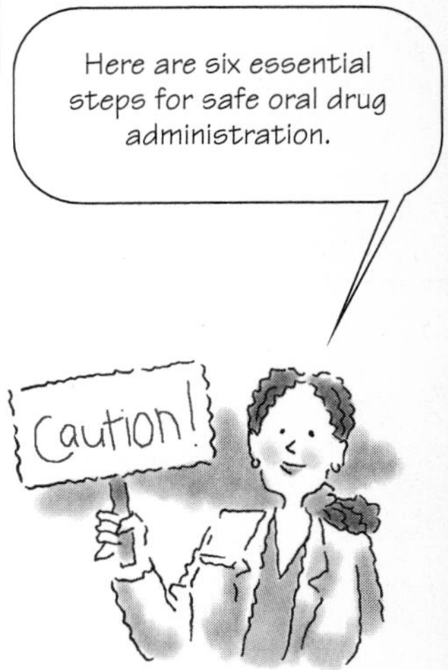

Here are six essential steps for safe oral drug administration.
Caution!

The doctor has ordered *nebivolol (Bystolic) 10 mg P.O. once daily* for your patient. Before giving the drug, follow this procedure to the letter:

1. Open the patient's medication drawer, find the drug labeled *nebivolol (Bystolic) 10 mg*, and note that it's in oral tablet form.
2. Place the labeled drug next to the transcribed order on the administration record and carefully compare each part of the label to the order.
3. If the drug is supplied in bulk, transfer one tablet from the supply to a medication container, pouring from the supply to the lid and then into the container without handling the tablet.

Unit-dose packaging

Tablets or capsules in unit doses may be dispensed on a card with the drugs sealed in bubbles or in strips with each drug separated by a tear line. Unit doses of liquids may be packaged in small sealed cups with identifying information on the cover.

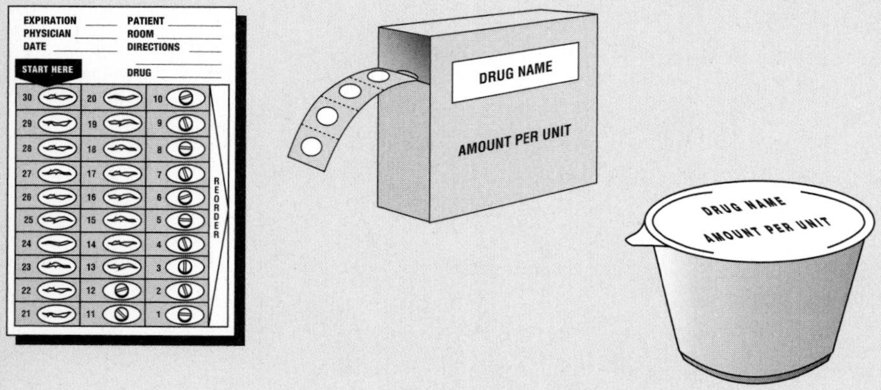

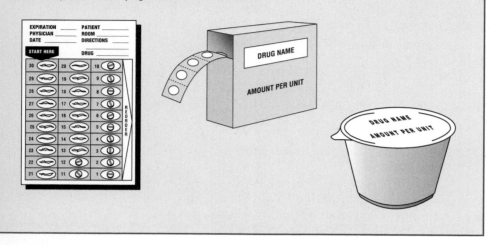

Before returning the supply to the drawer or shelf, once again compare the label to the order on the administration record, and note whether this is the right administration time. *When you've removed a drug from its container, you can't ever be certain that it's the correct drug unless you've carefully compared the label to the administration record while pouring.*

Now, go to the patient's bedside, verify the patient's identity using two patient identifiers, and do your third drug check, comparing the label to the order and checking the administration time again. Then give the drug.

If the drug comes in a unit-dose packet, don't remove it from the packet until you're at the patient's bedside and ready to administer it. Then do your third drug check. Remove the drug from the packet and give it to the patient, using the packet label for comparison when recording your administration information. (See *Unit-dose packaging.*)

Discovering discrepancies

If you notice discrepancies between the medication administration record and the drug label, check them out. For example, suppose the medication administration record specifies *Raniclor* and the drug packet is labeled *cefaclor*. Check your drug handbook and you'll find that Raniclor is a trade name for cefaclor.

Or, suppose the drug packet is labeled *Raniclor 250 mg* and the dose on the medication administration record is *500 mg*. In this case, you need to calculate the required dose. Scrupulous attention to details like these will help ensure safe, error-free drug administration.

Unit-dose systems

Many facilities use the unit-dose system, which provides prepackaged drugs in single-dose containers and decreases the need for dosage calculations. (See *Save time with the unit-dose system*.)

Calculating dosages

Despite the prevalence of unit-dose systems, calculations are still necessary in many patient situations. For example, you may have to determine individualized dosages for special patients. You also must know how to convert between measurement systems to determine how many tablets, capsules, or other dosage forms to administer. (See *Special delivery drug dosages*, page 176.)

You'll often use ratios and fractions in proportions to calculate drug dosages and to convert between measurement systems. The following section reviews these mathematical concepts and shows step-by-step calculations.

Using ratios, fractions, and proportions

Ratios and fractions are two ways to express the numerical relationship between things. A proportion expresses equality between two ratios or fractions. Proportions may be written using ratios, as in:

$$1:3::2:6$$

or using fractions, as in:

$$\frac{1}{3}=\frac{2}{6}$$

Save time with the unit-dose system

Using the unit-dose drug distribution system gives you more time for evaluating patient responses to drugs and for teaching patients about their drug regimens.

More exact (that's a fact)
This timesaving system provides the exact dose of medication needed for each patient. The pharmacist computes the number of tablets or the volume of liquid and prepares the proper dose for administration. Errors are decreased because the drug remains in its labeled container until you give it to the patient.

Don't throw away your calculator yet
Does this mean your dosage calculation days are over? Not by a long shot. Some facilities don't use the unit-dose system, and others have systems that don't operate 24 hours per day. So your dosage calculation skills are still vitally important.

When proportions are expressed using ratios, the product of the means (the inside numbers), equals the product of the extremes (the outside numbers):

means

$$2 : 4 :: 1 : 2$$

extremes

so,

$$4 \times 1 = 2 \times 2$$

When proportions are expressed as fractions, their cross products are equal:

$$\frac{3}{6} = \frac{6}{12}$$

so,

$$3 \times 12 = 6 \times 6$$

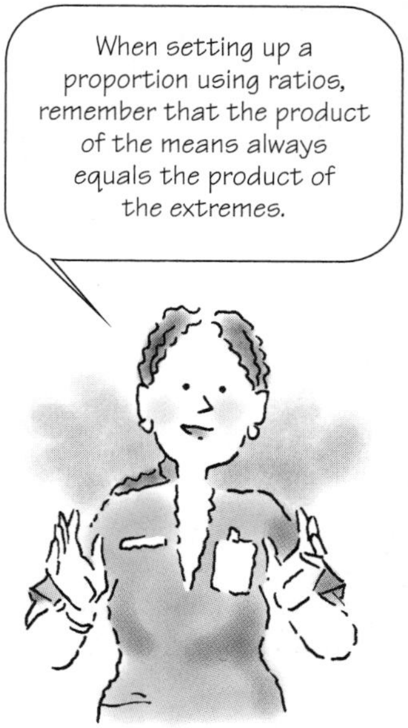

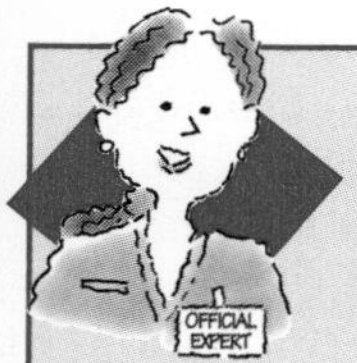

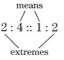

Advice from the experts

Special delivery drug dosages

Even if your facility uses the unit-dose system, you'll still need to calculate dosages for some patients. For example, patients on critical care units, pediatric patients, and geriatric patients require individualized medication dosages that may be unusually large or small.

The nearest milligram

Some patients need dosages that are calculated to the nearest milligram instead of the nearest 10 mg. For them, the correct calculation of the exact dosage can mean the difference between an underdose or overdose and the correct dose. A few examples of drugs that are measured to the nearest milligram or microgram include digoxin, levothyroxine sodium, and many pediatric drugs.

Changing the delivery route

Some people can't handle drugs that are delivered by the usual route because their ability to absorb, distribute, metabolize, or excrete drugs is impaired. Some patients can't absorb drugs from the GI tract because of upper GI disorders or surgery; deficiencies of gastric, pancreatic, or intestinal secretions; or passive congestion of GI blood vessels from severe heart failure. These patients may need drugs in parenteral form. Smaller doses of a drug can be used when the drug is given I.V. because it may be delivered to the bloodstream more efficiently and is more readily absorbed.

Don't forget these special patients

Other patients who need individualized dosages include those with conditions that cause abnormal drug distribution from the GI tract or from parenteral sites to the sites of action. Premature infants and patients with low serum protein levels or severe liver or kidney disease who can't metabolize or excrete drugs as readily as normal patients also require special drug dosages. You can help individualize drug regimens for these patients by assessing their kidney or liver function, monitoring blood levels of drugs, and calculating exact dosages.

Equally mean and extreme

When a proportion is expressed using ratios, the units of the mean on one side of the proportion must match the units of the extreme on the other side, and vice versa:

$$\text{mg} : \text{tablet} :: \text{mg} : \text{tablet}$$

When a proportion is expressed using fractions, the units of measure in the numerators must be the same, and the units of measure in the denominators must be the same:

$$\frac{\text{mg}}{\text{tablet}} = \frac{\text{mg}}{\text{tablet}}$$

Numerators are the same.

Denominators are the same.

Four rules for calculating drug dosages

To help you prevent calculation and medication errors and simplify your calculations, remember these four rules. (See *Helpful hints to minimize math mistakes.*)

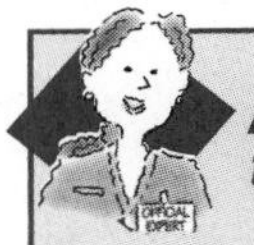

Advice from the experts

Helpful hints to minimize math mistakes

To avoid math mistakes when computing dosages, use these helpful hints:

- Write out all calculations, using the proper formula.
- Recheck your calculations with another nurse or the pharmacist.

Rule 1: Use correct units of measure

Using the incorrect unit of measure is one of the most common dosage calculation errors. When calculating doses, matching units of measure in the numerator and denominator cancel each other, leaving the correct unit of measure in the answer. Here's an example:

How many milligrams of a drug are in two tablets if one tablet contains 5 mg of the drug?

State the problem as a proportion:

$$5 \text{ mg} : 1 \text{ tablet} :: X : 2 \text{ tablets}$$

Remember that the product of the means equals the product of the extremes:

$$1 \text{ tablet} \times X = 5 \text{ mg} \times 2 \text{ tablets}$$

Multiply the means.

Multiply the extremes.

Solve for *X*. Divide each side of the equation by the known value, 1 tablet, and cancel units that appear in both the numerator and denominator:

$$\frac{\cancel{1 \text{ tablet}} \times X}{\cancel{1 \text{ tablet}}} = \frac{5 \text{ mg} \times 2 \cancel{\text{ tablets}}}{1 \cancel{\text{ tablet}}}$$

$$X = 10 \text{ mg}$$

Rule 2: Double-check decimals and zeros

An error in the number of decimal places or zeros in a dosage calculation can cause a tenfold or greater dosage error. Here's an example using decimals and zeros: The doctor orders *0.05 mg Synthroid P.O.*, but the only Synthroid on hand is in tablets that contain 0.025 mg each. How many tablets should you give?

- State the problem as a proportion:

$$0.025 \text{ mg} : 1 \text{ tablet} :: 0.05 \text{ mg} : X$$

- The product of the means equals the product of the extremes:

$$1 \text{ tablet} \times 0.05 \text{ mg} = 0.025 \text{ mg} \times X$$

- Solve for X by dividing each side of the equation by 0.025 mg and canceling units that appear in both the numerator and denominator, carefully checking decimal placement:

$$\frac{1 \text{ tablet} \times 0.05 \cancel{\text{mg}}}{0.025 \cancel{\text{mg}}} = \frac{\cancel{0.025 \text{ mg}} \times X}{\cancel{0.025 \text{ mg}}}$$

$$X = 2 \text{ tablets}$$

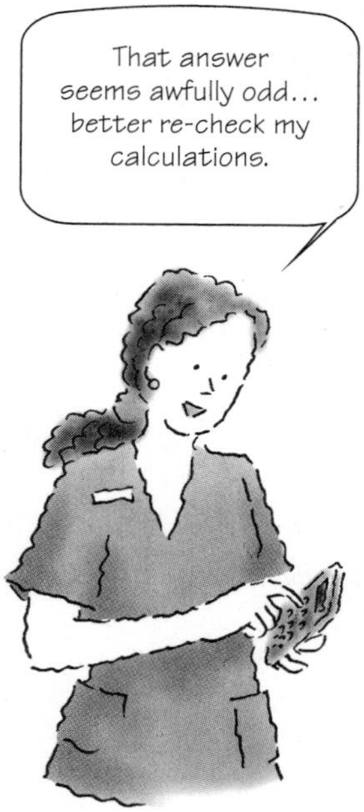

That answer seems awfully odd... better re-check my calculations.

Rule 3: Question strange answers

Be especially careful to recheck suspicious-looking calculations. For example, if a dosage calculation suggests giving 25 tablets or 200 ml of suspension, assume that you've made an error and check your figures. If you're still unsure about your results, have another nurse check your calculation.

Rule 4: Get out the calculator

A handheld calculator can improve the accuracy and speed of your calculations, *but it can't guarantee accuracy.* You still must set up proportions carefully and double-check units of measure and decimal places.

Special considerations

Occasionally when administering oral drugs, you may come across unusual situations that require you to take a few extra steps.

Divided doses

Most tablets, capsules, and similar dose forms are available in only a few strengths. Usually, you'll administer one tablet or one-half of a scored tablet.

Breaking a scored tablet in portions smaller than one-half usually creates inaccurate doses. If a dose smaller than one-half of a

Before you give that drug!

Be cautious with tablets and capsules

Before you break or crush a tablet or capsule, call the pharmacist to see if the drug is available in smaller dosage strengths or in liquid form for patients who have difficulty swallowing. Also check your drug handbook — or check with the pharmacist — to see if altering the drug will affect its action. Drugs that shouldn't be broken or crushed include:

- sustained-release drugs, also called *extended-release, timed-release,* or *controlled-release* (Suffixes such as "SR," "CR," "DUR," and "LA" in a drug name usually indicate that the drug is sustained-release.)
- capsules that contain tiny beads of medication (In some cases, you may empty the contents of these capsules into a beverage, pudding, or applesauce.)
- enteric-coated tablets, which have a hard coating (usually shiny or glossy) that's designed to protect the upper GI tract from irritation
- buccal and sublingual tablets.

Tips for crushing and breaking

If you need to crush a tablet, use a chewable form, which is softer. The easiest method is to crush the tablet while it's still in its package, using a pill crusher. Or, you can remove it from the package and crush it with a mortar and pestle.

If you need to break a tablet, use one that's scored. Carefully cut the tablet on the score line with a scalpel or pill cutter. Enlist the pharmacist's help when you need to break a tablet into smaller pieces than the score allows or when you must administer a portion of a capsule. If you need to break an unscored tablet, have the pharmacist crush, weigh, and dispense it in two equal doses.

scored tablet or any portion of an unscored tablet is needed, you should substitute a commercially available solution or suspension or have one prepared by the pharmacist.

You can also ask the pharmacist to crush the tablet and measure an exact dose. However, some oral preparations shouldn't be opened, broken, scored, or crushed because those actions change the drug's effect. (See *Be cautious with tablets and capsules.*)

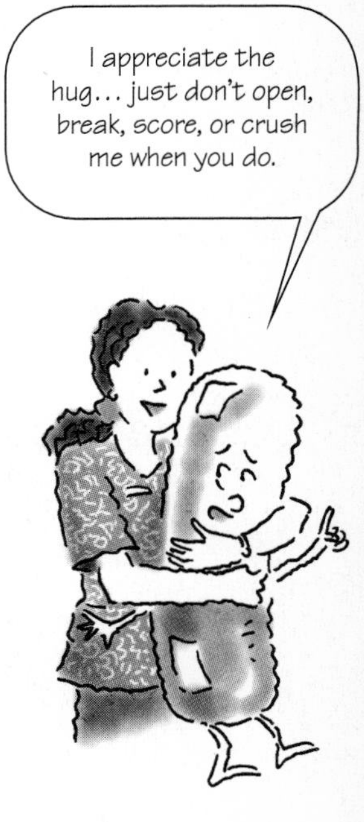

I appreciate the hug... just don't open, break, score, or crush me when you do.

All things being equianalgesic

At times, you may need to convert a dose of an analgesic from the parenteral route to the oral route. If so, equianalgesic charts provide the information you need to recalculate the dose necessary to produce the desired pain control. These charts use morphine sulfate as the gold standard for comparing pain control. (See *Equianalgesic charts: A painless path for converting dosages*, page 180.)

Equianalgesic charts: A painless path for converting dosages

When substituting one analgesic for another, equianalgesic charts provide the information you need to calculate the dose necessary to produce the desired pain control (equianalgesic effect).

These charts use morphine sulfate as the *gold standard* for comparison. On most charts, doses for many drugs are listed; each dose provides pain relief equivalent to 10 mg of I.M. morphine. Here's an example of an equianalgesic chart.

Medication	I.M. dose	P.O. dose
Morphine	10 mg	30 mg
Codeine	1.5 mg	7.5 mg
Hydromorphone	2 mg	4 mg
Levorphanol	130 mg	200 mg
Meperidine	75 mg	300 mg

Remember: Every dose on the equianalgesic chart provides an equivalent amount of pain control, and any change in medication requires a doctor's order.

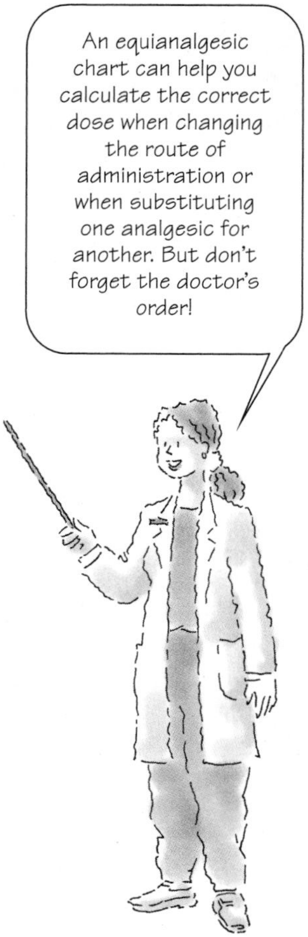
An equianalgesic chart can help you calculate the correct dose when changing the route of administration or when substituting one analgesic for another. But don't forget the doctor's order!

Real world problems

When calculating the number of tablets to administer, use proportions. Set up the first ratio or fraction with the known tablet strength. Set up the second ratio or fraction with the prescribed dose and the unknown quantity of tablets or capsules. Then solve for X to determine the correct dose. To illustrate, here are some typical patient situations.

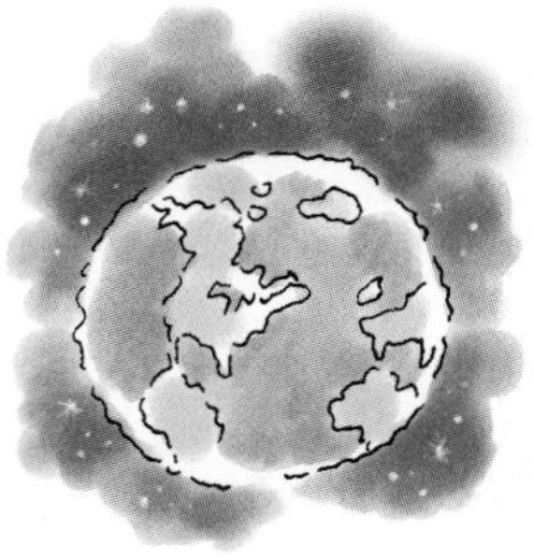

The acetaminophen answer

The doctor orders *650 mg acetaminophen P.O. STAT* for your patient, but the drug is available only in 325-mg tablets. How many tablets should you give?

Here's the calculation using ratios.

- Set up the first ratio with the known tablet strength:

$$325 \text{ mg} : 1 \text{ tablet}$$

• Set up the second ratio with the desired dose and the unknown number of tablets:

$$650 \text{ mg} : X$$

• Put these ratios into a proportion:

$$325 \text{ mg} : 1 \text{ tablet} :: 650 \text{ mg} : X$$

• Set up the equation by multiplying the means and extremes:

$$1 \text{ tablet} \times 650 \text{ mg} = 325 \text{ mg} \times X$$

• Solve for X by dividing both sides of the equation by 325 mg and canceling units that appear in both the numerator and denominator:

$$\frac{1 \text{ tablet} \times 650 \cancel{\text{mg}}}{325 \cancel{\text{mg}}} = \frac{\cancel{325 \text{ mg}} \times X}{\cancel{325 \text{ mg}}}$$

$$X = 2 \text{ tablets}$$

The clozapine clue

Your patient is prescribed *250 mg clozapine P.O. daily*. How many tablets should he take if each tablet contains 100 mg?

Here's the calculation using ratios.

• Set up the first ratio with the known tablet strength:

$$100 \text{ mg} : 1 \text{ tablet}$$

• Set up the second ratio with the desired dose and the unknown number of tablets:

$$250 \text{ mg} : X$$

• Put these ratios into a proportion:

$$100 \text{ mg} : 1 \text{ tablet} :: 250 \text{ mg} : X$$

• Multiply the means and the extremes:

$$1 \text{ tablet} \times 250 \text{ mg} = 100 \text{ mg} \times X$$

• Divide each side of the equation by 100 mg and cancel units that appear in both the numerator and denominator:

$$\frac{1 \text{ tablet} \times 250 \cancel{\text{mg}}}{100 \cancel{\text{mg}}} = \frac{\cancel{100 \text{ mg}} \times X}{\cancel{100 \text{ mg}}}$$

$$X = 2.5, \text{ or } 2\tfrac{1}{2} \text{ tablets}$$

Dosage drill

Test your math skills with this drill.

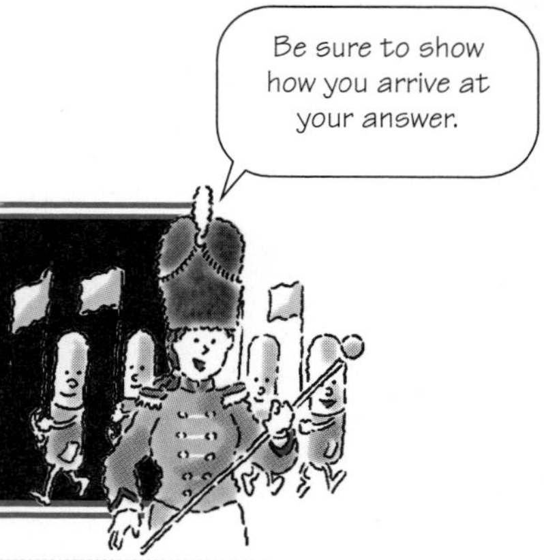
Be sure to show how you arrive at your answer.

A patient has been taking 0.5 g tablets of acetaminophen (Tylenol) P.O. for postoperative pain after an inguinal hernia repair. If the patient took a total of 1,500 mg in 72 hours, how many 0.5-g tablets were taken?

Your answer: ______________________

To find the answer, set up ratios and a proportion and solve for X.

$$1{,}000 \text{ mg} : 1 \text{ g} :: 1{,}500 \text{ mg} \times X \text{ g}$$

$$1{,}000 \text{ mg} \times X \text{ g} = 1 \text{ g} \times 1{,}500 \text{ mg}$$

$$1{,}000X = 1{,}500$$

$$X = \frac{1{,}500}{1{,}000}$$

$$X = 1.5 \text{ g}$$

$$0.5 \text{ g} : 1 \text{ tab} :: 1.5 \text{ g} : X \text{ tab}$$

$$0.5 \text{ g} \times X = 1 \times 1.5 \text{ g}$$

$$0.5X = 1.5$$

$$X = \frac{1.5}{0.5}$$

$$X = 3 \text{ tablets}$$

The patient took 3 tablets.

Gliding through glyburide

The doctor's order reads *glyburide 1.5 mg 3 tablets P.O. daily.* What's the total dose in milligrams?

Here's the solution using fractions.

- Set up the first fraction with the known tablet strength:

$$\frac{1.5 \text{ mg}}{1 \text{ tablet}}$$

- Set up the second fraction with the desired dose and the unknown number of milligrams:

$$\frac{X}{3 \text{ tablets}}$$

- Put these fractions into a proportion:

$$\frac{X}{3 \text{ tablets}} = \frac{1.5 \text{ mg}}{1 \text{ tablet}}$$

- Cross-multiply the fractions:

$$X \times 1 \text{ tablet} = 3 \text{ tablets} \times 1.5 \text{ mg}$$

- Divide both sides of the equation by 1 tablet and cancel units that appear in both the numerator and denominator:

$$\frac{X \times \cancel{1 \text{ tablet}}}{\cancel{1 \text{ tablet}}} = \frac{3 \cancel{\text{ tablets}} \times 1.5 \text{ mg}}{1 \cancel{\text{ tablet}}}$$

$$X = 4.5 \text{ mg}$$

Calculating liquid dosages

In addition to administering tablets to your patients, you'll also give them liquid medications in suspension or elixir form. Before calculating a dosage, read the label carefully to identify the dose strength in a specified amount of solution. Then check the label for the expiration date.

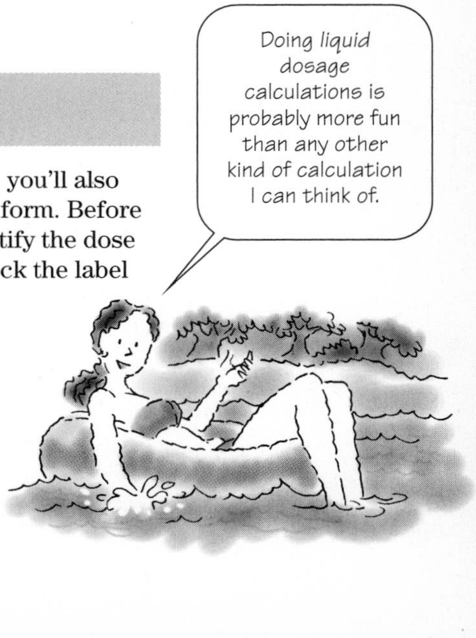
Doing liquid dosage calculations is probably more fun than any other kind of calculation I can think of.

More real world problems

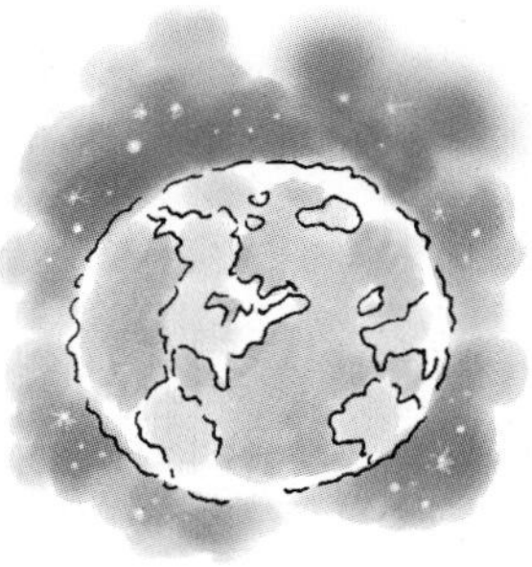

In each of the following problems, use the proportion method to calculate the amount of solution. Set up the first ratio or fraction with the known solution strength, and set up the second ratio or fraction with the desired dose and the unknown quantity. Then solve for *X* to find the correct dose.

Here are some typical patient situations.

Pay attention to the suspension

Your patient is receiving 500 mg of cefaclor oral suspension. The label reads *cefaclor 250 mg/5 ml*, and the bottle contains 100 ml. How many milliliters of cefaclor should you give?

Here's the solution using fractions.

- Set up the first fraction with the known solution strength:

$$\frac{5 \text{ ml}}{250 \text{ mg}}$$

- Set up the second fraction with the desired dose and the unknown number of milliliters:

$$\frac{X}{500 \text{ mg}}$$

- Put these fractions into a proportion:

$$\frac{X}{500 \text{ mg}} = \frac{5 \text{ ml}}{250 \text{ mg}}$$

- Cross-multiply the fractions:

$$X \times 250 \text{ mg} = 5 \text{ ml} \times 500 \text{ mg}$$

- Solve for *X* by dividing both sides of the equation by 250 mg and canceling units that appear in both the numerator and denominator:

$$\frac{X \times \cancel{250 \text{ mg}}}{\cancel{250 \text{ mg}}} = \frac{5 \text{ ml} \times 500 \cancel{\text{ mg}}}{250 \cancel{\text{ mg}}}$$

$$X = \frac{2{,}500 \text{ ml}}{250}$$

$$X = 10 \text{ ml}$$

Dosage drill

Test your math skills with this drill.

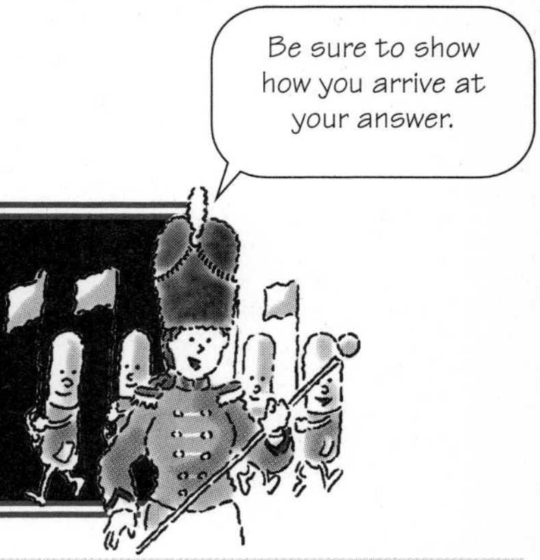
Be sure to show how you arrive at your answer.

The doctor orders 0.125 mg of digoxin (Lanoxin) elixir for a patient developing heart failure and pulmonary edema. The bottle is labeled 0.05 mg/ml. How many milliliters should the nurse administer?

Your answer: ____________________

To find the answer, set up ratios and a proportion and solve for *X*.

$$0.05 \text{ mg} : 1 \text{ ml} :: 0.125 \text{ mg} : X \text{ ml}$$

$$0.05 \text{ mg} \times X \text{ ml} = 0.125 \text{ mg} \times 1 \text{ ml}$$

$$\frac{\cancel{0.05 \text{ mg}} \times X \text{ ml}}{\cancel{0.05 \text{ mg}}} = \frac{0.125 \cancel{\text{mg}} \times 1 \text{ ml}}{0.05 \cancel{\text{mg}}}$$

$$X = \frac{0.125}{0.05}$$

$$X = 2.5 \text{ ml}$$

The nurse should administer 2.5 ml.

Erythromycin enigma

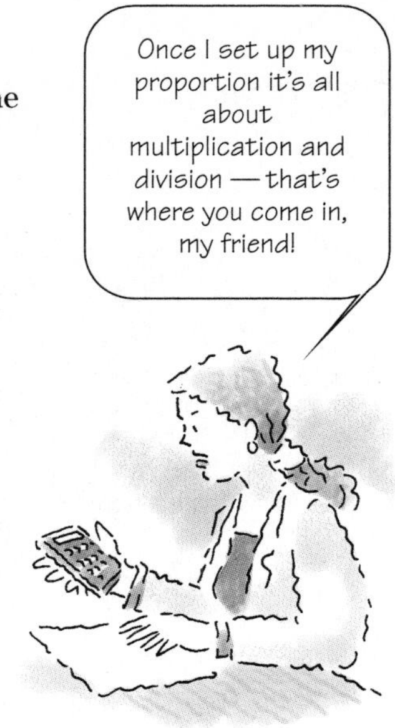

Once I set up my proportion it's all about multiplication and division — that's where you come in, my friend!

Your patient needs 400 mg of erythromycin oral suspension. The label reads *erythromycin 200 mg/5 ml.* How many milliliters should you give?

Here's the calculation using ratios.

- Set up the first ratio with the known solution strength:

$$5 \text{ ml} : 200 \text{ mg}$$

- Set up the second ratio with the unknown number of milliliters and the desired dose:

$$X : 400 \text{ mg}$$

- Put these ratios into a proportion:

$$5 \text{ ml} : 200 \text{ mg} :: X : 400 \text{ mg}$$

- Set up an equation by multiplying the means and extremes:

$$X \times 200 \text{ mg} = 5 \text{ ml} \times 400 \text{ mg}$$

- Solve for X by dividing both sides of the equation by 200 mg and canceling units that appear in both the numerator and denominator:

$$\frac{X \times \cancel{200 \text{ mg}}}{\cancel{200 \text{ mg}}} = \frac{5 \text{ ml} \times 400 \cancel{\text{mg}}}{200 \cancel{\text{mg}}}$$

$$X = \frac{2{,}000 \text{ ml}}{200}$$

$$X = 10 \text{ ml}$$

Don't dally over Dilantin doses

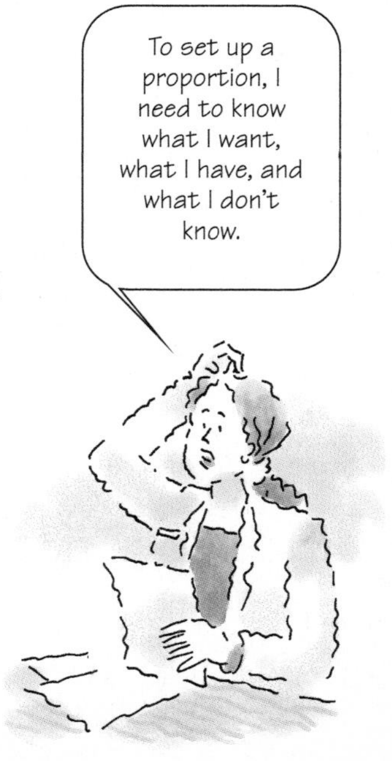

To set up a proportion, I need to know what I want, what I have, and what I don't know.

The doctor orders *100 mg Dilantin oral suspension t.i.d.* for your patient. The label reads *Dilantin 125 mg/5 ml.* How many milliliters should you give?

Here's the calculation using ratios.

- Set up the first fraction with the known solution strength:

$$5 \text{ ml} : 125 \text{ mg}$$

- Set up the second fraction with the unknown number of milliliters and the desired dose:

$$X : 100 \text{ mg}$$

- Put these ratios into a proportion:

$$X : 100 \text{ mg} :: 5 \text{ ml} : 125 \text{ mg}$$

Dosage drill

Test your math skills with this drill.

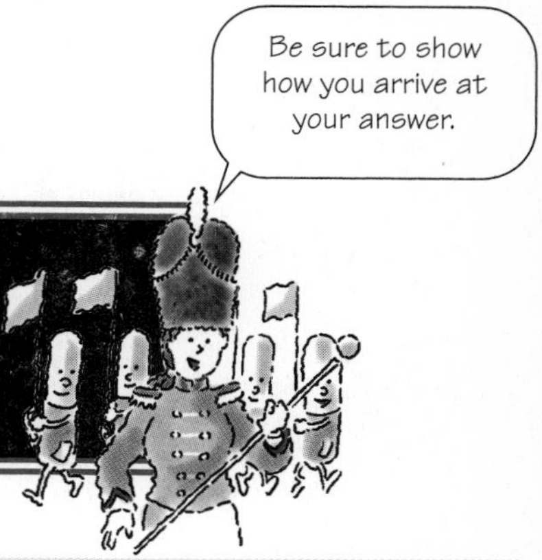
Be sure to show how you arrive at your answer.

A doctor orders 25 g of lactulose (Cephulac) for a patient entering a prehepatic coma. The bottle is labeled 10 g/15 ml. How many milliliters should the patient receive?

Your answer: ____________________

To find the answer, set up ratios and a proportion and solve for *X*.

$$10 \text{ g} : 15 \text{ ml} :: 25 \text{ g} : X \text{ ml}$$

$$10 \text{ g} \times X \text{ ml} = 15 \text{ ml} \times 25 \text{ g}$$

$$10X = 375$$

$$X = \frac{375}{10}$$

$$X = 37.5 \text{ ml}$$

The patient should receive 37.5 ml of the drug.

- Set up an equation by multiplying the means and extremes:

$$100 \text{ mg} \times 5 \text{ ml} = 125 \text{ mg} \times X$$

- Solve for X by dividing each side of the equation by 125 mg and canceling units that appear in both the numerator and denominator:

$$\frac{100 \cancel{\text{mg}} \times 5 \text{ ml}}{125 \cancel{\text{mg}}} = \frac{\cancel{125 \text{ mg}} \times X}{\cancel{125 \text{ mg}}}$$

$$\frac{500 \text{ ml}}{125} = X$$

$$X = 4 \text{ ml}$$

Diluting powders

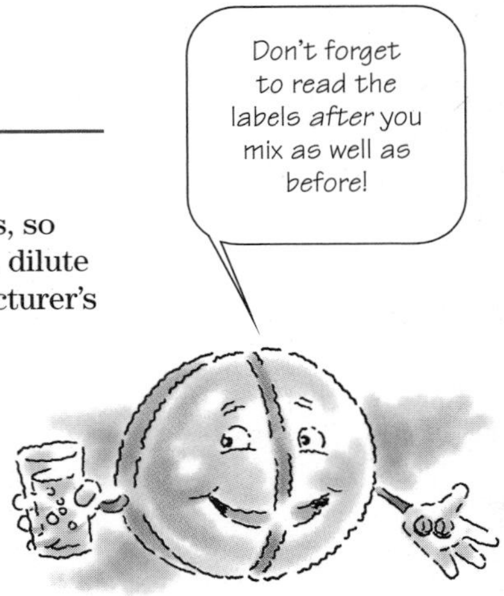

Don't forget to read the labels *after* you mix as well as before!

Some drugs become unstable when they're stored as liquids, so they're supplied in powder form. Before giving these drugs, dilute them with the appropriate diluent, according to the manufacturer's directions. Read the drug labels carefully to see how much diluent to add.

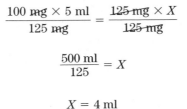

After adding the diluent and mixing thoroughly, read the labels again to determine the dose strengths contained in the volumes of fluid. To calculate the dosages, use the ratio or fraction and proportion method.

Weighing in

The dose concentration in oral solutions is expressed as the weight—or dose strength—of the drug contained in a volume of solution. For example, Lasix oral solution is provided as 10 mg/ml. So the solution contains 10 mg of Lasix (drug weight) in 1 ml (solution volume).

Measuring oral solutions

To administer an oral solution accurately, measure it with a medicine cup, dropper, or syringe.

Good to the last drop

Medicine cups are calibrated to measure solutions in milliliters, tablespoons, teaspoons, drams, and ounces. For accuracy, hold the cup at eye level while pouring the solution. Also, hold the solution container with the medication label turned toward the palm of your hand so that solution doesn't drip over the label when poured.

For good measure

Drugs that are prescribed in drops are usually packaged with a dropper. If they aren't, use a standard dropper. They can be used to measure solutions in milliliters or teaspoons. After measuring and administering a drug from a multiple-dose container, store it as directed on the drug label.

Syringe cringe

Syringes are handy for drawing up and measuring solutions accurately. However, never use a syringe to administer an oral drug. If you leave the plastic tip on by mistake, the patient can swallow or aspirate it.

Two-step dosage calculations

Most dosage calculations require more than one equation. For example, the doctor may order a drug in grains, but it may be available only in tablet, capsule, or liquid form in milligrams. When this happens, you need to convert from one measurement system to another before determining how much medication to administer. (See *When you need a new measure.*)

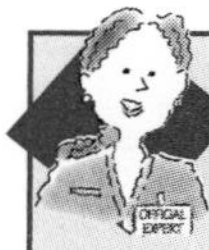

Advice from the experts

When you need a new measure

To easily determine a dose when you must first convert to a different measurement system, remember these tips:

- Read the drug order thoroughly, paying close attention to decimal places and zeros.
- Convert the dose from the system in which it's ordered to the system in which it's available.
- Calculate the number of capsules or tablets or the amount of solution needed to obtain the desired dose.

Keeping in step

When converting between measurement systems, first consult a conversion table to find the standard equivalent value — the equivalent between the two measurement systems. Then use the ratio and proportion or fraction method to calculate the correct dose. Put the standard equivalent values in the first ratio or fraction, and put the quantity ordered and the unknown quantity in the second ratio or fraction.

Still more real world problems

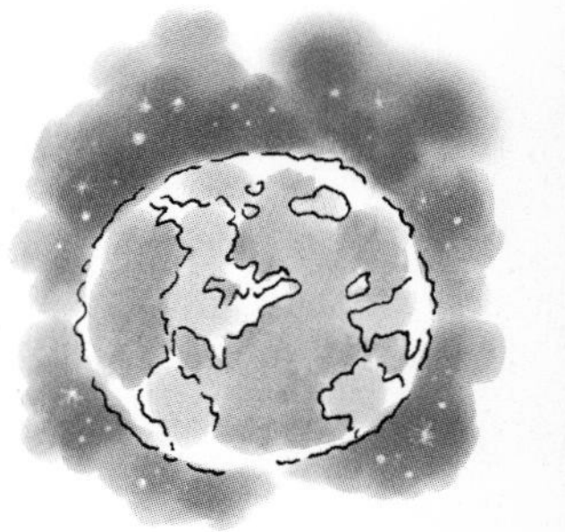

The following examples show how to convert from one measurement system to another and then how to calculate the correct dose.

Wary of apothecaries' units?

Your patient's order, written in apothecaries' units, reads *aspirin gr x P.O. daily,* but the unit-dose package says *aspirin 325 mg.* How many tablets should you administer daily?

Here's how to solve this problem using fractions.

- Recall that in apothecaries' units, "aspirin gr x" indicates 10 gr of aspirin. Refer to *Measure for measure,* page 109, to find that

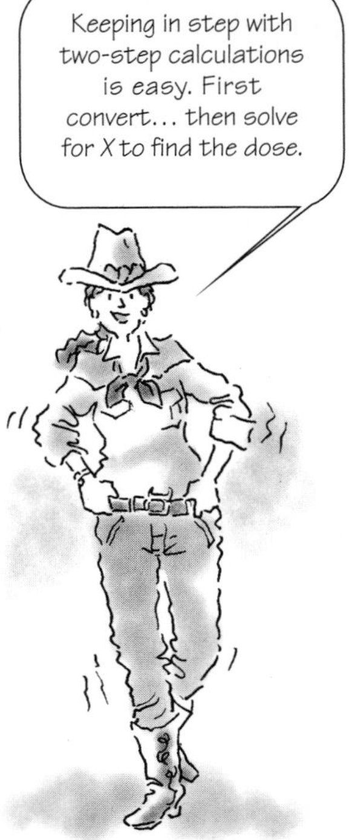

Keeping in step with two-step calculations is easy. First convert… then solve for X to find the dose.

1 gr is equivalent to approximately 60 mg. Then set up the first fraction with the standard equivalent values:

$$\frac{60 \text{ mg}}{1 \text{ grain}}$$

- Set up the second fraction with the unknown quantity in the appropriate position:

$$\frac{X}{10 \text{ grains}}$$

- Put these fractions into a proportion:

$$\frac{60 \text{ mg}}{1 \text{ grain}} = \frac{X}{10 \text{ grains}}$$

- Cross-multiply the fractions to set up an equation:

$$60 \text{ mg} \times 10 \text{ grains} = X \times 1 \text{ grain}$$

- Solve for X by dividing both sides of the equation by 1 gr and canceling units that appear in the numerator and denominator:

$$\frac{60 \text{ mg} \times 10 \cancel{\text{grains}}}{1 \cancel{\text{grain}}} = \frac{X \times \cancel{1 \text{ grain}}}{\cancel{1 \text{ grain}}}$$

$$X = 600 \text{ mg}$$

- The dose to be given is 600 mg. Now determine the number of tablets to give by setting up a proportion:

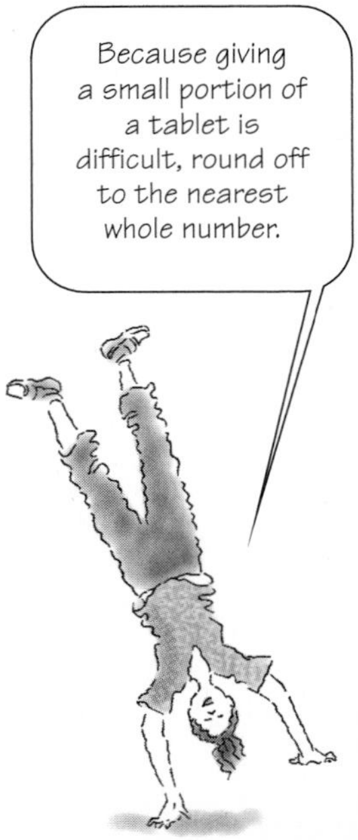

Because giving a small portion of a tablet is difficult, round off to the nearest whole number.

$$\frac{X}{600 \text{ mg}} = \frac{1 \text{ tablet}}{325 \text{ mg}}$$

- Cross-multiply the fractions:

$$X \times 325 \text{ mg} = 1 \text{ tablet} \times 600 \text{ mg}$$

- Solve for X by dividing each side of the equation by 325 mg and canceling units that appear in both the numerator and denominator:

$$\frac{X \times \cancel{325 \text{ mg}}}{\cancel{325 \text{ mg}}} = \frac{1 \text{ tablet} \times 600 \cancel{\text{mg}}}{325 \cancel{\text{mg}}}$$

$$X = \frac{600 \text{ tablets}}{325}$$

$$X = 1\tfrac{4}{5} \text{ tablets}$$

- Because giving $1\frac{4}{5}$ tablets would be very difficult, round off the dose to 2 tablets.

Pondering a prescription

A prescription reads *phenobarbital gr ¼ take gr ½ t.i.d. P.O. daily*. How many milligrams of phenobarbital should this patient receive?

Here's how to solve this problem using fractions.

- Convert "gr ¼" to milligrams by consulting a conversion table such as that in *Measure for measure*, page 109. You'll see that 1 gr equals approximately 60 mg.
- Set up the first fraction with the standard equivalent values:

$$\frac{60 \text{ mg}}{1 \text{ grain}}$$

- Set up the second fraction with the unknown quantity in the appropriate position:

$$\frac{X}{\text{grain } \frac{1}{4}}$$

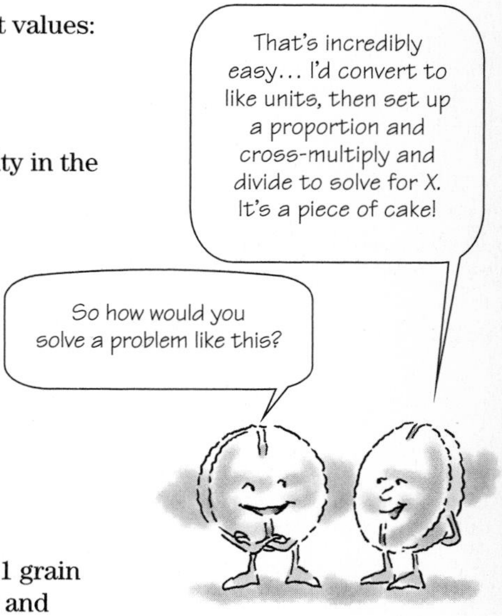

So how would you solve a problem like this?
That's incredibly easy... I'd convert to like units, then set up a proportion and cross-multiply and divide to solve for X. It's a piece of cake!

- Put these fractions into an equation:

$$\frac{60 \text{ mg}}{1 \text{ grain}} = \frac{X}{\text{grain } \frac{1}{4}}$$

- Cross-multiply the fractions:

$$60 \text{ mg} \times \text{grain } \tfrac{1}{4} = X \times 1 \text{ grain}$$

- Solve for X by dividing each side of the equation by 1 grain and canceling units that appear in both the numerator and denominator:

$$\frac{X \times \cancel{1 \text{ grain}}}{\cancel{1 \text{ grain}}} = \frac{60 \text{ mg} \times \cancel{\text{grain}} \tfrac{1}{4}}{1 \cancel{\text{grain}}}$$

$$X = 60 \text{ mg} \times \tfrac{1}{4}$$

$$X = 15 \text{ mg}$$

- Now we know that grain ¼ equals 15 mg. However, the prescribed dose is grain ½. Calculate the number of milligrams to give the patient by setting up a proportion:

$$\frac{X}{\text{grain } \frac{1}{2}} = \frac{15 \text{ mg}}{\text{grain } \frac{1}{4}}$$

- Cross-multiply the fractions:

$$X \times \text{grain } \tfrac{1}{4} = 15 \text{ mg} \times \text{grain } \tfrac{1}{2}$$

• Solve for X by dividing both sides of the equation by grain ¼ and canceling units that appear in both the numerator and denominator:

$$\frac{X \times \cancel{\text{grain } 1/4}}{\cancel{\text{grain } 1/4}} = \frac{15 \text{ mg} \times \cancel{\text{grain}}\ 1/2}{\cancel{\text{grain}}\ 1/4}$$

$$X = \frac{15 \text{ mg} \times 1/2}{1/4}$$

$$X = \frac{7\,1/2 \text{ mg}}{1/4}$$

$$X = 30 \text{ mg}$$

The dose to be given is 30 mg.

Digoxin dilemma

Your patient receives a prescription for *62.5 mcg of digoxin elixir P.O. daily.* The elixir label reads *0.05 mg/ml.* How many milliliters of digoxin should you give?

Here's how to solve this problem using ratios.

• Convert micrograms to milligrams. Recall that 1,000 mcg equals 1 mg.

• Set up the first ratio with the standard equivalent value:

$$1 \text{ mg} : 1{,}000 \text{ mcg}$$

• Set up the second ratio with the unknown quantity in the appropriate position:

$$X : 62.5 \text{ mcg}$$

• Put these ratios into a proportion:

$$1 \text{ mg} : 1{,}000 \text{ mcg} :: X : 62.5 \text{ mcg}$$

• Multiply the means and the extremes:

$$X \times 1{,}000 \text{ mcg} = 1 \text{ mg} \times 62.5 \text{ mcg}$$

• Solve for X by dividing both sides of the equation by 1,000 mcg and canceling units that appear in both the numerator and denominator:

$$\frac{X \times \cancel{1{,}000 \text{ mcg}}}{\cancel{1{,}000 \text{ mcg}}} = \frac{1 \text{ mg} \times 62.5\ \cancel{\text{mcg}}}{1{,}000\ \cancel{\text{mcg}}}$$

$$X = \frac{62.5 \text{ mg}}{1{,}000}$$

$$X = 0.0625 \text{ mg}$$

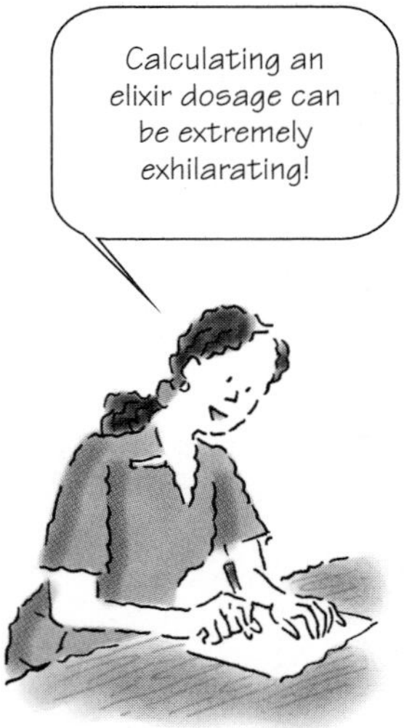

Calculating an elixir dosage can be extremely exhilarating!

Dosage drill

Test your math skills with this drill.

Be sure to show how you arrive at your answer.

A patient is to receive 0.25 mg of Synthroid. The medication is only available in tablets that contain 125 mcg each. How many tablets should the nurse administer?

Your answer: ______________________

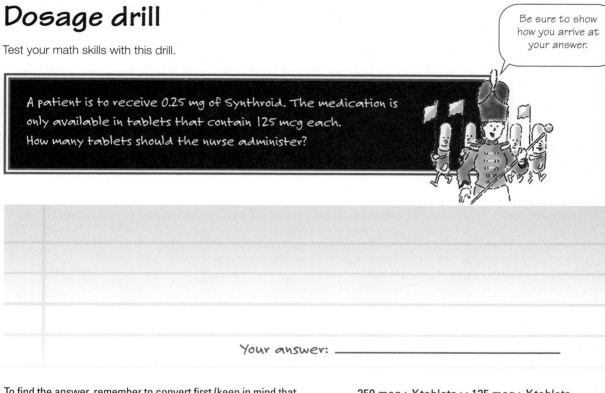

To find the answer, remember to convert first (keep in mind that 1 mg equals 1,000 mcg). Then use ratios and a proportion to solve for *X*.

$$1 \text{ mg} : 1{,}000 \text{ mcg} :: 0.25 \text{ mg} : X \text{ mcg}$$

$$1 \text{ mg} \times X \text{ mcg} = 1{,}000 \text{ mcg} \times 0.25 \text{ mg}$$

$$X = 250 \text{ mcg}$$

$$250 \text{ mcg} : X \text{ tablets} :: 125 \text{ mcg} : X \text{ tablets}$$

$$250 = 125X$$

$$X = \frac{250}{125}$$

$$X = 2 \text{ tablets}$$

The nurse should administer 2 tablets.

• The prescribed dose is 62.5 mcg, or 0.0625 mg. Calculate the number of milliliters to be given by setting up a proportion:

$$0.0625 \text{ mg} : X :: 0.05 \text{ mg} : 1 \text{ ml}$$

• Set up an equation by multiplying the means and extremes:

$$X \times 0.05 \text{ mg} = 1 \text{ ml} \times 0.0625 \text{ mg}$$

• Solve for X by dividing each side of the equation by 0.05 mg and canceling units that appear in both the numerator and denominator:

$$\frac{X \times \cancel{0.05 \text{ mg}}}{\cancel{0.05 \text{ mg}}} = \frac{1 \text{ ml} \times 0.0625 \cancel{\text{mg}}}{0.05 \cancel{\text{mg}}}$$

$$X = 1.25 \text{ ml}$$

The dose to be given is 1.25 ml.

The desired-over-have method

The desired-over-have method is another way to solve two-step problems. This method uses fractions to express the known and unknown quantities in proportions:

$$\frac{\text{amount desired}}{\text{amount you have}} = \frac{\text{equivalent amount desired}}{\text{equivalent amount you have}}$$

Make sure the units of measure used in the numerator and denominator of the first fraction correspond to the units of measure in the numerator and denominator of the second fraction.

The following three problems show how to use the desired-over-have method.

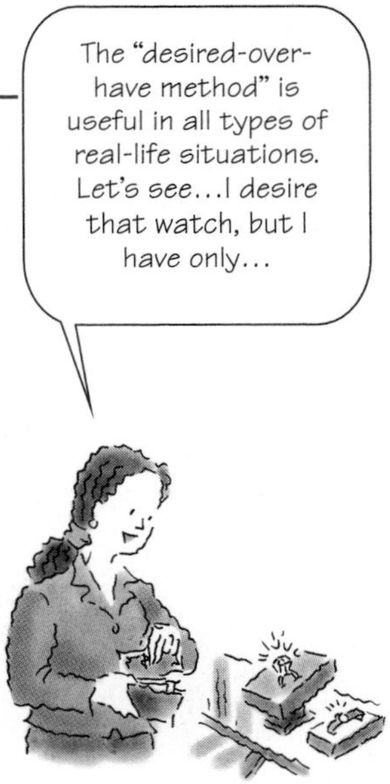

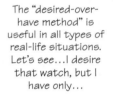

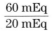

The potassium chloride puzzler

The doctor orders *60 mEq potassium chloride liquid* as a one-time dose, but the only solution on hand contains 20 mEq/15 ml. How many tablespoons should you give the patient?

Here's the calculation.

• Convert milliliters to tablespoons by consulting a conversion table such as that in *Measure for measure*, page 109. You'll see that 15 ml equals 1 tbs. Therefore, 20 mEq of the solution on hand equals 1 tbs.

• Set up the first fraction with the amount desired over the amount you have:

$$\frac{60 \text{ mEq}}{20 \text{ mEq}}$$

• Set up the second fraction with the unknown amount desired — represented by X — in the appropriate position:

$$\frac{X}{1 \text{ tbs}}$$

• Put these fractions into a proportion:

$$\frac{X \text{ desired}}{1 \text{ tbs have}} = \frac{60 \text{ mEq desired}}{20 \text{ mEq have}}$$

• Cross-multiply the fractions:

$$X \times 20 \text{ mEq} = 1 \text{ tbs} \times 60 \text{ mEq}$$

• Solve for X by dividing each side of the equation by 20 mEq and canceling units that appear in both the numerator and denominator:

$$\frac{X \times \cancel{20 \text{ mEq}}}{\cancel{20 \text{ mEq}}} = \frac{1 \text{ tbs} \times 60 \cancel{\text{ mEq}}}{20 \cancel{\text{ mEq}}}$$

$$X = 3 \text{ tbs}$$

The patient should receive 3 tbs of potassium chloride liquid.

Acetaminophen alley

The order reads *acetaminophen elixir 650 mg P.O. STAT.* The pharmacy sends you Tylenol 325 mg/5 ml. How many teaspoons do you give?

Here's the calculation.

• Convert milliliters to teaspoons by consulting a conversion table such as that in *Measure for measure*, page 109. You'll see that 1 tsp equals 5 ml.

• Set up the first fraction with the amount desired over the amount you have:

$$\frac{650 \text{ mg}}{325 \text{ mg}}$$

• Set up the second fraction with the unknown amount desired in the appropriate position:

$$\frac{X}{1 \text{ tsp}}$$

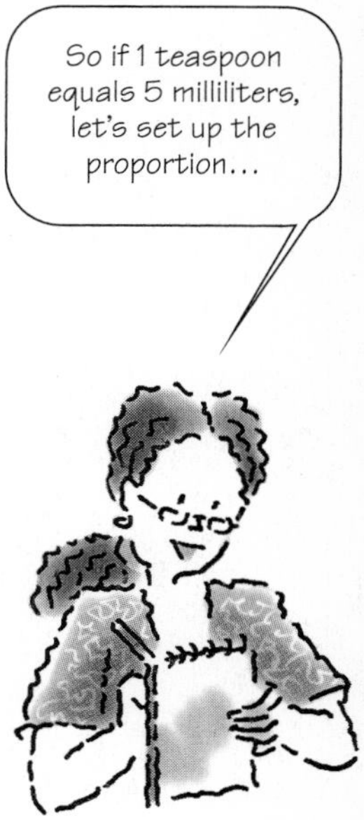

So if 1 teaspoon equals 5 milliliters, let's set up the proportion...

- Put these fractions into a proportion:

$$\frac{X \text{ desired}}{1 \text{ tsp have}} = \frac{650 \text{ mg desired}}{325 \text{ mg have}}$$

- Cross-multiply the fractions:

$$X \times 325 \text{ mg} = 1 \text{ tsp} \times 650 \text{ mg}$$

- Solve for X by dividing both sides of the equation by 325 mg and canceling units that appear in both the numerator and denominator:

$$\frac{X \times \cancel{325 \text{ mg}}}{\cancel{325 \text{ mg}}} = \frac{1 \text{ tsp} \times 650 \cancel{\text{mg}}}{325 \cancel{\text{mg}}}$$

$$X = 2 \text{ tsp}$$

The patient should receive 2 tsp of acetaminophen elixir.

Teaspoon teaser

The doctor orders *60 mg phenobarbital elixir at bedtime daily* for your patient, but the drug is available only as 20 mg/5 ml. How many teaspoons should you give?

Here's the calculation.

- Convert milliliters to teaspoons by consulting a conversion chart. You'll see that 1 tsp equals 5 ml.
- Set up the first fraction with the amount desired over the amount you have:

$$\frac{60 \text{ mg}}{20 \text{ mg}}$$

- Set up the second fraction with the unknown amount desired in the appropriate position:

$$\frac{X}{1 \text{ tsp}}$$

- Put these fractions into a proportion:

$$\frac{60 \text{ mg}}{20 \text{ mg}} = \frac{X}{1 \text{ tsp}}$$

- Cross-multiply the fractions:

$$60 \text{ mg} \times 1 \text{ tsp} = 20 \text{ mg} \times X$$

- Solve for X by dividing both sides of the equation by 20 mg and canceling units that appear in both the numerator and denominator:

$$\frac{60\ \cancel{\text{mg}} \times 1\ \text{tsp}}{20\ \cancel{\text{mg}}} = \frac{\cancel{20\ \text{mg}} \times X}{\cancel{20\ \text{mg}}}$$

$$\frac{60\ \text{tsp}}{20} = X$$

$$3\ \text{tsp} = X$$

You should give the patient 3 tsp of phenobarbital elixir.

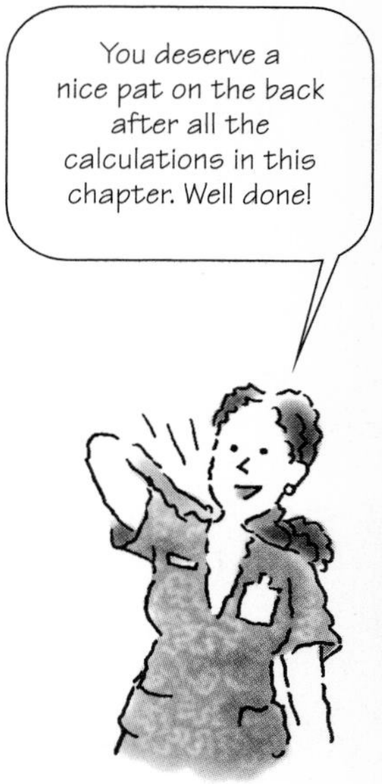

You deserve a nice pat on the back after all the calculations in this chapter. Well done!

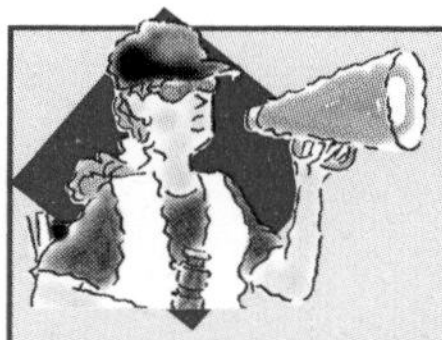

That's a wrap!

Calculating oral drug dosages review

Keep these important facts in mind when calculating doses of oral drugs.

Reading oral drug labels
- First, check the drug's generic name and trade name. Remember that combination drugs are usually ordered using the trade name.
- Then check the dose strength.
- Lastly, check the expiration date.

Safe oral drug administration
- Check the "six rights" of medication administration.
- Check drug names.
- Check the dosage, route, and medication administration record.
- Check orders and labels three times.

Dosage calculation key
- Use correct units of measure.
- Double-check units of measure and decimal places.
- Check answers that seem wrong.
- Use a calculator.

Liquid dosages
- Read drug labels carefully: the drug concentration is expressed as the dose strength contained in a volume of solution.
- Dilute powders with the appropriate diluent according to the manufacturer's directions.
- Measure oral solutions with a medicine cup, dropper, or syringe.

Calculating with different systems
- First, find the standard equivalent value with a conversion table.
- Then calculate the dosage using the ratio and proportion method.
- The standard equivalent values equal the unknown quantity over the quantity ordered.

Desired-over-have method
- The amount desired over the amount you have equals the equivalent amount desired over the equivalent amount you have.
- For both fractions, verify that the units of measure in the numerators and denominators correspond to one another.

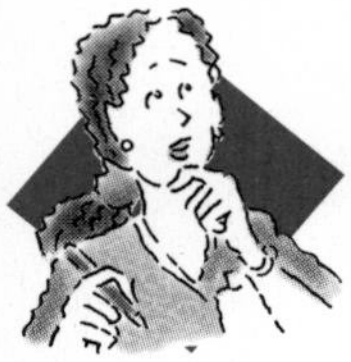

Quick quiz

1. If a patient needs 100 mcg of Synthroid P.O. and the available dose is 25 mcg/tablet, the number of tablets to give is:

A. 2.
B. 3.
C. 4.
D. 6.

Answer: C. If 1 tablet provides 25 mcg, divide 100 by 25 to get the answer: 4 tablets.

2. If 250 mg of Clozaril is ordered for a patient, but only 100-mg tablets are available, you should give:

A. 2 tablets.
B. 2½ tablets.
C. 3 tablets.
D. 3½ tablets.

Answer: B. By dividing 250 by 100, you get 2.5, or 2½ tablets.

3. If the doctor orders *640 mg Tylenol liquid P.O. STAT* and the bottle label reads *Tylenol 80 mg per ½ tsp*, you should give the patient:

A. 10 ml.
B. 15 ml.
C. 18 ml.
D. 20 ml.

Answer: D. First, consult a conversion table to find that 1 tsp equals 5 ml. Then use proportions to solve for *X*.

4. A patient needs 50 mg of Benadryl elixir P.O. STAT and the bottle label reads *Benadryl 12.5 mg/5 ml.* You should give:

A. 15 ml.
B. 18 ml.
C. 20 ml.
D. 25 ml.

Answer: C. Use fractions to solve for *X*. The known factor is 12.5 mg equals 5 ml.

Scoring

☆☆☆ If you answered all four items correctly, excellent! Expressed as a ratio it's 10 : 10 :: 100 : 100 (in other words, perfect).

☆☆ If you answered three items correctly, good job! Your calculation skills are almost perfect! (But, remember, a good calculator never hurt anybody.)

☆ If you answered fewer than three items correctly, don't worry! Keep on calculatin' (a little practice goes a long way).

11

Calculating topical and rectal drug dosages

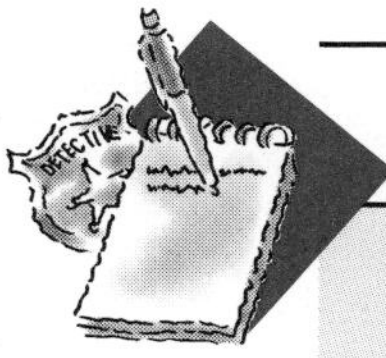

Just the facts

In this chapter, you'll learn:

- ♦ how to interpret topical and rectal drug labels
- ♦ what types of drugs are given topically and rectally and how they work
- ♦ how to perform dosage calculations for topical and rectal drugs.

A look at topical and rectal drugs

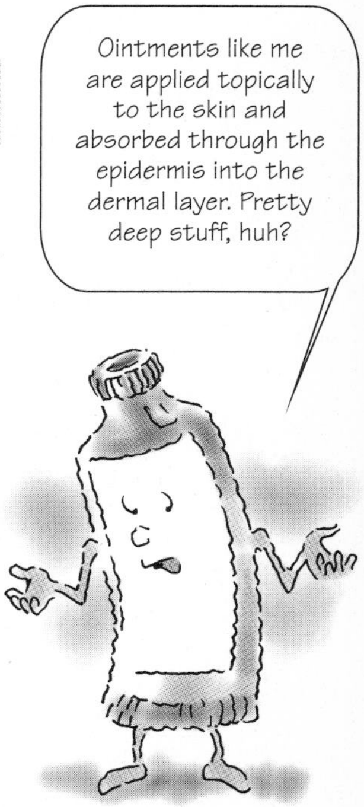
Ointments like me are applied topically to the skin and absorbed through the epidermis into the dermal layer. Pretty deep stuff, huh?

Some types of drugs must be administered by the topical, or dermal, route. These drugs include creams, lotions, ointments, and powders, which are commonly used for dermatologic treatment or wound care, or patches, which have various uses, including treating angina. Topical drugs are applied to the skin and absorbed through the epidermis into the dermis.

Drugs may also be given rectally. This route may be best for patients who can't take drugs orally, such as those with nasogastric tubes, nausea, or vomiting. It may also be used for unconscious patients who can't swallow and to achieve specific local and systemic effects. Rectal drugs include enemas and suppositories.

Are you label able?

When you read the labels on topical and rectal drugs, look for the same information you would look for on oral and parenteral drug labels. (See *Labeling a successful administration*, page 202.)

The trade name appears first, followed by the generic name, the dose strength, and the total volume of the package. Labels may also contain special administration instructions. Sometimes,

Before you give that drug!

Labeling a successful administration

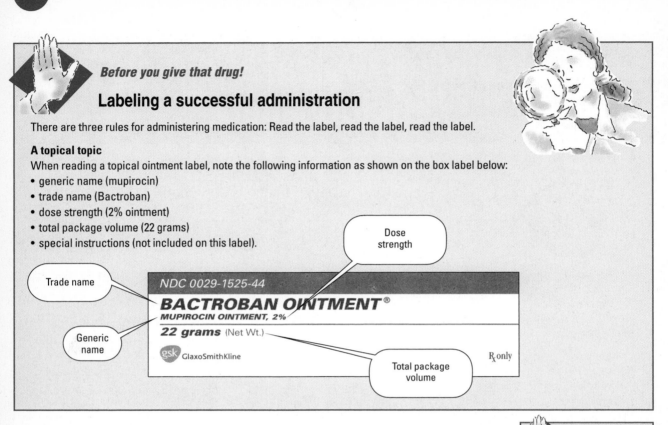

There are three rules for administering medication: Read the label, read the label, read the label.

A topical topic

When reading a topical ointment label, note the following information as shown on the box label below:

- generic name (mupirocin)
- trade name (Bactroban)
- dose strength (2% ointment)
- total package volume (22 grams)
- special instructions (not included on this label).

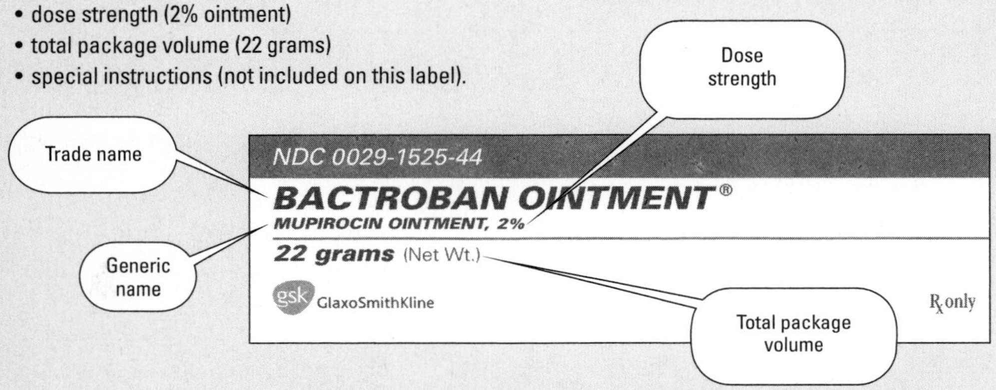

the print on the labels is quite small, so look carefully. (See *Combination product alert.*)

Transdermal patches

In the past, topical drugs were used almost solely for their local effects. Today, however, several topical drugs, such as transdermal patches, are used for their systemic effects as well.

I've got you under my skin

Transdermal patch drugs penetrate the outer layers of the skin by way of passive diffusion at a constant rate; then the drugs are absorbed into the circulation. Patches are a good way to administer drugs that aren't absorbed well in the GI tract as well as those that are metabolized and eliminated too quickly to be effective.

Patches are convenient and easy to use, and they maintain consistent blood levels of the drug. However, they also have disadvantages. Their onset of action is slow, so a therapeutic blood level takes hours or even days to achieve. Patches must also be checked frequently, especially if the patient is active, because they

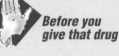

Before you give that drug

Combination product alert

Topical preparations may contain more than one drug. For example, Neosporin ointment contains bacitracin, neomycin, and polymyxin B. Carefully note all ingredients when checking labels and make sure that your patient isn't allergic to any of them.

Prescribed patches

These transdermal drugs allow you to topically administer systemic drugs.

Nitroglycerin
Transdermal nitroglycerin provides prophylactic treatment of chronic angina. Available brands include Nitro-Dur and Minitran. A new patch is applied daily (usually in the morning) and removed after 12 to 14 hours to prevent the patient from developing a tolerance to the drug.

Nicotine
Transdermal nicotine is used to treat smoking addiction. Brands include Habitrol, NicoDerm CQ, and ProStep. These drugs should be used only as adjuncts to behavioral therapy programs. A new patch is applied daily.

Fentanyl
Transdermal fentanyl is administered to treat severe chronic pain. Its brand name is Duragesic. Each patch may be worn up to 72 hours.

Clonidine
Clonidine is used to treat hypertension. The brand name for this drug is Catapres TTS. A new patch is applied every 7 days.

Scopolamine
Scopolamine is used to treat nausea, vomiting, and vertigo. Its brand name is Transderm-Scōp. The patch is applied to the skin behind the ear at least 4 hours before an antiemetic effect is needed. It can be worn for 3 days.

Estradiol
Transdermal estradiol provides hormone replacement to estrogen-deficient women. The brand names include Climara, Estraderm, and Vivelle. It's administered on an intermittent cyclic schedule (3 weeks of therapy followed by discontinuation for 1 week).

Testosterone
Transdermal testosterone provides hormone replacement for men with testosterone deficiency. The brand name is Androderm. The Androderm patch is applied once daily to clean intact, non-scrotal skin (back, abdomen, thighs, or upper arm).

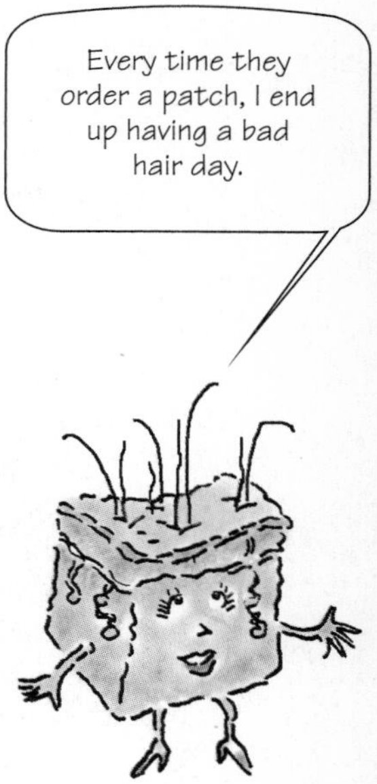

Every time they order a patch, I end up having a bad hair day.

may become displaced. In addition, reversing the toxic effects of patches can be difficult because the drug takes so long to be metabolized.

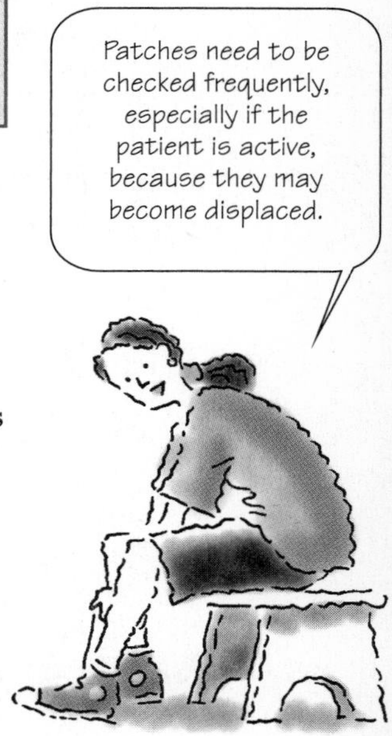

Release me

Drug concentrations in transdermal patches vary depending on the design of the patch, but the concentration isn't as important as the drug's rate of release. Two patches containing the same drug in different concentrations may actually release the same amount of drug per hour. (See *Prescribed patches*.)

Batches of patches

Patches are available for many conditions, including a nitroglycerin patch to prevent angina, a clonidine patch to control hypertension, and a fentanyl patch to manage chronic pain.

The fentanyl transdermal system, or Duragesic patch, is an example of a transdermal drug used systemically. It's held in a reservoir behind a membrane that allows controlled drug absorption through the skin. These patches are available in doses of 12.5, 25, 50, 75, and 100 mcg/hour, with the higher doses for use with opioid-resistant patients. To ensure that the patient receives the correct dose, change the patch every 72 hours and check the label to verify the fentanyl dosage.

Topical drug dosages

Determining topical drug dosages requires very little calculating. As previously discussed, transdermal patches are changed at regular intervals to ensure that the patient receives the correct dose. To apply a patch, simply remove the old patch and replace it with a new one at the appropriate time, following the manufacturer's guidelines.

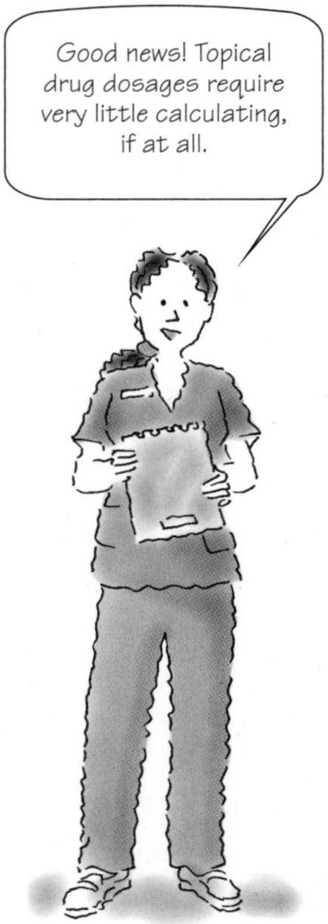
Good news! Topical drug dosages require very little calculating, if at all.

Measuring a topical dose

To measure a specified amount of ointment from a tube, squeeze the prescribed length of ointment in inches or centimeters onto a paper ruler. Then use the ruler to apply the ointment to the patient's skin at the appropriate time, following the manufacturer's guidelines for administration.

Applying your judgment (along with the ointment)

When the doctor prescribes an ointment as part of wound care or dermatologic treatment, he usually leaves the amount to apply up to you. He may give general guidance, such as "use a thin layer" or "apply thickly." When an ointment contains a drug intended for a systemic effect, more specific administration guidelines are necessary.

Many ointments, including nitroglycerin, are available in tubes. To apply ointment from a tube, use a paper ruler applicator, if available, to measure the correct dose. (See *Measuring a topical dose.*)

Rectal drug dosages

Rectal drugs include enemas and suppositories. Suppositories are the most common form of rectal drugs.

To calculate the number of suppositories to give, use the proportion method with ratios or fractions. The doctor usually prescribes drugs in the dose provided by one suppository, but occasionally you may need to insert two suppositories. (See *Check and check again*, page 206.)

Real world problems

These problems illustrate how to calculate suppository dosages.

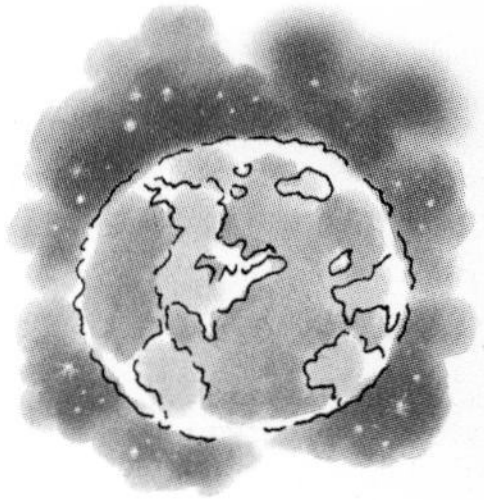

Arriving at an acetaminophen answer

Your pediatric patient needs 240 mg of acetaminophen by suppository. The package label reads *acetaminophen suppositories 120 mg.* How many suppositories should you give?

This is how to solve this problem using fractions.

- Set up the first fraction with the known suppository dose:

$$\frac{1 \text{ supp}}{120 \text{ mg}}$$

- Set up the second fraction with the desired dose and the unknown number of suppositories:

$$\frac{X}{240\text{ mg}}$$

- Put these fractions into a proportion:

$$\frac{1\text{ supp}}{120\text{ mg}} = \frac{X}{240\text{ mg}}$$

- Cross-multiply the fractions:

$$120\text{ mg} \times X = 1\text{ supp} \times 240\text{ mg}$$

- Solve for *X* by dividing each side of the equation by 120 mg and canceling units that appear in both the numerator and denominator:

$$\frac{\cancel{120\text{ mg}} \times X}{\cancel{120\text{ mg}}} = \frac{1\text{ supp} \times 240\ \cancel{\text{mg}}}{120\ \cancel{\text{mg}}}$$

$$X = 2\text{ suppositories}$$

Dealing with a Dulcolax dilemma

The doctor's order states *Dulcolax 10 mg per rectum at 6 a.m.* You only have 5-mg suppositories on hand. How many suppositories should you give this patient?

This is how to solve this problem using fractions.

- Set up the first fraction with the known suppository dose:

$$\frac{1\text{ supp}}{5\text{ mg}}$$

- Set up the second fraction with the desired dose and the unknown number of suppositories:

$$\frac{X}{10\text{ mg}}$$

- Put these fractions into a proportion:

$$\frac{1\text{ supp}}{5\text{ mg}} = \frac{X}{10\text{ mg}}$$

Before you give that drug

Check and check again

Occasionally you may need to insert more than one or a portion of one suppository. Here's what to do.

More than one

Do your dosage calculations indicate a need for more than one suppository? If so, check your figures and ask another nurse to check them, too. Then ask the pharmacist whether the suppository is available in other dosage strengths.

More than two

If more than two suppositories are needed, confirm the dose with the doctor. Then check with the pharmacist. He may be able to give you one suppository with an adequate amount of the drug.

A portion of one

If less than one suppository is needed, check your calculations and have another nurse do the same. Then ask the pharmacist if the dose is available in one suppository. This ensures the most accurate dose.

Dosage drill

Test your math skills with this drill.

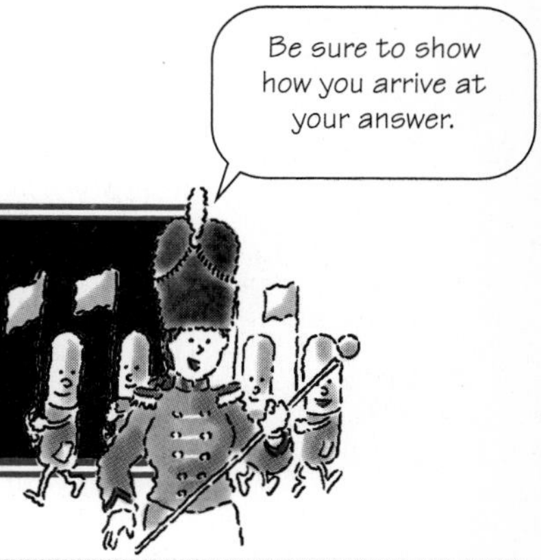
Be sure to show how you arrive at your answer.

The doctor orders a 650-mg aspirin suppository for a patient. The pharmacy is closed and the only aspirin on hand contains 325 mg per suppository. How many suppositories should you give?

Your answer: ______________________

To find the answer, set up the equation using ratios and a proportion. Then solve for *X*.

$$1 \text{ supp} : 325 \text{ mg}$$

$$X \text{ supp} : 650 \text{ mg}$$

$$1 \text{ supp} : 325 \text{ mg} :: X \text{ supp} : 650 \text{ mg}$$

$$325 \text{ mg} \times X \text{ supp} = 650 \text{ mg} \times 1 \text{ supp}$$

$$\frac{\cancel{325 \text{ mg}} \times X \text{ supp}}{\cancel{325 \text{ mg}}} = \frac{650 \cancel{\text{ mg}} \times 1 \text{ supp}}{325 \cancel{\text{ mg}}}$$

$$X = 2 \text{ supp}$$

You should give the patient 2 suppositories.

• Cross-multiply the fractions:

$$1 \text{ supp} \times 10 \text{ mg} = X \times 5 \text{ mg}$$

• Solve for X by dividing each side of the equation by 5 mg and canceling units that appear in both the numerator and denominator:

$$\frac{1 \text{ supp} \times 10 \cancel{\text{mg}}}{5 \cancel{\text{mg}}} = \frac{X \times \cancel{5 \text{ mg}}}{\cancel{5 \text{ mg}}}$$

$$X = 2 \text{ suppositories}$$

Don't compro–mize your calculations

The doctor orders a 10-mg Compro suppository for your patient. The pharmacy is closed, and the only Compro on hand contains 5 mg per suppository. How many suppositories should you give?

This is how to solve this problem using ratios.

• Set up the first ratio with the known suppository dose:

$$1 \text{ supp} : 5 \text{ mg}$$

• Set up the second ratio with the desired dose and the unknown number of suppositories:

$$X : 10 \text{ mg}$$

• Put these ratios into a proportion:

$$1 \text{ supp} : 5 \text{ mg} :: X : 10 \text{ mg}$$

• Multiply the means and the extremes:

$$5 \text{ mg} \times X = 10 \text{ mg} \times 1 \text{ supp}$$

• Solve for X by dividing each side of the equation by 5 mg and canceling units that appear in both the numerator and denominator:

$$\frac{\cancel{5 \text{ mg}} \times X}{\cancel{5 \text{ mg}}} = \frac{10 \cancel{\text{mg}} \times 1 \text{ supp}}{5 \cancel{\text{mg}}}$$

$$X = 2 \text{ suppositories}$$

Dosage drill

Test your math skills with this drill.

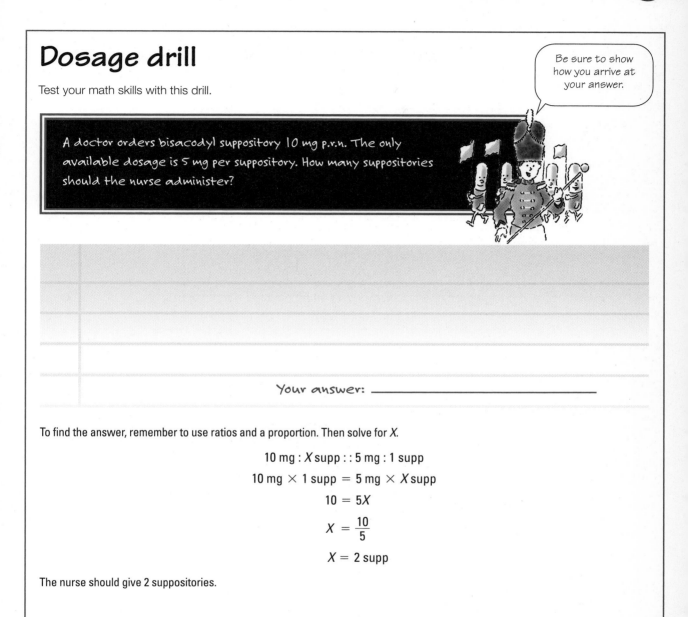

Be sure to show how you arrive at your answer.

A doctor orders bisacodyl suppository 10 mg p.r.n. The only available dosage is 5 mg per suppository. How many suppositories should the nurse administer?

Your answer: ______________________

To find the answer, remember to use ratios and a proportion. Then solve for X.

$$10 \text{ mg} : X \text{ supp} :: 5 \text{ mg} : 1 \text{ supp}$$

$$10 \text{ mg} \times 1 \text{ supp} = 5 \text{ mg} \times X \text{ supp}$$

$$10 = 5X$$

$$X = \frac{10}{5}$$

$$X = 2 \text{ supp}$$

The nurse should give 2 suppositories.

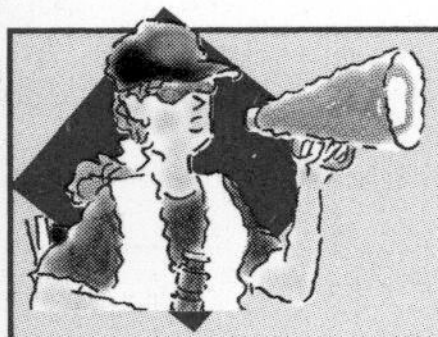

That's a wrap!

Topical and rectal drug dosages review

Review these key facts before giving topical and rectal drugs.

Transdermal patches

- Transdermal patch drugs penetrate the outer layers of the skin by passive diffusion and then are absorbed into the circulation.
- These drugs have a slow onset of action, so it may take hours or even days to achieve a therapeutic drug level.

Topical drug calculations

- Use your own judgment in accordance with the doctor's general instructions.
- Follow specific guidelines for drugs prescribed for a systemic effect.

Rectal drug calculations

- Use the proportion method with ratios or fractions.
- A dose is typically prescribed to be provided in one suppository (occasionally two).

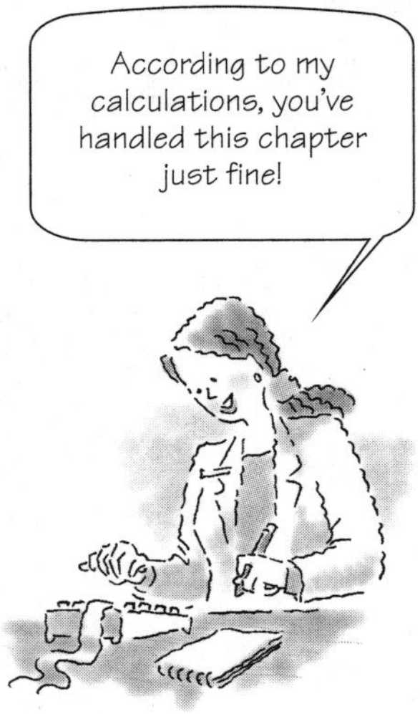

According to my calculations, you've handled this chapter just fine!

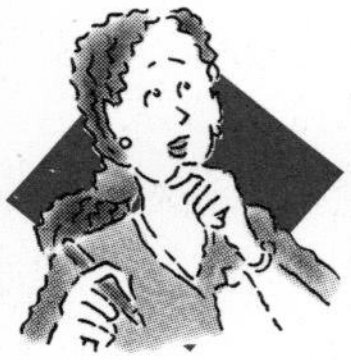

Quick quiz

1. Transdermal patches used to relieve chronic pain are effective for many hours due to:

A. controlled absorption through the skin.
B. an enhanced effect on local tissue.
C. rapid then slow release of analgesics.
D. sustained-release dosing.

Answer: A. These drugs are slowly released and absorbed through the skin over time.

2. A commonly used transdermal drug is:

A. Anectine.
B. nitroglycerin.
C. MS Contin.
D. morphine.

Answer: B. Nitroglycerin patches are used to prevent angina.

3. If a drug label reads *Compro (prochlorperazine) suppositories 5 mg, Paddock Laboratories, for rectal use only,* the drug's proprietary name is:

A. Compro.
B. prochlorperazine.
C. Paddock Laboratories.
D. suppositories.

Answer: A. The proprietary name, or trade name, usually appears first on a drug label, just before or above the generic name.

4. If the doctor's order reads *Nitrol Ointment 1″ q6h,* you should measure this dose:

A. on a paper ruler applicator.
B. by using your own judgment to approximate 1″ of ointment.
C. by holding a wooden ruler to the patient's skin to measure the ointment.
D. by dispensing it into a syringe.

Answer: A. Nitrol Ointment comes with its own paper ruler. Squeeze the prescribed length of ointment onto the ruler and then use the ruler to apply the ointment to the patient's skin.

5. If a patient needs 500 mg of aminophylline by suppository, but all you have are 250-mg suppositories, you should insert:

A. 1 suppository.
B. 2 suppositories.
C. 3 suppositories.
D. 4 suppositories.

Answer: B. A simple calculation tells you that the patient needs 2 suppositories. However, because more than 1 suppository is needed, you should check your calculations, have another nurse do the same, and then call the pharmacy to see if a 500-mg dose is available.

6. When a doctor prescribes an antibiotic ointment for a finger laceration, you should:

A. ask him to prescribe a specific amount.
B. use a paper applicator to apply the ointment.
C. use your own judgment about the amount of ointment to apply.
D. call the pharmacist for the recommended amount of ointment to apply.

Answer: C. Unless the ointment has a systemic effect, the doctor will usually leave the amount to apply up to you.

7. If a child needs 2.5 mg of Compro, and the package label reads *Compro suppositories 5 mg*, you should give:

A. 2 suppositories.
B. 1½ suppositories.
C. 1 suppository.
D. ½ suppository.

Answer: D. By setting up a proportion and solving for *X*, you'll find that the child needs ½ of a 5-mg suppository. You could also call the pharmacist to see if this dose is available in one suppository to ensure the most accurate dose.

8. Your patient is receiving transdermal nitroglycerin to treat angina. Which action is necessary when administering this drug?

A. Remove the patch after 7 days.
B. Remove the patch after 72 hours.
C. Remove the patch after 12 to 14 hours.
D. Remove the patch after 1 to 2 hours.

Answer: C. Transdermal nitroglycerin should be removed after 12 to 14 hours to prevent the patient from developing a tolerance to the drug.

Scoring

☆☆☆ If you answered all eight items correctly, wow! You know your routes better than AAA!

☆☆ If you answered six or seven items correctly, all right! You'll soon be top dog in topical drug administration.

☆ If you answered fewer than six items correctly, keep at it! You're absorbing information at an incredible rate.

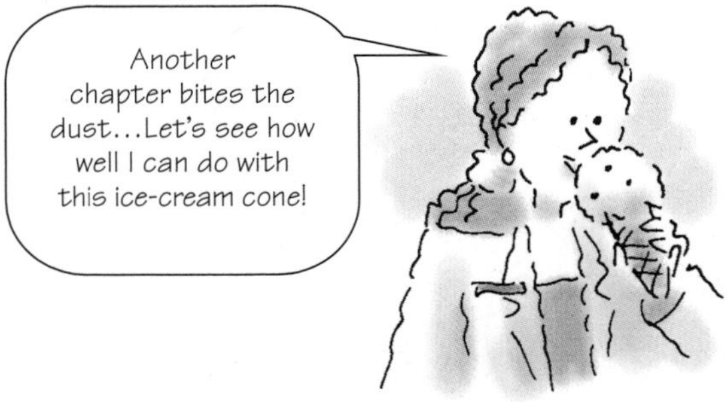

Another chapter bites the dust...Let's see how well I can do with this ice-cream cone!

Part V Parenteral administration

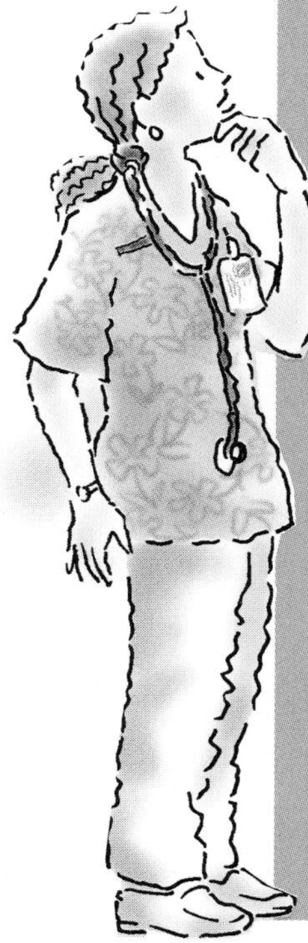

12

Calculating parenteral injections

Just the facts

In this chapter, you'll learn:

- about calculating intradermal, subcutaneous, and intramuscular injections
- about different types of syringes and needles
- how to interpret parenteral drug labels
- how to administer insulin and other unit-based drugs
- how to reconstitute powders.

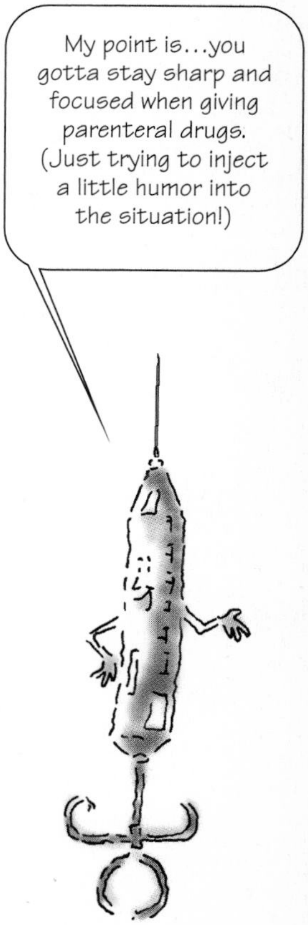
My point is…you gotta stay sharp and focused when giving parenteral drugs. (Just trying to inject a little humor into the situation!)

A look at parenteral injections

Parenteral is a term that refers to "outside the intestines." Drugs may be administered parenterally through direct injection into the skin, subcutaneous tissue, muscle, or vein. They may be supplied as liquids or as powders that require reconstitution. When using either form, you need to perform calculations to determine the amount of liquid medication to inject.

This chapter shows how to use the ratio or fraction and proportion method to calculate liquid parenteral dosages as well as how to reconstitute powdered drugs. Another parenteral drug administration route, I.V. infusion, is discussed in the next chapter. I.V. injections are discussed in chapter 16, Calculating critical care dosages.

Types of injections

Parenteral drugs are administered by four types of injections:

- intradermal
- subcutaneous (subQ)
- intramuscular (I.M.)
- I.V. (See chapter 13, Calculating I.V. infusions.)

Giving parenteral drugs safely depends on choosing the right syringe and needle for the type of injection ordered.

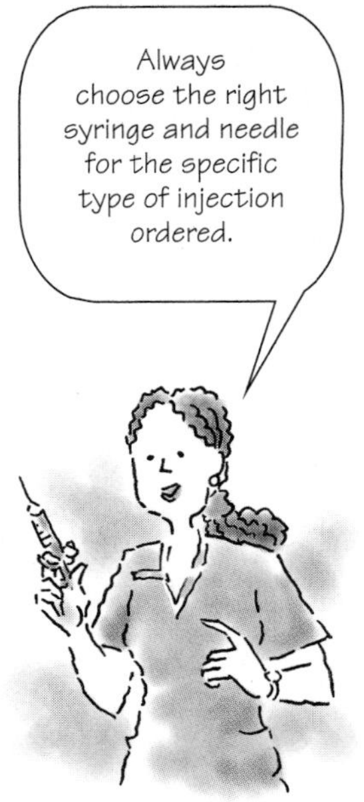

Intradermal injections

In an intradermal injection, medication is injected into the dermis—the layer of skin beneath the epidermis, or the outermost layer of skin. This type of injection is used to anesthetize the skin for invasive procedures and to test for allergies, tuberculosis, histoplasmosis, and other diseases.

I've got you intra my skin

The volume of a drug that's given by intradermal injection is less than 0.5 ml. A 1-ml syringe, calibrated in 0.01-ml increments, is usually used, along with a 25- to 27-gauge (G) needle that's 3/8″ to 5/8″ long.

To perform an intradermal injection, use this basic procedure:

1. Clean the skin thoroughly using an antiseptic swab.
2. Stretch the skin taut with one hand.
3. With your other hand, insert the needle quickly at a 10- to 15-degree angle to a depth of about 0.5 cm.
4. Inject the drug. A small wheal forms where the drug is injected into the skin.

Subcutaneous injections

In a subQ injection, the drug is injected into the subcutaneous tissue, which is beneath the dermis and above the muscle. Drugs are absorbed faster in this layer than in the dermis because the subcutaneous layer has more capillaries. Insulin, heparin, tetanus toxoid, and some opioid analgesics are injected through this route.

More than skin *deep*

Only 0.5 to 1 ml of a drug can be injected subQ. The needles used for subQ injections are 23G to 28G and 1/2″ to 5/8″ long. SubQ injection sites include the:

- anterior aspect of the thighs
- lateral areas of the upper arms and thighs
- abdomen (above, below, and lateral to the umbilicus)
- upper back.

To perform a subQ injection, use this basic procedure:

- Choose the injection site.
- Clean the skin with an antiseptic swab.
- If the patient is thin, pinch the skin between your index finger and thumb, and insert the needle at a 45-degree angle.
- If the patient is obese, insert the needle into the fatty tissue at a 90-degree angle.
- Administer the injection.
- Apply gentle pressure or massage the site after removing the needle; this may enhance absorption. Don't massage the site if you're giving heparin or insulin.

Intramuscular injections

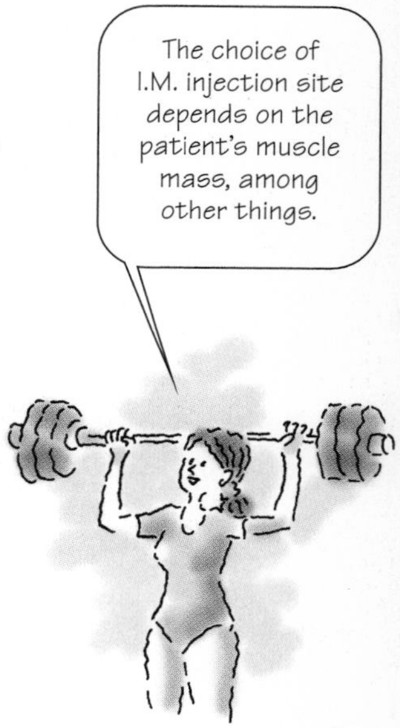
The choice of I.M. injection site depends on the patient's muscle mass, among other things.

An I.M. injection, which goes into a muscle, is used for drugs that need to be absorbed quickly, that are given in a large volume, or that irritate the tissues if given by a shallow route. The volume for these injections ranges from 0.5 to 3 ml. I.M. injection sites include the:

- ventral gluteal or vastus lateralis muscle (for 3-ml injections)
- deltoid muscle (for injections of less than 2 ml).

The choice of injection site depends on the patient's muscle mass and overlying tissue and the volume of the injection. The needles are 1″ to 3″ long and are 18G to 23G in diameter.

Use a little muscle

To administer an I.M. injection, use this basic procedure:

- Choose the injection site.
- Clean the skin with an antiseptic swab.
- Using a quick, dartlike action, insert the needle at a 75- to 90-degree angle.
- Before injecting the drug, aspirate for blood to make sure that the needle isn't in a vein.
- Push the plunger and keep the syringe steady.
- After the drug is injected, pull the needle straight out and apply pressure to the site.

Syringes and needles

The many types of syringes and needles used to administer parenteral drugs are designed for specific purposes.

Types of syringes

To measure and administer parenteral drugs, three basic types of syringes are used, including:

- standard syringes
- tuberculin syringes
- prefilled syringes.

Although these syringes are sometimes calibrated in cubic centimeters, the drugs they're used to measure are commonly ordered in milliliters. (Recall that 1 cc equals 1 ml and that milliliters and cubic centimeters are used interchangeably.)

Standard syringes

Standard syringes are available in 3, 5, 10, 20, 30, 50, and 60 ml. Each syringe consists of a plunger, a barrel, a hub, a needle, a safety device, and dead space. The dead space holds fluid that remains in the syringe and needle after the plunger is completely depressed. Some syringes, such as insulin syringes, don't have dead space. (See *Anatomy of a syringe.*)

Marked for good measure

The calibration marks on syringes allow you to accurately measure drug doses. The 3-ml syringe, the most commonly used, is calibrated in tenths of a milliliter on the right and minims on the left. It has large marks for every 0.5 ml on the right. The large-volume syringes are calibrated in 2- to 10-ml increments.

Anatomy of a syringe

Standard syringes come in many different sizes, but each syringe has the same components. This illustration shows the parts of a standard syringe.

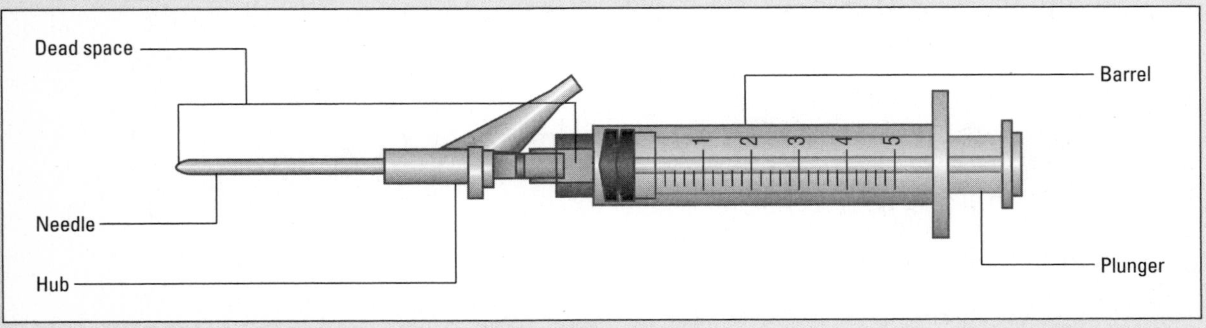

To administer a drug, remember the "six rights" of medication administration — right drug, right route, right dose, right time, right patient, right documentation — and then follow these basic steps:

- Use aseptic technique.
- Calculate the dose.
- Draw the drug into the syringe.
- Pull the plunger back until the top ring of the plunger's black portion aligns with the correct calibration mark.
- Double-check the dose measurement.
- Administer the drug.

Double the fun (well, not exactly fun)

Parenteral drugs come in various dose strengths or concentrations so that the usual adult dose can be contained in 1 to 3 ml of solution. If a patient needs a dose larger than 3 ml, give it in two injections at two different sites to ensure proper drug absorption.

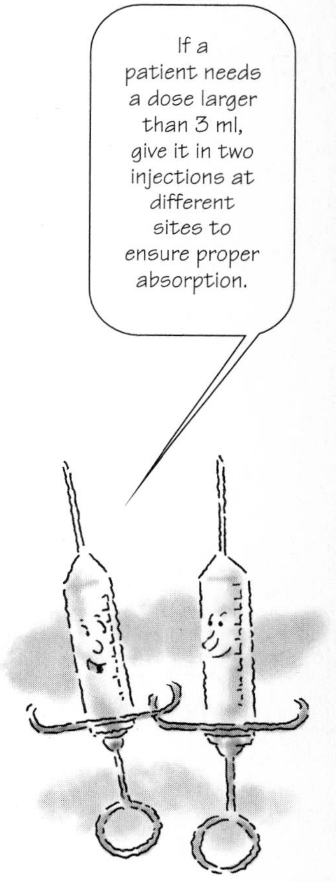
If a patient needs a dose larger than 3 ml, give it in two injections at different sites to ensure proper absorption.

Tuberculin syringes

Tuberculin syringes are commonly used for intradermal injections and to administer small amounts of drugs, such as those given to pediatric patients or those on intensive care units. Each syringe is calibrated in hundredths of a milliliter, allowing you to accurately administer doses as small as 0.25 ml. (See *Touring a tuberculin syringe*, page 220.)

Read the fine print

Measure drugs in a tuberculin syringe as you would those in a standard syringe. Take extra care when reading the dose, however, because the measurements on the tuberculin syringe are very small.

Prefilled syringes

A sterile syringe filled with a premeasured dose of drug is called a *prefilled syringe.* These syringes usually come with a cartridge-needle unit and require a special holder called a *Carpuject* to release the drug from the cartridge. Each cartridge is calibrated in tenths of a milliliter and has larger marks for half and full milliliters. (See *Perusing a prefilled syringe*, page 221.)

Room for one more

Some cartridges are designed so that a diluent or a second drug can be added when a combined dose is ordered. For example, the antianxiety drug lorazepam (Ativan) comes from the manufacturer in prefilled syringes. Because lorazepam requires the addition of a diluent, the lorazepam cartridge allows for the addition of the

Touring a tuberculin syringe

A tuberculin syringe has the same components as a standard syringe. However, size and calibration of the syringe are distinct. Because the measurements on the tuberculin syringe are so small, take extra care when reading the dose.

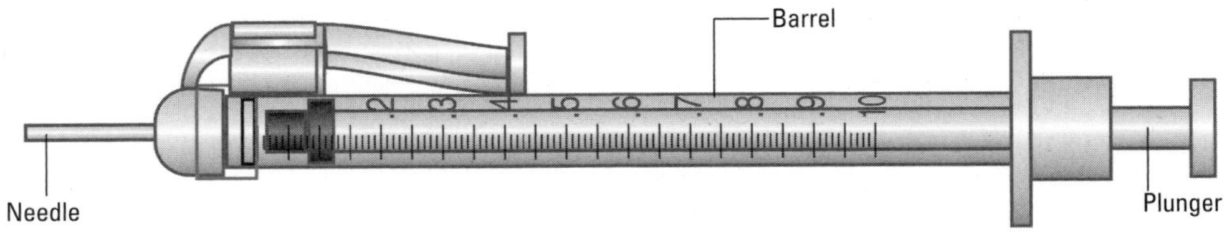

diluent. Remember to always check a compatibility chart when adding a diluent or mixing more than one drug in a syringe.

First, the good news...

Prefilled syringes have many advantages over multiple-dose vials. Because they're labeled with the drug name and dose, preparation time is reduced and so is the risk of drug errors. This labeling also makes it easier to record the amount of drug used and eliminates the need to figure out how much drug is left in a vial after you've given an injection, which is especially important with opioid doses because the law says that they must be recorded exactly.

The most obvious advantage of prefilled syringes is that you don't have to measure each drug dose. The manufacturer has already done this and placed the dose in the syringe. However, be aware that most manufacturers add a little extra drug to the syringe in case some is wasted when the syringe is purged of air.

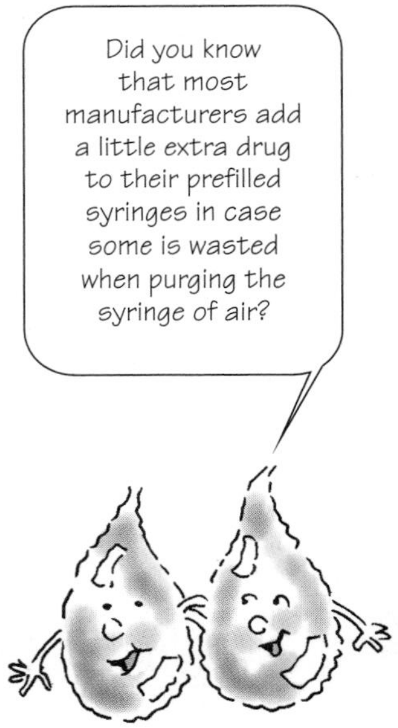

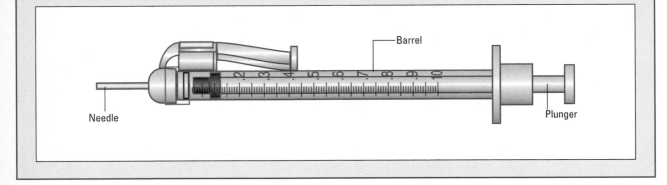

...Now, the bad news

Unfortunately, prefilled syringes aren't available in all doses. When the ordered dose doesn't match the amount in the prefilled syringe, you'll need to calculate the correct amount of drug needed.

Before giving the injection, discard the extra drug by expelling it from the syringe. If the drug is an opioid, carefully document the amount of drug you discard. Have another nurse witness the expulsion of the drug and then co-sign the controlled substances record.

Perusing a prefilled syringe

This illustration shows the parts of a prefilled syringe. Take note of the holder at right. The most commonly used brand of prefilled syringe is Carpuject.

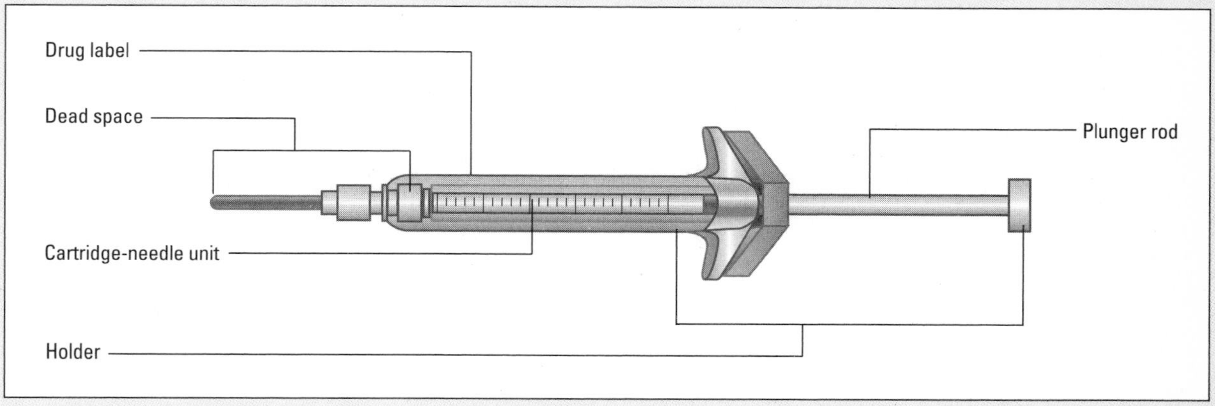

Closed-system devices

Another type of prefilled syringe, a closed-system device, comes with a needle and syringe in place and a separate prefilled drug chamber. Emergency drugs, such as atropine and lidocaine, come in this type of prefilled syringe.

To prepare a closed-system device, hold the drug chamber in one hand and the syringe and needle in the other. Flip the protective caps off both ends. Insert the drug chamber into the syringe section. Then remove the needle cap and expel air and extra medication.

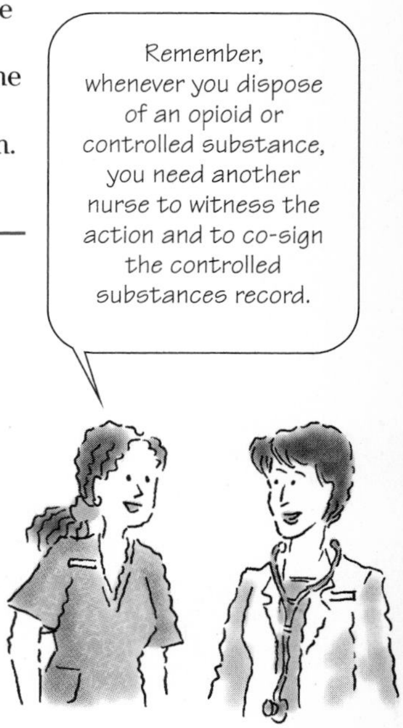
Remember, whenever you dispose of an opioid or controlled substance, you need another nurse to witness the action and to co-sign the controlled substances record.

Types of needles

Although most safety syringes come with a preattached needle, you may need to choose a needle on occasion.

Five types of needles are used to inject drugs: intradermal, subQ, I.M., I.V., and filter. Each type of needle is designed for a different purpose. (See *Choosing the right needle*, page 222.)

When choosing a needle, consider the gauge, bevel, and length:

- Gauge refers to the inside diameter of the needle; the smaller the gauge, the larger the diameter. For example, a 14G needle has a larger diameter than a 25G needle.
- Bevel refers to the angle at which the needle tip is opened. The bevel may be short, medium, or long.
- Length describes the distance from needle tip to needle hub. It ranges from ⅜″ to 3″.

Choosing the right needle

When choosing a needle, consider its purpose as well as its gauge, bevel, and length. Use this selection guide to choose the right needles for your patients.

Intradermal needles

Intradermal needles are $\frac{3}{8}$″ to $\frac{5}{8}$″ long, usually have short bevels, and are 25G to 27G in diameter.

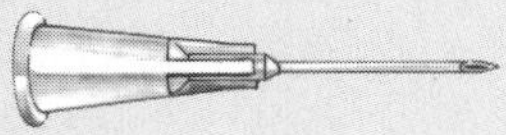

Subcutaneous needles

Subcutaneous needles are $\frac{1}{2}$″ to $\frac{5}{8}$″ long, have medium bevels, and are 23G to 28G in diameter.

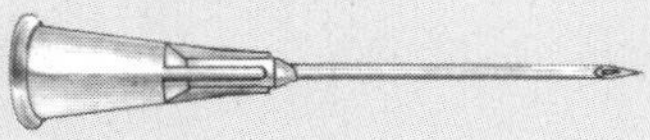

I.M. needles

I.M. needles are 1″ to 3″ long, have medium bevels, and are 18G to 23G in diameter.

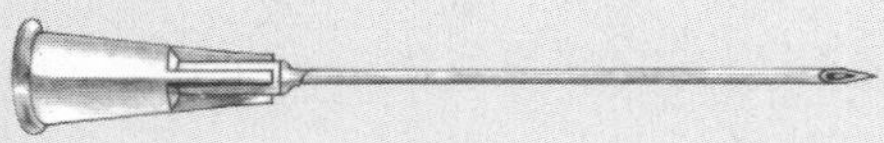

I.V. needles

I.V. needles are 1″ to 3″ long, have long bevels, and are 14G to 25G in diameter.

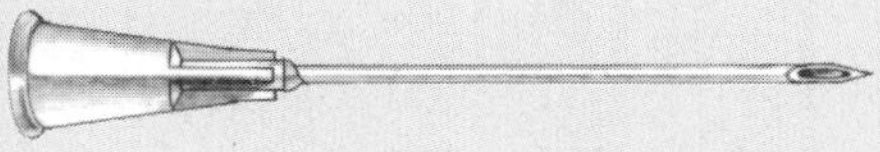

Filter needles

Filter needles are used for preparing a solution from a vial or ampule and shouldn't be used for injections. They're $1\frac{1}{2}$″ long, have medium bevels, and are 20G in diameter.

Microscopic pieces of rubber or glass can enter the solution when you puncture the diaphragm of a vial with a needle or snap open an ampule. You can use a filter needle with a screening device in the hub to remove minute particles of foreign material from a solution. *Remember:* After the medication is prepared, discard the filter needle!

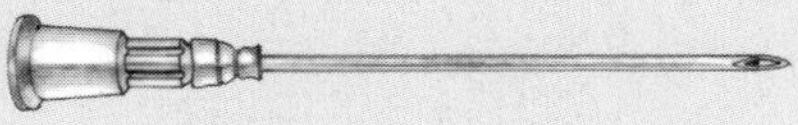

Real world problems

The following examples show how to use the ratio or fraction and proportion method to calculate doses given by injection.

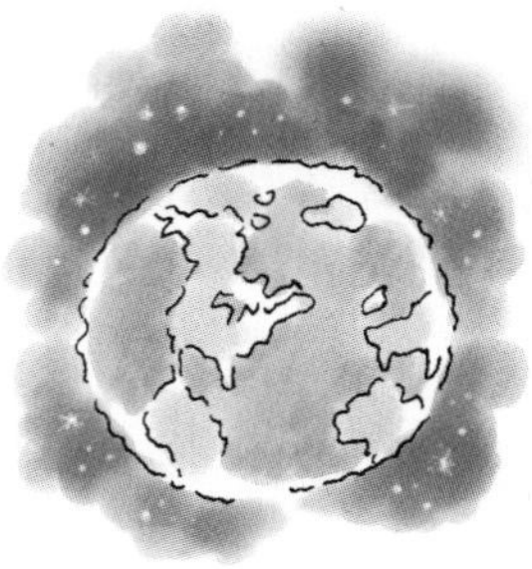

Prefilled painkiller problem

The doctor prescribes *4 mg of I.M. morphine q3h* for your patient's pain. The drug is available in a prefilled syringe containing 10 mg of morphine/ml. How many milliliters of morphine should you discard?

This is how to solve this problem using fractions.

- Set up the first fraction using the known morphine concentration:

$$\frac{10 \text{ mg}}{1 \text{ ml}}$$

• Set up the second fraction with the desired dose and the unknown amount of morphine:

$$\frac{4\text{ mg}}{X}$$

• Put these fractions into a proportion:

$$\frac{10\text{ mg}}{1\text{ ml}} = \frac{4\text{ mg}}{X}$$

• Cross-multiply the fractions:

$$10\text{ mg} \times X = 4\text{ mg} \times 1\text{ ml}$$

• Solve for X by dividing each side of the equation by 10 mg and canceling units that appear in both the numerator and denominator:

$$\frac{\cancel{10\text{ mg}} \times X}{\cancel{10\text{ mg}}} = \frac{4\cancel{\text{ mg}} \times 1\text{ ml}}{10\cancel{\text{ mg}}}$$

$$X = \frac{4\text{ ml}}{10}$$

$$X = 0.4\text{ ml}$$

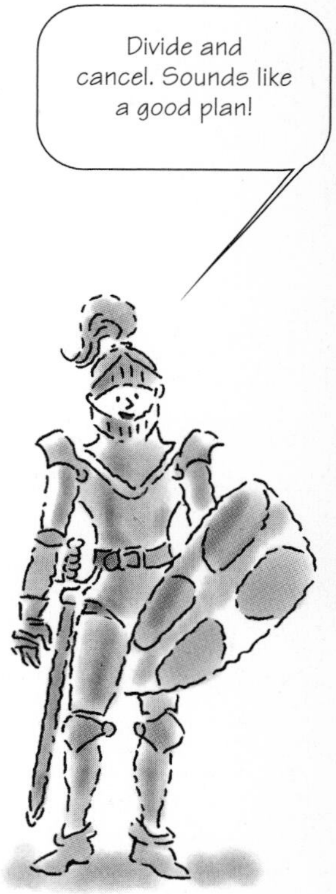
Divide and cancel. Sounds like a good plan!

• The amount of morphine to give the patient is 0.4 ml. To calculate the amount to be wasted, subtract the ordered dose from the entire contents of the syringe:

$$\begin{array}{rl} 1.0\text{ ml} = & 10\text{ mg morphine} \\ -\ 0.4\text{ ml} = & 4\text{ mg morphine} \\ \hline 0.6\text{ ml} = & 6\text{ mg morphine} \end{array}$$

The amount of morphine to be discarded is 0.6 ml. (Remember to have another nurse witness the drug's disposal and co-sign the controlled substances record, following your facility's protocol.)

Medrol milligram mystery

The doctor orders *100 mg methylprednisolone (Solu-Medrol) I.M. q4h* for your patient with asthma. The vial contains 120 mg/ml. How much Solu-Medrol should you give?

Here's how to solve this problem using ratios.

• Set up the first ratio with the known Solu-Medrol concentration:

$$120\text{ mg} : 1\text{ ml}$$

• Set up the second ratio with the desired dose and the unknown amount of Solu-Medrol:

$$100\text{ mg} : X$$

- Put these ratios into a proportion:

$$120 \text{ mg} : 1 \text{ ml} :: 100 \text{ mg} : X$$

- Set up an equation by multiplying the means and extremes:

$$100 \text{ mg} \times 1 \text{ ml} = 120 \text{ mg} \times X$$

- Solve for X by dividing each side of the equation by 120 mg and canceling units that appear in both the numerator and denominator:

$$\frac{100 \cancel{\text{mg}} \times 1 \text{ ml}}{120 \cancel{\text{mg}}} = \frac{\cancel{120 \text{ mg}} \times X}{\cancel{120 \text{ mg}}}$$

$$\frac{100 \text{ ml}}{120} = X$$

$$X = 0.83 \text{ ml}$$

You should give the patient 0.83 ml of Solu-Medrol.

Vial trial

The doctor prescribes *100 mg of gentamicin I.M.* for your patient. The vial available contains 40 mg/ml. How much gentamicin should you give?

Here's how to solve this problem using ratios:

- Set up the first ratio with the known gentamicin concentration:

$$40 \text{ mg} : 1 \text{ ml}$$

- Set up the second ratio with the desired dose and the unknown amount of gentamicin:

$$100 \text{ mg} : X$$

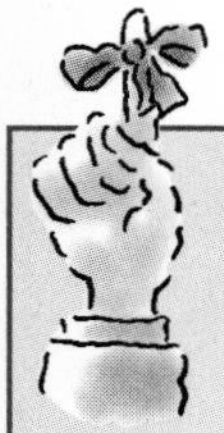

Memory jogger

When you're working with ratios and proportions, the trick is to keep like units in the same position on both sides of the proportion:

120 **mg** : 1 **ml** :: 100 **mg** : ***X*** **ml**

Remember to multiply the means and extremes:

means = **m**iddle numbers

extremes = **e**nd numbers.

Finally, isolate ***X*** to solve the problem:

Divide each side of the equation by the number you want to eliminate so that ***X*** is by itself, then cancel units that appear in both the numerator and denominator.

Dosage drill

Test your math skills with this drill.

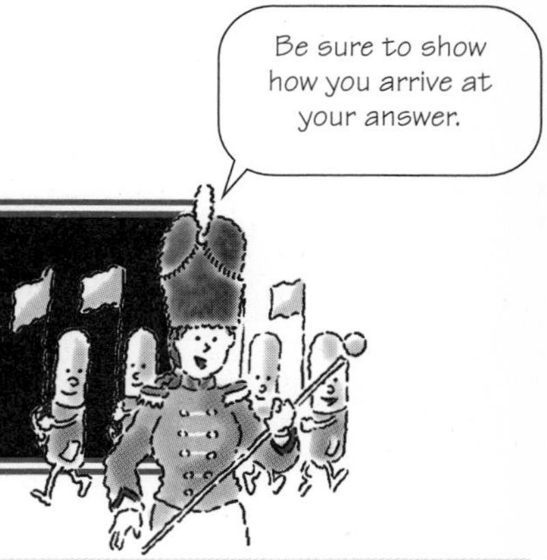
Be sure to show how you arrive at your answer.

The doctor orders furosemide (Lasix) 40 mg I.V. STAT for your patient with heart failure. The vial contains 10 mg/ml. How much furosemide should you give?

Your answer: ____________________

To find the answer, first set up a proportion.

$$10 \text{ mg} : 1 \text{ ml} :: 40 \text{ mg} : X$$

Set up the equation by multiplying the means and extremes.

$$10 \text{ mg} \times X = 40 \text{ mg} \times 1 \text{ ml}$$

Solve for *X*.

$$\frac{\cancel{10 \text{ mg}} \times X}{\cancel{10 \text{ mg}}} = \frac{40 \cancel{\text{ mg}} \times 1 \text{ ml}}{10 \cancel{\text{ mg}}}$$

$$\frac{40 \text{ ml}}{10} = X$$

$$X = 4 \text{ ml}$$

• Put these ratios into a proportion:

$$40 \text{ mg} : 1 \text{ ml} :: 100 \text{ mg} : X$$

• Set up an equation by multiplying the means and extremes:

$$1 \text{ ml} \times 100 \text{ mg} = 40 \text{ mg} \times X$$

• Solve for X by dividing each side of the equation by 40 mg and canceling units that appear in both the numerator and denominator:

$$\frac{1 \text{ ml} \times 100 \cancel{\text{mg}}}{40 \cancel{\text{mg}}} = \frac{\cancel{40 \text{ mg}} \times X}{\cancel{40 \text{ mg}}}$$

$$\frac{100 \text{ ml}}{40} = X$$

$$X = 2.5 \text{ ml}$$

You should give the patient 2.5 ml of gentamicin.

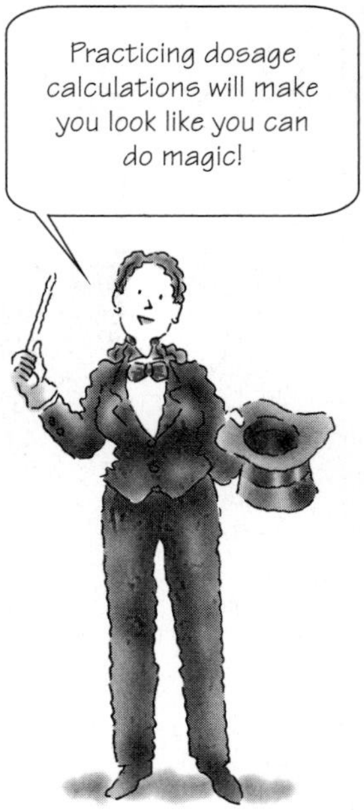

Practicing dosage calculations will make you look like you can do magic!

Interpreting drug labels

Before you can safely administer a parenteral drug, you must know how to read its label. (See *A close look at a label.*) Parenteral drugs are packaged in glass ampules, in single- or multiple-dose vials with rubber stoppers, and in prefilled syringes and cartridges. The packaging will clearly state that the drugs are used for injection.

A close look at a label

The label below shows the information you need to know to safely administer a parenteral drug.

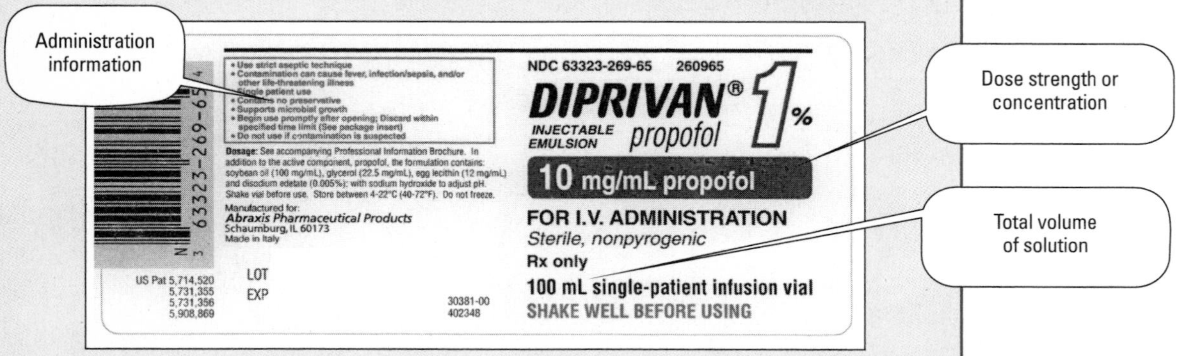

Dosage drill

Test your math skills with this drill.

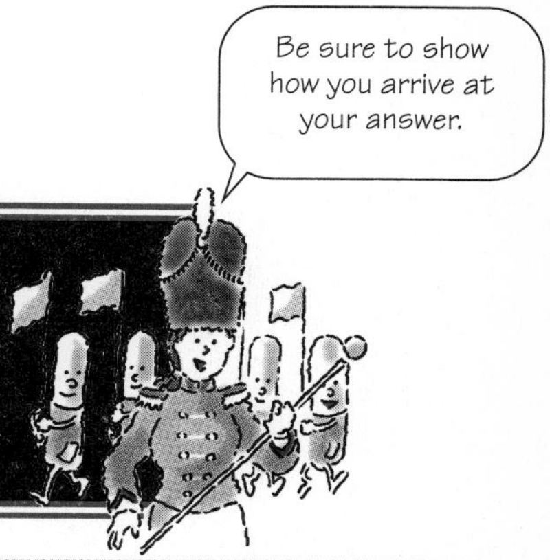
Be sure to show how you arrive at your answer.

The doctor orders metoprolol (Lopressor) 5 mg I.V. q 2 minutes for three doses for your patient with an acute myocardial infarction. The ampule contains 1 mg/ml. How many milliliters of metoprolol should you administer with each dose?

Your answer: ______________________

To find the answer, first set up a proportion, substituting X for the unknown amount of medication in milliliters.

$$5 \text{ mg} : X :: 1 \text{ mg} : 1 \text{ ml}$$

Set up an equation by multiplying the means and extremes.

$$1 \text{ mg} \times X = 5 \text{ mg} \times 1 \text{ ml}$$

Now solve for X.

$$\frac{1 \cancel{\text{mg}} \times X}{1 \cancel{\text{mg}}} = \frac{5 \cancel{\text{mg}} \times 1 \text{ ml}}{1 \cancel{\text{mg}}}$$

$$\frac{5 \text{ ml}}{1} = X$$

$$X = 5 \text{ ml}$$

Looking at labels

Reading the label of a parenteral solution is a lot like reading an oral solution label. Here's the information you'll see:

- trade name
- generic name
- total volume of solution in the container
- dose strength or concentration (drug dose present in a volume of solution)
- approved routes of administration
- expiration date
- special instructions, as needed.

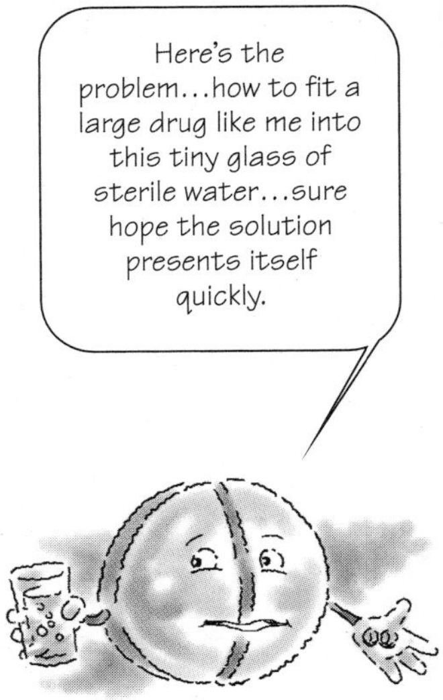

Here's the problem...how to fit a large drug like me into this tiny glass of sterile water...sure hope the solution presents itself quickly.

Solution components

A solute is a liquid or solid form of a drug. A solution is a liquid that contains a solute dissolved in a diluent or solvent, most commonly sterile water. Normal saline solution is a solution of salt (the solute) in purified water (the solvent).

Solution strengths

Solutions come in different strengths, which are expressed on the drug label as percentage solutions or ratio solutions. (See *Interpreting percentage solutions.*)

Interpreting percentage solutions

You can determine the contents of a weight per volume (W/V) or volume per volume (V/V) percentage solution by reading the label, as shown here.

What the label says	What the solution contains
0.9% (W/V) NaCl	0.9 g of sodium chloride in 100 ml of finished solution
5% (W/V) boric acid solution	5 g of boric acid in 100 ml of finished solution
5% (W/V) dextrose	5 g of dextrose in 100 ml of finished solution
2% (V/V) hydrogen peroxide	2 ml of hydrogen peroxide in 100 ml of finished solution
70% (V/V) isopropyl alcohol	70 ml of isopropyl alcohol in 100 ml of finished solution
10% (V/V) glycerin	10 ml of glycerin in 100 ml of finished solution

Percentage solutions: Always part of 100

A clear way to label or describe a solution is as a percentage. Providing information in percentages makes it easy to make dosage calculations, dilutions, or alterations.

On the label, a solution may be expressed either as weight per volume (W/V) or volume per volume (V/V).

In a W/V solution, the percentage or strength refers to the number of grams (the weight) of solute per 100 ml (the volume) of finished, or reconstituted, solution. With a V/V solution, the percentage refers to the number of milliliters of solute per 100 ml of finished solution.

Here's how to express these two relationships mathematically:

$$\% = \frac{\text{weight}}{\text{volume}} = \text{grams solute/100 ml finished solution}$$

$$\% = \frac{\text{volume}}{\text{volume}} = \text{milliliters solute/100 ml finished solution}$$

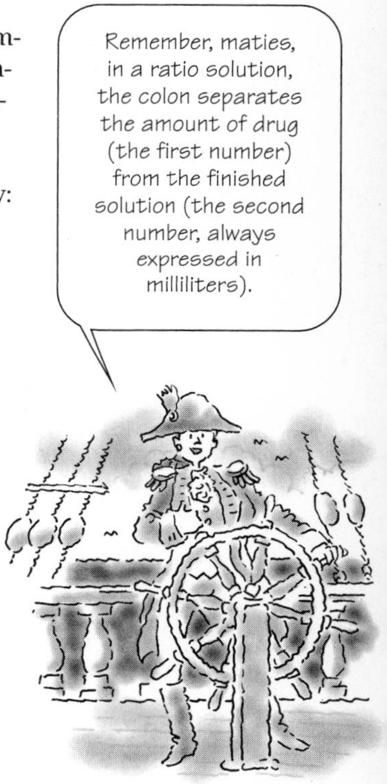
Remember, maties, in a ratio solution, the colon separates the amount of drug (the first number) from the finished solution (the second number, always expressed in milliliters).

Horatio ratio solutions: Parts one and two

Another way to label or describe a solution is as a ratio. (See *Interpreting ratio solutions.*) The strength of a ratio solution is usually expressed as two numbers separated by a colon. In a weight per volume (W:V) solution, the first number signifies the amount of a drug in grams. In a volume per volume (V:V) solution, the first number signifies the amount of drug in milliliters; the second signifies the volume of finished solution in milliliters.

This relationship is expressed as:

$$\text{Ratio} = \text{amount of drug : amount of finished solution}$$

Interpreting ratio solutions

You can determine the contents of a weight per volume (W : V) or volume per volume (V : V) ratio solution from what's on the label, as shown here.

What the label says	What the solution contains
benzalkonium chloride 1 : 750 (W : V)	1 g of benzalkonium chloride in 750 ml of finished solution
silver nitrate 1 : 100 (W : V)	1 g of silver nitrate in 100 ml of finished solution
hydrogen peroxide 2 : 100 (V : V)	2 ml of hydrogen peroxide in 100 ml of finished solution
glycerin 10 : 100 (V : V)	10 ml of glycerin in 100 ml of finished solution

Insulin and unit-based drugs

Some drugs, such as insulin, heparin, and penicillin G, are measured in units. The unit system is based on an international standard of drug potency, not on weight. The number of units appears on the drug label. (See *Look for the unit label.*)

Insisting on insulin

The body needs insulin, a potent hormone produced by the pancreas, to regulate carbohydrate metabolism. The effect of insulin's activity is reflected in blood glucose levels. A lack of insulin or insulin resistance causes diabetes. (See *Differentiating diabetes.*)

Each year, about 1.5 million patients are diagnosed with diabetes in the United States. Chances are, at some point, you'll need to give an insulin injection or teach a patient how to inject himself.

Insulin is injected subQ in patients with chronic diabetes or I.V. in patients with acute diabetic ketoacidosis or in those who are critically ill and require tight glycemic control. You must calculate and administer insulin doses carefully because even a small error can cause a hypoglycemic or hyperglycemic reaction.

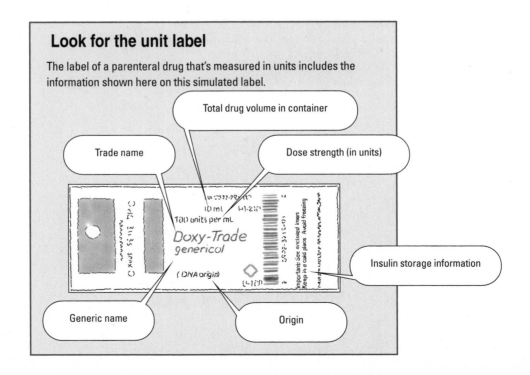

Look for the unit label

The label of a parenteral drug that's measured in units includes the information shown here on this simulated label.

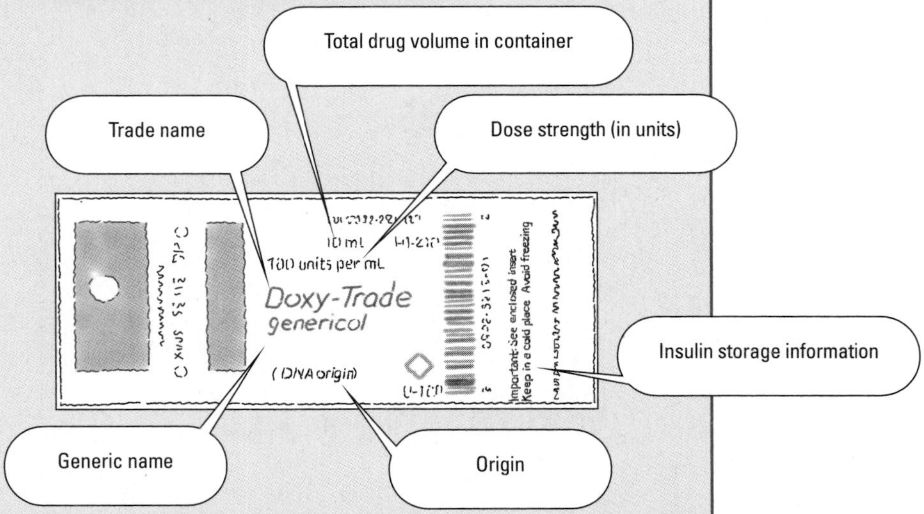

Differentiating diabetes

Diabetes is classified according to two major types: type 1 and type 2.

Type 1

In type 1 diabetes (also known as *juvenile or insulin-dependent diabetes*), the pancreas makes little or no insulin. Patients are typically diagnosed before age 20 and require long-term insulin therapy.

Type 2

In type 2 diabetes, the pancreas produces some insulin, but it's either too little or ineffective. This type of diabetes (also known as *adult-onset* or *non-insulin-dependent diabetes*) commonly affects patients older than age 40, although the incidence among children is rising. Type 2 diabetes can be controlled by diet and oral antidiabetic agents; however, insulin may be needed to stabilize blood glucose levels.

Before you give that drug

Heparin hazards

Heparin comes in many concentrations. Make sure that the heparin concentration is appropriate for the intended use.

Dosage calculation errors with heparin can cause excessive bleeding or undertreatment of a clotting disorder.

Hip to heparin

The anticoagulant heparin is used in moderate doses to prevent thrombosis and embolism, and in large doses to treat these disorders. Like insulin, it requires careful calculation and administration to prevent complications. (See *Heparin hazards.*)

Types of insulin

Several types of insulin are available. The doctor chooses a particular type based on the patient's diet and activity level and disease severity.

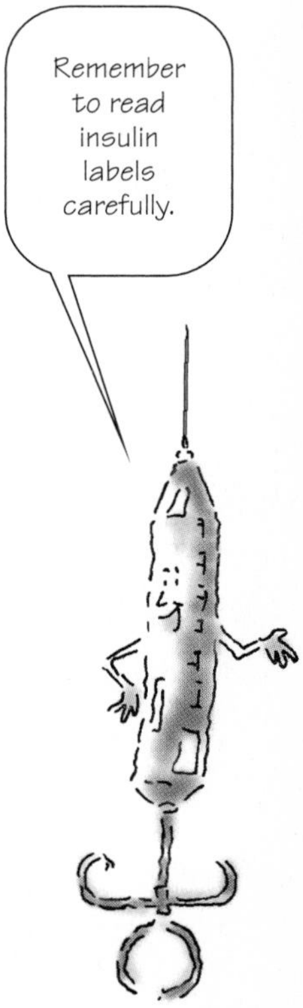
Remember to read insulin labels carefully.

Deducing the derivation

Insulin is classified according to its action time and origin. Insulins are identical to human insulin or are produced by recombinant deoxyribonucleic acid techniques. The origin appears on the drug label.

Insulin initials

Some insulin labels also contain an initial after the trade name, indicating the type of insulin. These different types of insulin vary in onset, peak, and duration of action. The initials are:

- R for regular insulin
- N for neutral protamine Hagedorn (NPH) insulin.

Each in its own time

Insulin preparations are modified by combination with larger, insoluble protein molecules to slow absorption and prolong activity. Thus, the different types of insulin vary in pharmacokinetic properties.

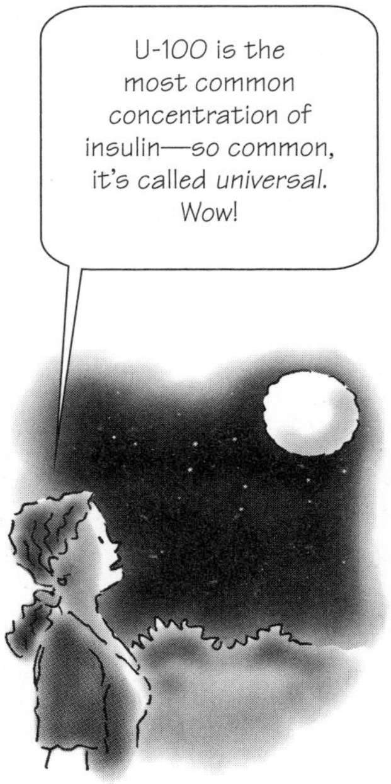
U-100 is the most common concentration of insulin—so common, it's called *universal*. Wow!

What dose do U want?

Insulin doses, expressed in units, are available in two concentrations. U-100 insulin, which contains 100 units of insulin per milliliter, is called universal because it's the most common concentration. U-500 insulin, which contains 500 units/ml, is used on rare occasions when a patient needs an unusually large dose.

Insulin syringes

A U-100 syringe, the only type of insulin syringe available in the United States, is calibrated so that 1 ml holds 100 units of insulin. A low-dose U-100 syringe, holding 50 units of insulin or less, is also used for some patients. Another low-dose U-100 syringe holds 30 units of insulin or less.

Selecting an insulin syringe

These syringes are examples of the different dose-specific insulin syringes that are available. The 1-ml U-100 syringe delivers up to 100 units of insulin. The low-dose 3⁄10-ml and 1⁄2-ml syringes deliver up to 30 or 50 units of U-100 insulin.

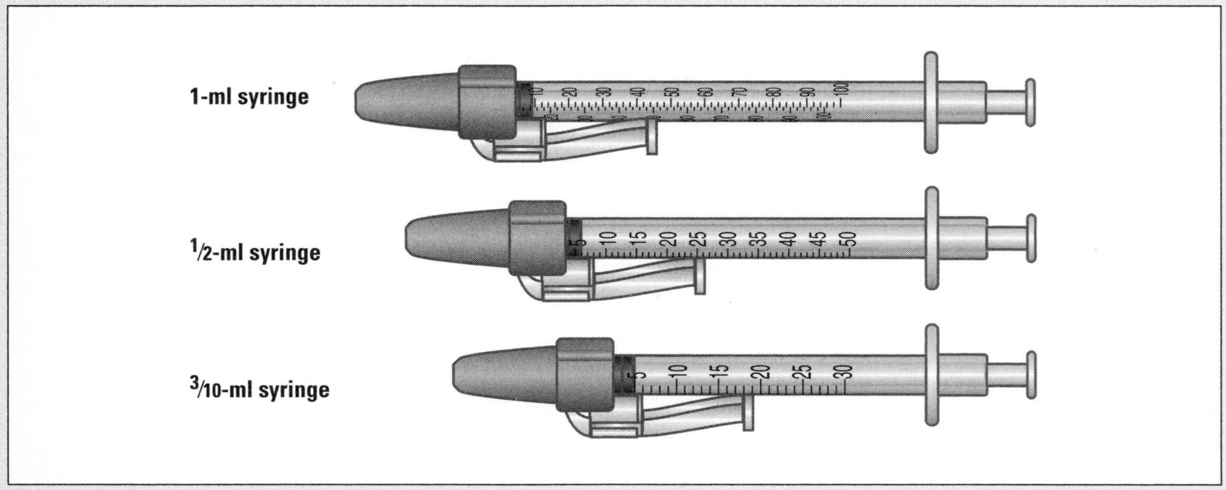

Because no syringes are made for it, U-500 insulin must also be administered with a U-100 syringe. Therefore, exercise caution when administering this drug. (See *Selecting an insulin syringe.*)

Reading insulin orders

Sometimes insulin doses are based on home monitoring of the patient's blood glucose values with glucometers. When a diagnosis of diabetes is first made, however, the patient undergoes tests to determine blood and urine glucose levels. Usually, he's enrolled in an outpatient center where he can be educated about diet, exercise, monitoring blood glucose levels, and insulin administration. Blood and urine glucose baselines are established.

Based on these determinations, the doctor may order small doses of rapid-acting insulin to be given at set times, such as every 4 hours or before meals and at bedtime, for several days. After a stable 24-hour dosage has been determined, the doctor may order dosage adjustments, such as one or two daily doses of intermediate-

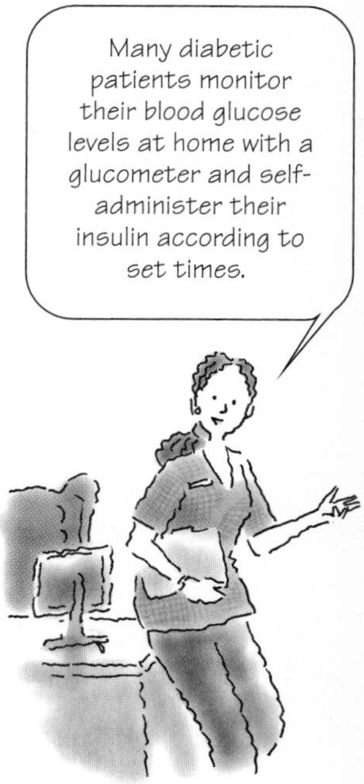

Many diabetic patients monitor their blood glucose levels at home with a glucometer and self-administer their insulin according to set times.

Insulin action times

Insulin preparations are modified through combination with larger insoluble protein molecules to slow absorption and prolong activity. An insulin preparation may be rapid acting, regular acting, intermediate acting, or long acting, as shown in the table below.

Drug	Onset	Peak	Duration
Rapid acting			
insulin lispro, insulin aspart, insulin glulisine	Less than 15 min	1 to 2 hr	3 to 4 hr
Regular acting			
regular insulin	30 min to 1 hr	2 to 3 hr	3 to 6 hr
Intermediate acting			
isophane insulin suspension (NPH)	1 to 2 hr	4 to 12 hr	18 to 24 hr
Long acting			
insulin detemir	1 to 2 hr	Flat	Up to 24 hr
insulin glargine (Lantus)	1 to 2 hr	None	24 hr

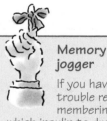

acting insulin, possibly accompanied by small doses of rapid-acting insulin. (See *Insulin action times*, page 233.)

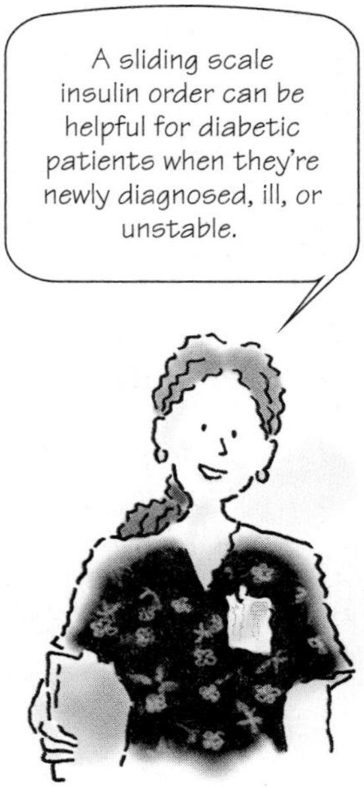
A sliding scale insulin order can be helpful for diabetic patients when they're newly diagnosed, ill, or unstable.

Insulin on a sliding scale

For a newly diagnosed, ill, or unstable diabetic patient, the doctor may write an order on a sliding scale. This type of order individualizes the insulin doses and administration times according to the patient's age, activity level, work habits, desired degree of blood glucose level control, and response to insulin preparations.

This is an example of such an order:

Start regular insulin sliding scale:

Blood glucose values:	*Insulin dose:*
Less than 180 mg/dl	*No insulin*
180 to 240 mg/dl	*10 units regular insulin subQ*
241 to 400 mg/dl	*20 units regular insulin subQ*
Greater than 400 mg/dl	*Call doctor for orders.*

Making connections with the dots

When reading insulin orders, check closely for decimal points that indicate unusual doses.

If an order doesn't include the dose strength, then administer U-100 insulin, the universal strength. If U-500 insulin is needed, the doctor specifies this on the order.

Combining insulins

Sometimes the doctor will order regular insulin mixed with NPH insulin to be injected together at the same site. When you receive an order for these drugs, draw them into the same syringe, following this procedure:

- Read the insulin order carefully.
- Read the vial labels carefully, noting the type, concentration, source, and expiration date of the drugs.
- Roll the NPH vial between your palms to mix it thoroughly.
- Choose the appropriate syringe.
- Clean the tops of both vials of insulin with an antiseptic swab.
- Inject air into the NPH vial equal to the amount of insulin you need to give. Withdraw the needle and syringe, but don't withdraw any NPH insulin.
- Inject into the regular insulin vial an amount of air equal to the dose of the regular insulin. Then invert or tilt the vial and withdraw the prescribed amount of regular insulin into the syringe. Draw the clear, regular insulin first to avoid contamination by the cloudy, longer-acting insulin.
- Clean the top of the NPH vial again with an antiseptic swab. Then insert the needle of the syringe containing the regular insulin into the vial, and withdraw the prescribed amount of NPH insulin.

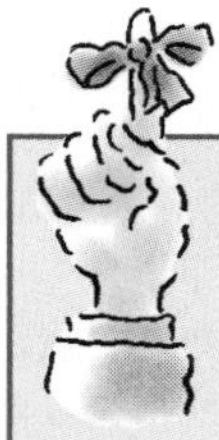

Memory jogger

If you have trouble remembering which insulin to draw first, think of the phrase "clear before cloudy." (Who doesn't prefer a clear day to a cloudy day?)

This phrase also reminds you how these drugs work: A clear day seems short, but a cloudy day seems to go on forever. Clear, regular insulin is short-acting and cloudy, NPH insulin is long-acting.

- Mix the insulins in the syringe by pulling back slightly on the plunger and tilting the syringe back and forth.
- Recheck the drug order.
- Have a second nurse verify the withdrawn dose and co-sign the medication administration record.
- Verify the patient's identity using two patient identifiers.
- Administer the insulin immediately.

Real world problems

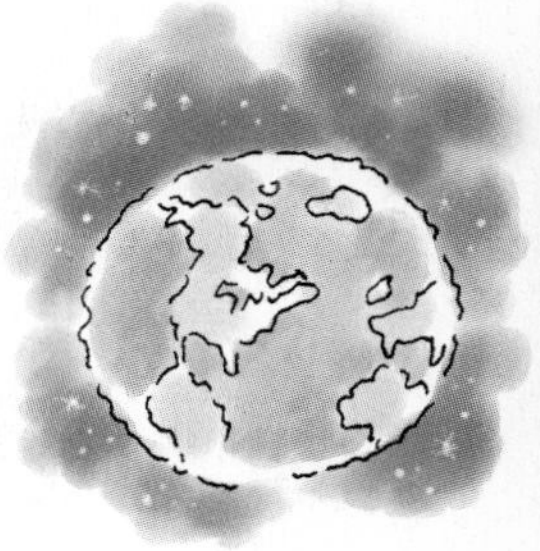

Before drawing up and administering insulin, heparin, or other drugs measured in units, check all your calculations for accuracy. The following examples show how to use the proportion method and a sliding scale to calculate insulin and heparin doses.

Help! How much heparin?

The doctor orders *7,000 units of heparin subQ q12h.* The heparin you have available contains 10,000 units/ml. How many milliliters of heparin should you give?

This is the calculation using ratios.

- Set up the first ratio with the known heparin concentration:

$$10{,}000 \text{ units} : 1 \text{ ml}$$

- Set up the second ratio with the desired dose and the unknown amount of heparin:

$$7{,}000 \text{ units} : X$$

- Put these ratios into a proportion:

$$10{,}000 \text{ units} : 1 \text{ ml} :: 7{,}000 \text{ units} : X$$

- Set up an equation by multiplying the means and extremes:

$$1 \text{ ml} \times 7{,}000 \text{ units} = 10{,}000 \text{ units} \times X$$

- Solve for X by dividing each side of the equation by 10,000 units and canceling units that appear in both the numerator and denominator:

$$\frac{1 \text{ ml} \times 7{,}000 \cancel{\text{units}}}{10{,}000 \cancel{\text{units}}} = \frac{\cancel{10{,}000 \text{ units}} \times X}{\cancel{10{,}000 \text{ units}}}$$

$$X = 0.7 \text{ ml}$$

You should give the patient 0.7 ml of heparin.

U-nsure about insulin?

The doctor prescribes *20 units of U-100 regular insulin.* What is the equivalent in milliliters?

Dosage drill

Test your math skills with this drill.

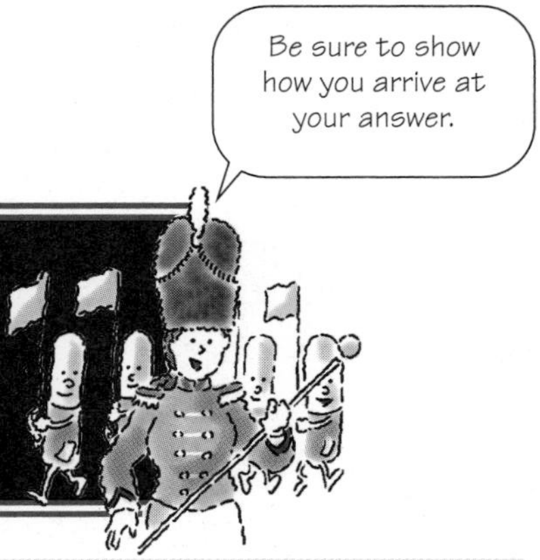
Be sure to show how you arrive at your answer.

The doctor orders heparin 5,000 units I.V. now for your patient admitted with a deep vein thrombosis. The heparin you have available contains 1,000 units/ml. How many milliliters of heparin should you give?

Your answer: ______________________

To find the answer, first set up a proportion, substituting X for the unknown amount of medication in milliliters.

$$5{,}000 \text{ units} : X :: 1{,}000 \text{ units} : 1 \text{ ml}$$

Set up an equation by multiplying the means and extremes.

$$1{,}000 \text{ units} \times X = 5{,}000 \text{ units} \times 1 \text{ ml}$$

Solve for X.

$$\frac{\cancel{1{,}000 \text{ units}} \times X}{\cancel{1{,}000 \text{ units}}} = \frac{5{,}000 \cancel{\text{ units}} \times 1 \text{ ml}}{1{,}000 \cancel{\text{ units}}}$$

$$\frac{5{,}000 \text{ ml}}{1{,}000} = X$$

$$X = 5 \text{ ml}$$

The nurse should give 5 ml.

Insulin sliding scale

Insulin doses may be based on blood glucose levels, as shown in this table.

Blood glucose level	Insulin dose
Less than 200 mg/dl	No insulin
201 to 250 mg/dl	2 units regular insulin
251 to 300 mg/dl	4 units regular insulin
301 to 350 mg/dl	6 units regular insulin
351 to 400 mg/dl	8 units regular insulin
Greater than 400 mg/dl	Call doctor for insulin order.

This is the calculation using fractions.

- Set up the first fraction with the known insulin concentrations:

$$\frac{100 \text{ units}}{1 \text{ ml}}$$

- Set up the second fraction with the unknown amount of insulin in milliliters and the desired dose:

$$\frac{20 \text{ units}}{X}$$

- Put these fractions into a proportion:

$$\frac{100 \text{ units}}{1 \text{ ml}} = \frac{20 \text{ units}}{X}$$

- Cross-multiply the fractions:

$$100 \text{ units} \times X = 20 \text{ units} \times 1 \text{ ml}$$

- Solve for X by dividing each side of the equation by 100 units and canceling units that appear in both the numerator and denominator:

$$\frac{\cancel{100 \text{ units}} \times X}{\cancel{100 \text{ units}}} = \frac{20 \cancel{\text{ units}} \times 1 \text{ ml}}{100 \cancel{\text{ units}}}$$

$$X = 0.2 \text{ ml}$$

The equivalent is 0.2 ml of regular insulin.

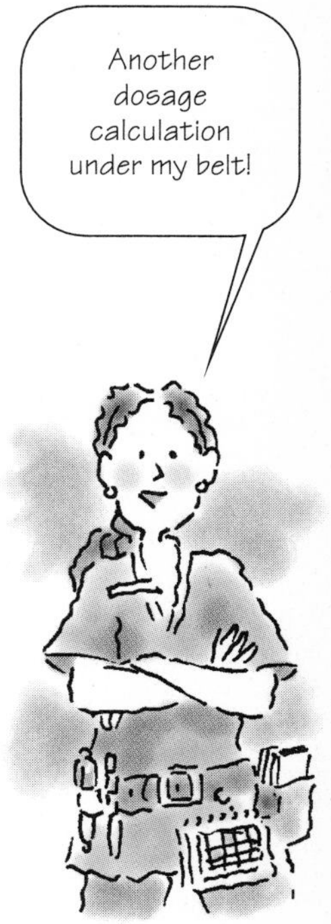
Another dosage calculation under my belt!

Insulin on a sliding scale

Your patient's blood glucose is 384 mg/dl. Based on the sliding scale above, how much insulin should you give him? (See *Insulin sliding scale.*)

You should administer 8 units of regular insulin.

Reconstituting powders

Some drugs — such as levothyroxine sodium (Synthroid) and penicillins — are manufactured and packaged as powders because they become unstable quickly when they're in solution. When the doctor prescribes such a drug, either you or the pharmacist must reconstitute it before it can be administered.

The strength of one or many

Powders come in single-strength or multiple-strength formulations. A single-strength powder — such as levothyroxine sodium — may be reconstituted to only one dose strength per administration route, as specified by the manufacturer. A multiple-strength powder — such as penicillin — can be reconstituted to various dose strengths by adjusting the amounts of diluent.

When reconstituting a multiple-strength powder, check the drug label or package insert for the dose-strength options and choose the one that's closest to the ordered dose strength.

How to reconstitute

Follow the general guidelines described here when reconstituting a powder for injection.

Learn from the label

Begin by checking the label of the powder container. The label tells you the quantity of drug in a vial or ampule, the amount and type of diluent to add to the powder, and the strength and expiration date of the resulting solution.

Fluid out exceeds fluid in

When a diluent is added to a powder, the fluid volume increases. That's why the label calls for less diluent than the total volume of the prepared solution. For example, the instructions may say to add 1.7 ml of diluent to a vial of powdered drug to obtain 2 ml of prepared solution.

Check out the chambers

Some drugs that need reconstitution are packaged in vials with two chambers separated by a rubber stopper. The upper chamber contains the diluent, and the lower chamber contains the powdered drug. (See *Two chambers [one's a powder room!].*)

When you depress the top of the vial, the stopper dislodges, allowing the diluent to flow into the lower chamber, where it can mix with the powdered drug. Then you can remove the correct amount of solution with a syringe.

Two chambers (one's a powder room!)

Some drugs that require reconstitution are packaged in vials with two chambers separated by a rubber stopper. In the illustration below, note that the upper chamber contains the diluent and the lower chamber contains the powder. The plunger is depressed to inject the diluent into the powder.

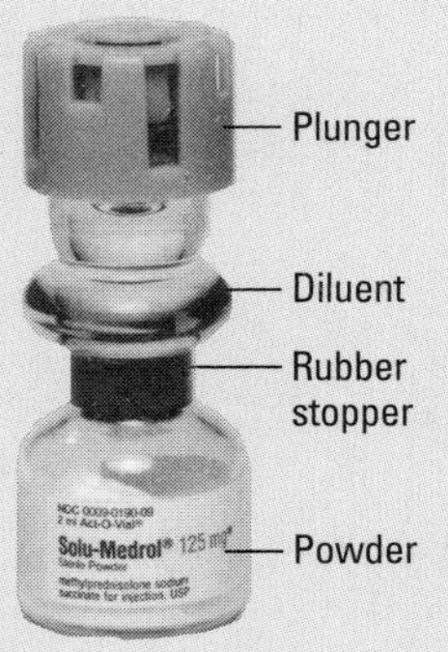

Say it with an equation

To determine how much solution to give, refer to the drug label for information about the dose strength of the prepared solution. For example, to give 500 mg of a drug when the dose strength of the solution is 1 g (or 1,000 mg)/10 ml, set up a proportion with fractions as follows:

$$\frac{X}{500 \text{ mg}} = \frac{10 \text{ ml}}{1{,}000 \text{ mg}}$$

If information about a drug's dose strength isn't on the label, check the package insert. The label or insert will also list the type and amount of diluent needed, the dose strength after reconstitution, and special instructions about administration and storage after reconstitution. (See *Inspect the insert,* page 240.)

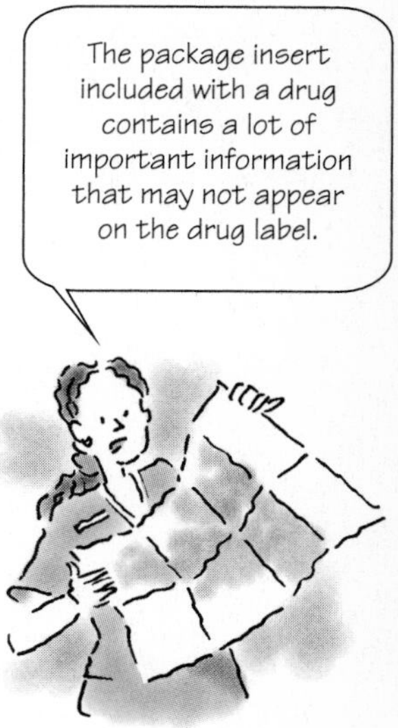
The package insert included with a drug contains a lot of important information that may not appear on the drug label.

Special considerations

When you reconstitute a powder that comes in multiple strengths, be especially careful in choosing the most appropriate strength for the prescribed dose.

Label logic

After you have reconstituted a drug, make sure you label it with the following information:

- your initials
- reconstitution date
- expiration date
- dose strength.

Real world problems

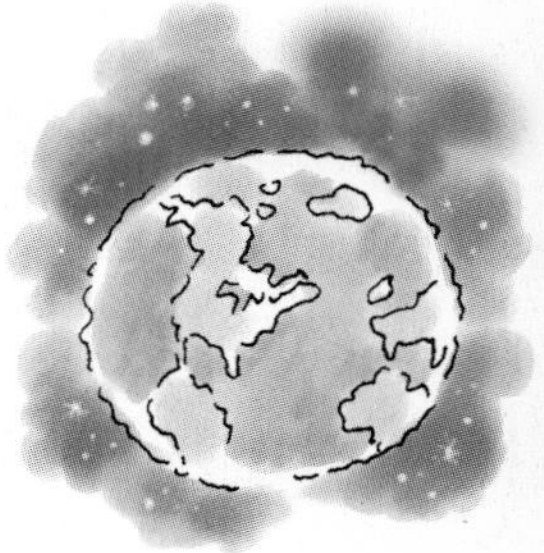

The following problems show how to calculate the amount of reconstituted drug to give a patient.

Penicillin puzzler (the solution is in the solution)

The doctor prescribes *100,000 units penicillin* for your patient, but the only available vial holds 1 million units. The drug label says to add 4.5 ml of normal saline solution to yield 1 million units/5 ml. How much solution should you administer after reconstitution?

Here's how to solve this problem using fractions.

- First, dilute the powder according to the instructions on the label. Then set up the first fraction with the known penicillin concentration:

$$\frac{1{,}000{,}000 \text{ units}}{5 \text{ ml}}$$

Before you give that drug!

Inspect the insert

The package inserts that are included with drugs commonly provide a great deal of information that may not be on the outer label. For example, the drug label for ceftazidime provides no information about reconstitution, but the package insert does. These are the possible diluent combinations as they appear in the package insert that comes with this drug.

Vial size	Diluent to be added	Approximate available	Approximate average concentration
I.M. or I.V. direct (bolus) injection			
500 mg	1.5 ml	1.8 ml	280 mg/ml
1 g	3 ml	3.6 ml	280 mg/ml
I.V. infusion			
500 mg	5.3 ml	5.7 ml	100 mg/ml
1 g	10 ml	10.8 ml	100 mg/ml
2 g	10 ml	11.5 ml	170 mg/ml

- Set up the second fraction with the desired dose and the unknown amount of solution:

$$\frac{100{,}000 \text{ units}}{X}$$

- Put these fractions into a proportion:

$$\frac{1{,}000{,}000 \text{ units}}{5 \text{ ml}} = \frac{100{,}000 \text{ units}}{X}$$

- Cross-multiply the fractions:

$$5 \text{ ml} \times 100{,}000 \text{ units} = X \times 1{,}000{,}000 \text{ units}$$

- Solve for X by dividing each side of the equation by 1 million units and canceling units that appear in both the numerator and denominator:

$$\frac{5 \text{ ml} \times 100{,}000 \cancel{\text{units}}}{1{,}000{,}000 \cancel{\text{units}}} = \frac{X \times \cancel{1{,}000{,}000 \text{ units}}}{\cancel{1{,}000{,}000 \text{ units}}}$$

$$X = \frac{500{,}000 \text{ ml}}{1{,}000{,}000}$$

$$X = 0.5 \text{ ml}$$

The amount of solution that yields 100,000 units of penicillin after reconstitution is 0.5 ml.

Deciphering diluents

Your patient needs 25 mg of gentamicin I.M. The label says to add 1.3 ml sterile diluent to yield 50 mg/1.5 ml. How many milliliters of reconstituted solution should you give the patient?

Here's how to solve this problem using ratios.

- First, dilute the powder according to the label instructions. Then set up the first ratio with the known gentamicin concentration:

$$50 \text{ mg} : 1.5 \text{ ml}$$

- Set up the second ratio with the desired dose and the unknown amount of solution:

$$25 \text{ mg} : X$$

- Put these ratios into a proportion:

$$50 \text{ mg} : 1.5 \text{ ml} :: 25 \text{ mg} : X$$

- Set up an equation by multiplying the means and extremes:

$$1.5 \text{ ml} \times 25 \text{ mg} = X \times 50 \text{ mg}$$

- Solve for X. Divide each side of the equation by 50 mg and cancel units that appear in both the numerator and denominator:

$$\frac{1.5 \text{ ml} \times 25 \cancel{\text{mg}}}{50 \cancel{\text{mg}}} = \frac{X \times \cancel{50 \text{ mg}}}{\cancel{50 \text{ mg}}}$$

$$X = \frac{37.5 \text{ ml}}{50}$$

$$X = 0.75 \text{ ml}$$

The patient should receive 0.75 ml of the solution.

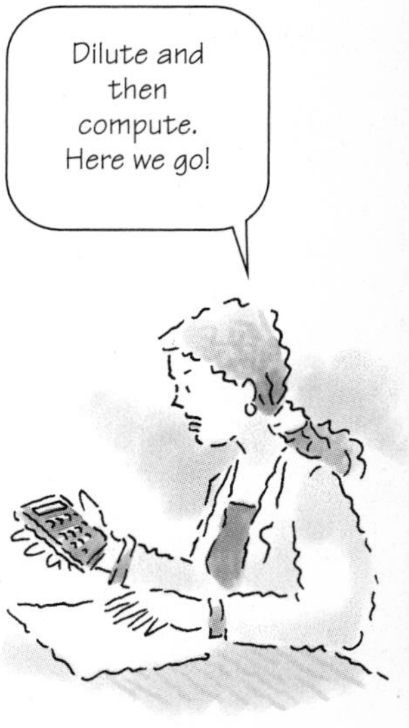
Dilute and then compute. Here we go!

Attaining the ampicillin answer

The doctor orders *500 mg ampicillin* for your patient. A 1-g vial of powdered ampicillin is available. The label says to add 4.5 ml sterile water to yield 1 g/5 ml. How many milliliters of reconstituted ampicillin should you give?

Here's how to solve this problem using fractions.

- First, dilute the powder according to the instructions on the label. Then set up the first fraction with the known ampicillin concentration (recall that 1 g equals 1,000 mg):

$$\frac{1{,}000 \text{ mg}}{5 \text{ ml}}$$

- Set up the second fraction with the desired dose and the unknown amount of solution:

$$\frac{500 \text{ mg}}{X}$$

Dosage drill

Test your math skills with this drill.

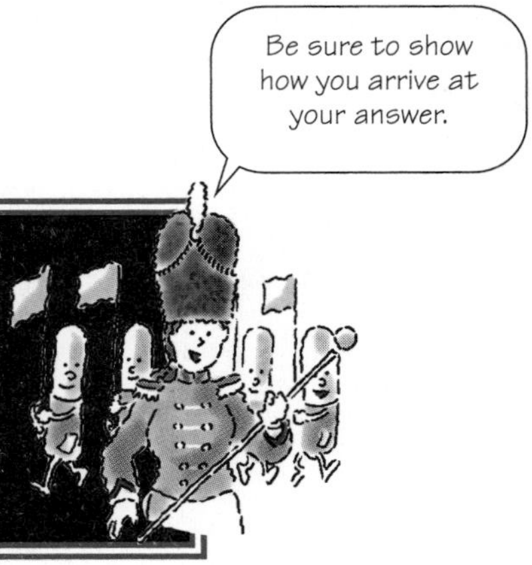
Be sure to show how you arrive at your answer.

The doctor orders acetazolamide 250 mg I.V. now to lower your patient's intraocular pressure. A 500-mg vial of powdered acetazolamide is available. The label says to add 5 ml of sterile water for injection to yield 100 mg/ml. How many milliliters of reconstituted acetazolamide should you give?

Your answer: ____________________

To find the answer, first set up a proportion, substituting *X* for the unknown amount of medication in milliliters.

$$250 \text{ mg} : X :: 100 \text{ mg} : 1 \text{ ml}$$

Set up an equation by multiplying the means and extremes.

$$100 \text{ mg} \times X = 250 \text{ mg} \times 1 \text{ ml}$$

Solve for *X*.

$$\frac{\cancel{100 \text{ mg}} \times X}{\cancel{100 \text{ mg}}} = \frac{250 \cancel{\text{ mg}} \times 1 \text{ ml}}{100 \cancel{\text{ mg}}}$$

$$\frac{2.5 \text{ ml}}{1} = X$$

$$X = 2.5 \text{ ml}$$

- Put these fractions into a proportion, making sure the same units of measure appear in both numerators. In this case, the units must be grams or milligrams. If you use milligrams, the proportion would be:

$$\frac{1{,}000 \text{ mg}}{5 \text{ ml}} = \frac{500 \text{ mg}}{X}$$

- Cross-multiply the fractions:

$$1{,}000 \text{ mg} \times X = 500 \text{ mg} \times 5 \text{ ml}$$

- Solve for X by dividing each side of the equation by 1,000 mg and canceling units that appear in both the numerator and denominator:

$$\frac{\cancel{1{,}000 \text{ mg}} \times X}{\cancel{1{,}000 \text{ mg}}} = \frac{500 \cancel{\text{ mg}} \times 5 \text{ ml}}{1{,}000 \cancel{\text{ mg}}}$$

$$X = \frac{2{,}500 \text{ ml}}{1{,}000}$$

$$X = 2.5 \text{ ml}$$

You should give the patient 2.5 ml of the solution, which will deliver 500 mg of ampicillin.

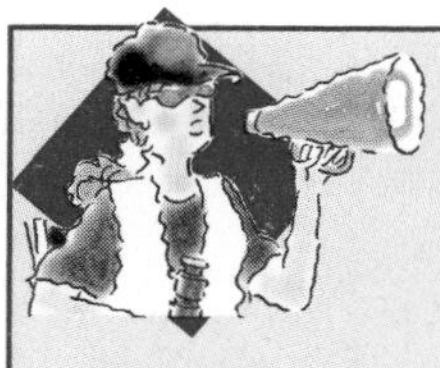

That's a wrap!

Calculating parenteral injections review

Keep these important points in mind when giving parenteral injections.

Intradermal injections

- This route is used to anesthetize the skin for invasive procedures and to test for allergies, tuberculosis, histoplasmosis, and other diseases.
- Amount of drug injected is less than 0.5 ml.
- Syringe and needle are a 1-ml syringe with a 25G to 27G needle that's ⅜″ to ⅝″ long.

SubQ injections

- Drugs commonly given subQ include insulin, heparin, tetanus toxoid, and some opioids.
- Amount of drug injected is 0.5 to 1 ml.
- Needle is 23G to 28G and ½″ to ⅝″ long.

I.M. injections

- This route is used for drugs that require quick absorption or those that are irritating to tissue.
- Amount of drug injected is 0.5 to 3 ml.
- Needles are 18G to 23G and 1″ to 3″ long.
- Before injection, aspirate for blood to make sure that the needle isn't in a vein.

Syringe types

- Standard syringes come in a variety of sizes (3, 5, 10, 20, 30, 50, and 60 ml).
- Tuberculin syringes (commonly used for intradermal injections) are 1-ml syringes marked to hundredths of a milliliter, allowing for accurate measurement of very small doses.

(continued)

Calculating parenteral injections review *(continued)*

- Prefilled syringes — sterile syringes that contain a premeasured drug dose — require a special holder (Carpuject) to release the drug from the cartridge.

Needle terminology
- Gauge: inside diameter of the needle (the smaller the gauge, the larger the diameter)
- Bevel: angle at which the needle tip is open (may be short, medium, or long)
- Length: distance from needle tip to hub (ranges from ⅜″ to 3″)

Important parts of a parenteral drug label
- Trade name
- Generic name
- Total volume of solution in the container
- Dose strength or concentration
- Approved routes of administration
- Expiration date
- Special instructions

Ratio solutions
- Solute is a drug in liquid or solid form that's added to a solvent (diluent) to make a solution.
- Solution is a liquid (usually sterile water) containing a dissolved solute.
- W:V solution: First number represents the amount of drug in grams; second number is the volume of finished solution in milliliters.
- V:V solution: First number is the amount of drug in milliliters; second number is the volume of finished solution in milliliters.

Insulin doses
- Measured in units
- Based on drug potency (not weight)
- Classified by origin (human or animal) and action time
- Most common (universal) concentration is U-100 insulin

Insulin action times
- Rapid acting: lispro, aspart, glulisine
- Regular acting
- Intermediate acting: lente, NPH
- Long acting: insulin detemir, insulin glargine

Powders for reconstitution
- The fluid volume increases with the added diluent.
- Single-strength powders are reconstituted to one dose strength per administration route.
- Multiple-strength powders are reconstituted to appropriate strengths by adjusting the amount of diluent.

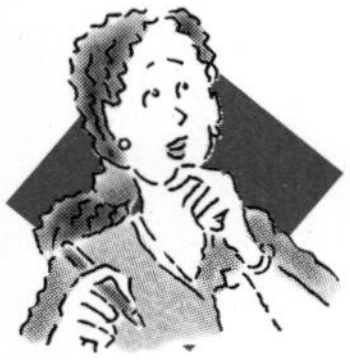

Quick quiz

1. To administer the medication in a prefilled syringe, you need:
  A. a Carpuject.
  B. a standard syringe.
  C. dead space.
  D. a tuberculin syringe.

Answer: A. Prefilled syringes come with a cartridge-needle unit and require a special holder called a Carpuject to release the drug from the cartridge.

2. You need to purge a prefilled syringe before administering a drug because:

A. the cartridge won't work otherwise.
B. the syringe may contain air.
C. doing so ensures needle patency.
D. doing so ensures more accurate dosing.

Answer: B. You must purge the air from a prefilled syringe. Because a small amount of drug is wasted during purging, most manufacturers add a little extra drug to prefilled syringes.

3. The only insulin that can be given I.V. is:

A. NPH.
B. insulin glargine.
C. lispro.
D. regular.

Answer: D. Regular insulin can be given I.V. NPH, insulin glargine, and lispro insulin must be given subQ.

4. The longest-acting insulin is:

A. regular.
B. insulin glargine.
C. lispro.
D. NPH.

Answer: B. Insulin glargine has a duration of 24 hours. Regular insulin lasts 6 to 8 hours, lispro lasts 3 to 4 hours, and NPH insulin lasts 18 to 24 hours.

5. The needle used for an intradermal injection is:

A. 25G to 27G and ⅜″ to ⅝″ long.
B. 14G to 18G and 1″ to 1½″ long.
C. 22G and ¾″ long.
D. 18G to 23G and 1″ to 3″ long.

Answer: A. A 1-ml syringe, calibrated in 0.01-ml increments, is usually used with this needle for an intradermal injection.

6. In a subQ injection, the drug is injected into the:

A. muscle.
B. tissue in the vastus lateralis.
C. tissue above the dermis.
D. tissue below the dermis.

Answer: D. A subQ injection delivers the drug into the subcutaneous tissue, located below the dermis but above the muscle.

7. A percentage solution can be expressed in terms of:

A. weight/volume and volume/volume.
B. weight/weight and volume/volume.
C. weight/weight and strength/volume.
D. grams/weight and milliliters/volume.

Answer: A. Percentage solutions are expressed as weight/volume or volume/volume. These are the clearest and most common ways to label or describe solutions.

8. When a diluent is added to a powder for injection, the fluid volume:

A. increases.
B. decreases.
C. stays the same.
D. always doubles.

Answer: A. When a diluent is added to a powder, the fluid volume increases. That's why the label calls for less diluent than the total volume of the prepared solution.

9. If information about a drug's dose strength isn't on the label:

A. call the doctor.
B. check the package insert.
C. mix it with 5 ml of normal saline solution.
D. ask your supervisor.

Answer: B. The package insert includes information about the drug's dose strength, the amount of diluent needed, the dose strength after reconstitution, and any special instructions.

Scoring

☆☆☆ If you answered all nine items correctly, bravo! You've earned the right to say to anyone, "This won't hurt a bit."

☆☆ If you answered six to eight items correctly, you're almost a parenteral powerhouse!

☆ If you answered fewer than six items correctly, okay! Remember the golden rule of dosage calculations: Keep things in proportion.

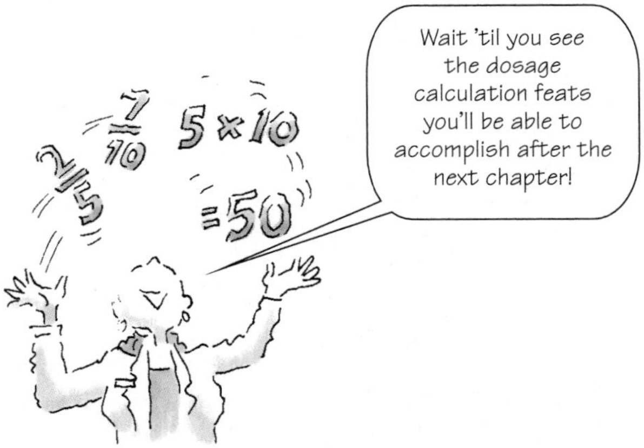

Wait 'til you see the dosage calculation feats you'll be able to accomplish after the next chapter!
7/10
5 × 10
= 50

13

Calculating I.V. infusions

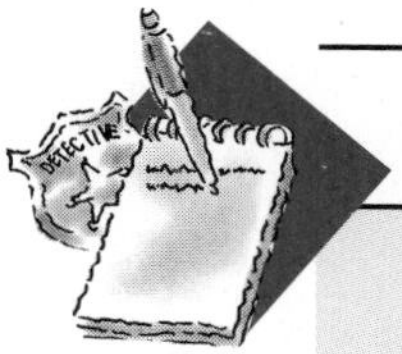

Just the facts

In this chapter, you'll learn:

- formulas for calculating drip rates and flow rates
- how to regulate an infusion manually and electronically
- how to calculate infusion time
- ways to calculate, monitor, and regulate infusions of blood, total parenteral nutrition, heparin, insulin, and electrolytes.

A look at I.V. infusions

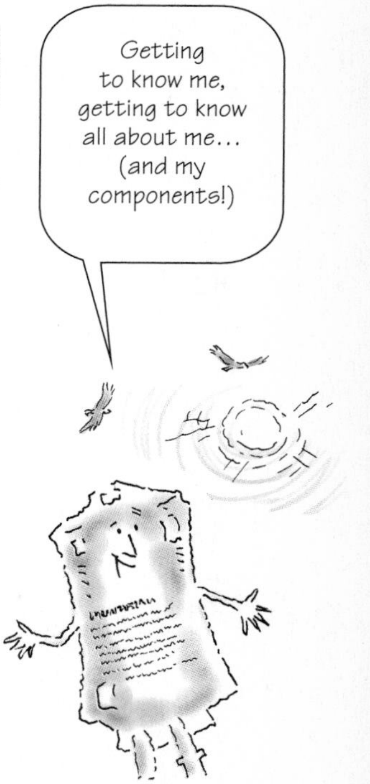

Getting to know me, getting to know all about me... (and my components!)

Careful administration of I.V. fluids is critical, especially when dealing with patients who are susceptible to fluid volume changes. Rapid infusion of I.V. fluids or blood products may seriously threaten your patient's health.

Work from the outside in

To administer I.V. fluids safely, you need information specifying how much fluid to give, the correct length of time for administration, the type of fluid, and what may be added to the fluid. Start by examining the outside of a full I.V. bag and learn to identify all its components. (See *Read the bag*, page 248.)

Next, you'll need to be able to select the proper tubing, calculate drip rates and flow rates, and become comfortable working with I.V. equipment such as electronic infusion devices. (See *Checking an I.V.*, page 248.)

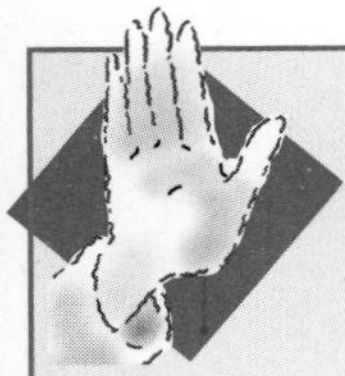

Before you give that drug!

Read the bag

The outside of an I.V. bag is an important source of information for calculating infusion rates and times. Read it carefully!

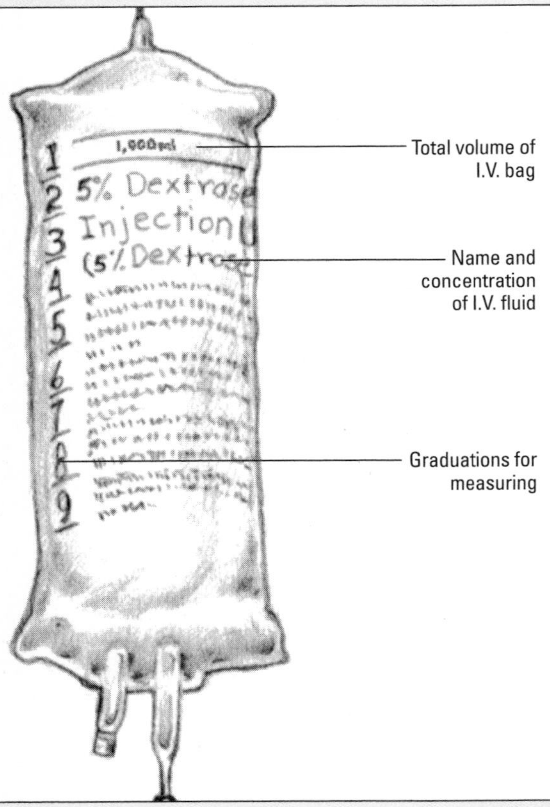

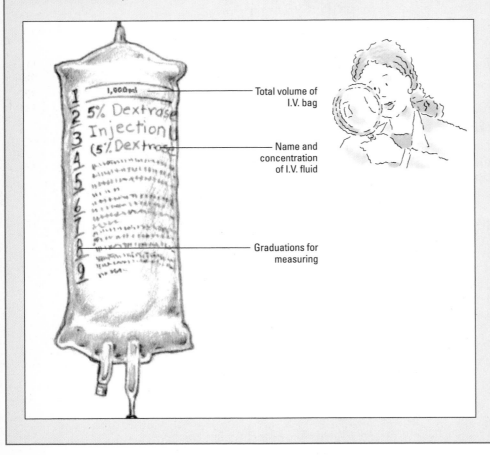

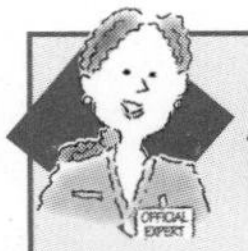

Advice from the experts

Checking an I.V.

You can save time by assessing your patient's I.V. infusion at the beginning of every shift. Performing checks early helps avoid confusion when your shift gets busy.

- Are the time, volume, and rate labeled correctly? If so, do they match the order?
- Check maintenance fluids and drug infusions, such as insulin, dopamine, and morphine. Are the additives correct? Are they in the right solutions?
- After calculating the drug dosage, check the bag again to verify that the solution is labeled with the time, name, and amount of drug added.
- If an electronic infusion device is being used, is it set correctly?
- Examine the tubing from the bag down to the patient to see whether the drug is infusing into the correct I.V. port. This is critical when a patient has multiple lines.

Administering I.V. fluids

To safely and accurately administer I.V. fluids to your patient, you must select the proper tubing. Selection of I.V. tubing plays an important role in calculating I.V. infusion rates.

Most facilities stock I.V. tubing in two sizes: microdrip and macrodrip. Microdrip tubing, as its name implies, delivers smaller drops than macrodrip. Microdrip also delivers more drops per minute.

Targeting the right tube

To decide the right size of tubing for your patient, you should first understand the purpose of the infusion and the desired infusion rate. If the infusion rate for a solution is relatively fast — for example, 125 ml/hour — select macrodrip tubing. If the infusion rate is relatively slow — for example, 40 ml/hour — select microdrip tubing. If you use macrodrip tubing for a slow infusion, maintaining accurate I.V. flow may be difficult if not impossible. (See *Tube tips*.)

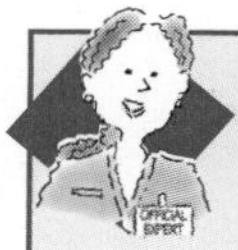

Advice from the experts

Tube tips

Follow these rules when selecting I.V. tubing:

- Use macrodrip tubing for infusions of at least 80 ml/hour.
- Use microdrip tubing for infusions of less than 80 ml/hour and for pediatric patients (to prevent fluid overload).
- With electronic infusion devices, select the tubing specifically made to work with those devices.

Calculating drip rates

Your next step is to determine the number of drops of solution you want to infuse per minute. In other words, you want to determine a *drip rate*.

To calculate the drip rate, you need to know the calibration for the I.V. tubing you've selected. Different I.V. solution sets deliver fluids at varying amounts per drop. The *drop factor* refers to the number of drops per milliliter of solution calibrated for an administration set.

The drop factor is listed on the package containing the I.V. tubing administration set. For a standard (macrodrip) administration set, the drop factor is usually 10, 15, or 20 gtt/ml (drops per milliliter). For a microdrip (minidrip) set, it's 60 gtt/ml. (See *Quick drip rate guide*, page 250.)

A formula dripping with success

One way to calculate the drip rate is to use the formula below:

$$\begin{array}{c}\text{Drip rate}\\\text{in drops/minute}\end{array} = \frac{\text{Total milliliters}}{\text{Total minutes}} \times \begin{array}{c}\text{Drop factor}\\\text{in drops/ml}\end{array}$$

The following two examples show how to calculate the drip rate using this formula.

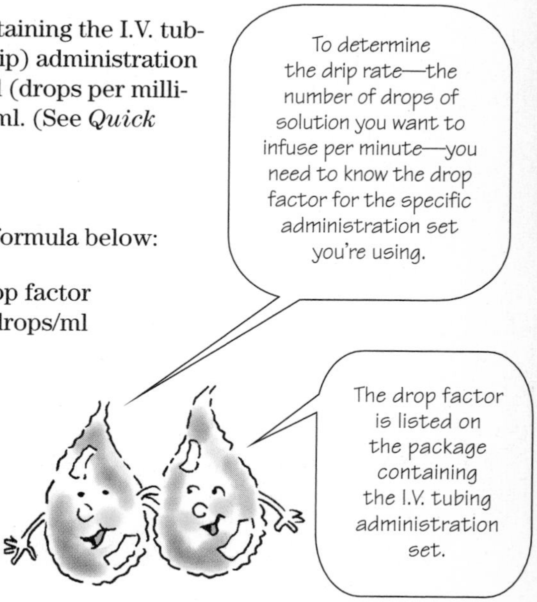
To determine the drip rate—the number of drops of solution you want to infuse per minute—you need to know the drop factor for the specific administration set you're using.
The drop factor is listed on the package containing the I.V. tubing administration set.

Doing the dextrose drip

Your patient needs an infusion of dextrose 5% in water (D_5W) at 125 ml/hour. If the tubing set is calibrated at 15 gtt/ml, what's the drip rate?

- First, convert 1 hour to 60 minutes to fit the formula.

Before you give that drug!

Quick drip rate guide

When calculating the drip rate of I.V. solutions, remember that the number of drops required to deliver 1 ml varies with the type of administration set and the manufacturer. To calculate the drip rate, you need to know the drop factor for each product. As a quick reference, consult the table below.

Manufacturer	**Drop factor**	**Drops/minute to infuse (drip rate)**					
		500 ml/24 hr	1,000 ml/24 hr	1,000 ml/20 hr	1,000 ml/10 hr	1,000 ml/8 hr	1,000 ml/6 hr
		21 ml/hr	42 ml/hr	50 ml/hr	100 ml/hr	125 ml/hr	166 ml/hr
Alaris	20 gtt/ml	7 gtt	14 gtt	17 gtt	34 gtt	42 gtt	56 gtt
Braun	15 gtt/ml	5 gtt	10 gtt	12 gtt	25 gtt	31 gtt	42 gtt
Hospira	15 gtt/ml	5 gtt	10 gtt	12 gtt	25 gtt	31 gtt	42 gtt

- Then set up a fraction. Place the volume of the infusion in the numerator. Place the number of minutes in which the volume is to be infused as the denominator:

$$\frac{125\text{ ml}}{60\text{ minutes}}$$

- To determine X—or the number of drops per minute to be infused— multiply the fraction by the drop factor. Cancel units that appear in both the numerator and denominator:

$$X = \frac{125\ \cancel{\text{ml}}}{60\text{ minutes}} \times \frac{15\text{ gtt}}{\cancel{\text{ml}}}$$

- Solve for X by dividing the numerator by the denominator:

$$X = \frac{125 \times 15\text{ gtt}}{60\text{ minutes}}$$

$$X = \frac{1{,}875\text{ gtt}}{60\text{ minutes}}$$

$$X = 31.25\text{ gtt/minute}$$

The drip rate is 31.25 gtt/minute, rounded to 31 gtt/minute.

Dosage drill

Test your math skills with this drill.

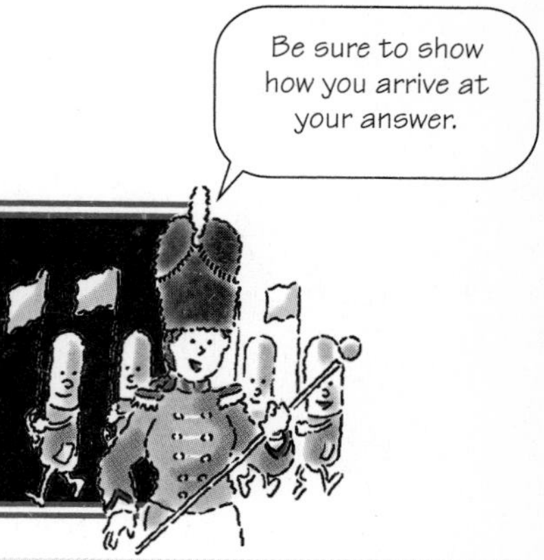
Be sure to show how you arrive at your answer.

A doctor orders 1 gram of vancomycin in 250 ml dextrose 5% in water over 1 hour as endocarditis prophylaxis. What's the drip rate for this medication if the macrodrip administration set delivers 15 gtt/ml?

Your answer: ______________________

To find the answer, change milliliters to drops using ratios and a proportion.

$$1 \text{ ml} : 15 \text{ gtt} :: 250 \text{ ml} : X \text{ gtt}$$

$$1 \text{ ml} \times X \text{ gtt} = 15 \text{ gtt} \times 250 \text{ ml}$$

$$\frac{\cancel{1 \text{ ml}} \times X \text{ gtt}}{\cancel{1 \text{ ml}}} = \frac{15 \text{ gtt} \times 250 \cancel{\text{ ml}}}{1 \cancel{\text{ ml}}}$$

$$X = 3{,}750 \text{ gtt}$$

Now, calculate the drip rate. (Remember to convert 1 hour to 60 minutes first.)

$$60 \text{ min} : 3{,}750 \text{ gtt} :: 1 \text{ min} : X \text{ gtt}$$

$$60 \text{ min} \times X \text{ gtt} = 3{,}750 \text{ gtt} \times 1 \text{ min}$$

$$\frac{\cancel{60 \text{ min}} \times X \text{ gtt}}{\cancel{60 \text{ min}}} = \frac{3{,}750 \text{ gtt} \times 1 \cancel{\text{ min}}}{60 \cancel{\text{ min}}}$$

$$X = \frac{3{,}750}{60}$$

$$X = 62.5 \text{ gtt/min}$$

The drip rate is 62.5 gtt/minute.

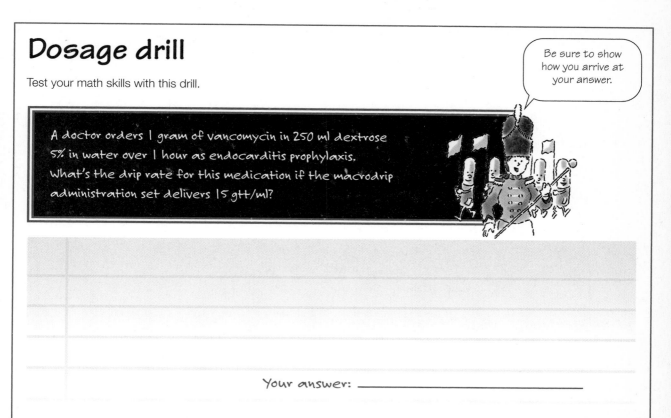

Vancomycin vanquisher

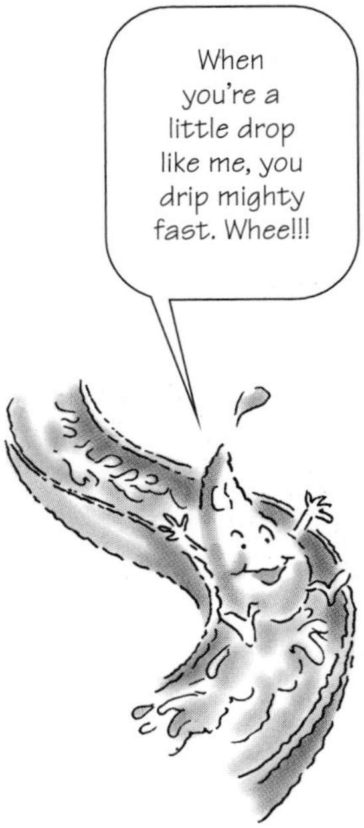

When you're a little drop like me, you drip mighty fast. Whee!!!

You receive an order that reads *Vancomycin 1 g in 200 ml NS over 60 minutes*. You decide to use a tubing set calibrated at 60 gtt/ml. What's the drip rate?

Here's how to solve this problem.

- Set up the fraction. Place the volume of the infusion in the numerator. Place the number of minutes for the infusion in the denominator:

$$\frac{200 \text{ ml}}{60 \text{ minutes}}$$

- To determine the number of drops per minute to be infused (solve for X), multiply the fraction by the drop factor. Cancel units that appear in both the numerator and denominator:

$$X = \frac{200 \cancel{\text{ml}}}{60 \text{ minutes}} \times \frac{60 \text{ gtt}}{\cancel{\text{ml}}}$$

- To solve for X, divide the numerator by the denominator:

$$X = \frac{200 \times 60 \text{ gtt}}{60 \text{ minutes}}$$

$$X = \frac{12{,}000 \text{ gtt}}{60 \text{ minutes}}$$

$$X = 200 \text{ gtt/minute}$$

The drip rate is 200 gtt/minute.

Calculating the flow rate

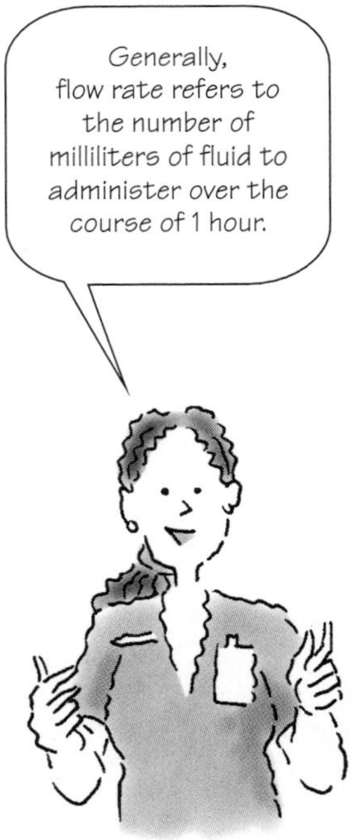

If your patient is receiving a large-volume infusion to maintain hydration or to replace fluids or electrolytes, you may need to calculate the flow rate. The *flow rate* is the number of milliliters of fluid to administer over 1 hour (it may also refer to the number of milliliters of fluid to administer per minute). To perform this calculation, you need to know the total volume to be infused in milliliters and the amount of time for the infusion.

Use this formula:

$$\text{Flow rate} = \frac{\text{total volume ordered}}{\text{number of hours}}$$

The next two examples illustrate how to determine the correct flow rate.

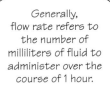

So, how flows it?

Your patient needs 1,000 ml of fluid over 8 hours. Find the flow rate by dividing the volume by the number of hours:

$$\text{Flow rate} = \frac{1{,}000 \text{ ml}}{8 \text{ hours}} = 125 \text{ ml/hour}$$

The flow rate is 125 ml/hour.

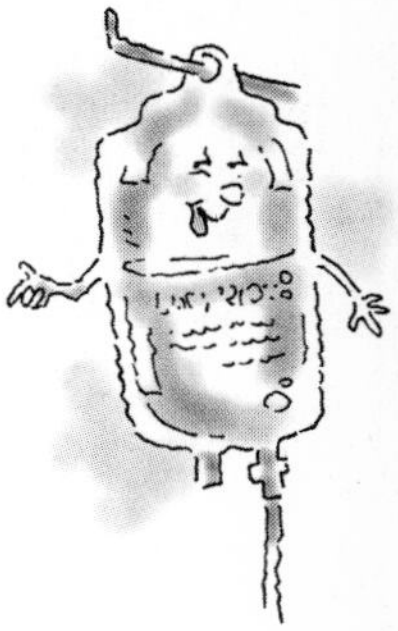
Calculating the flow rate? That's easy... divide the total volume of fluid by the number of hours.

Salient saline solution

Your patient needs 250 ml of normal saline solution over 2 hours. What's the infusion rate?

To solve this problem, first set up the equation. Then divide 250 ml by 2 hours to find the flow rate in milliliters per hour:

$$\text{Flow rate} = \frac{250 \text{ ml}}{2 \text{ hours}} = 125 \text{ ml/hour}$$

The flow rate is 125 ml/hour.

Quick calculation of drip rates

Here's a shortcut for calculating I.V. drip rates. It's based on the fact that all drop factors can be evenly divided into 60.

For macrodrip sets, use these rules to calculate drip rates:

- For sets that deliver 10 gtt/ml, divide the hourly flow rate by 6.
- For sets that deliver 15 gtt/ml, divide the hourly flow rate by 4.
- For sets that deliver 20 gtt/ml, divide the hourly flow rate by 3.

With a microdrip set (drop factor of 60 gtt/ml), simply remember that the drip rate is the same as the flow rate.

Why the microdrip flow rate equals the drip rate

Here's the equation for determining the drip rate for a solution with a flow rate of 125 ml/hour (125 ml/60 minutes) when using a microdrip set (drop factor of 60 gtt/ml). Note that the number of minutes and the number of drops per milliliter cancel each other out.

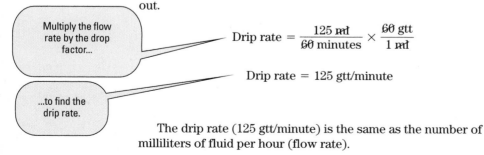

Multiply the flow rate by the drop factor...

$$\text{Drip rate} = \frac{125 \cancel{\text{ml}}}{\cancel{60} \text{ minutes}} \times \frac{\cancel{60} \text{ gtt}}{1 \cancel{\text{ml}}}$$

...to find the drip rate.

$$\text{Drip rate} = 125 \text{ gtt/minute}$$

The drip rate (125 gtt/minute) is the same as the number of milliliters of fluid per hour (flow rate).

Dosage drill

Test your math skills with this drill.

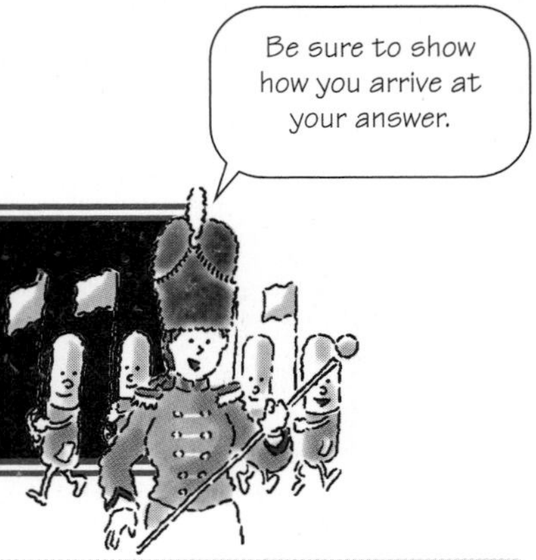
Be sure to show how you arrive at your answer.

A fluid challenge is ordered for a patient in hypovolemic shock. He needs 500 ml of normal saline solution over 2 hours. What should the nurse set the infusion rate at?

Your answer: ______________________

To find the answer, use ratios and a proportion and then solve for X.

$$2 \text{ hr} : 500 \text{ ml} :: 1 \text{ hr} : X \text{ ml}$$

$$2 \text{ hr} \times X \text{ ml} = 500 \text{ ml} \times 1 \text{ hr}$$

$$\frac{2 \cancel{\text{hr}} \times X \text{ ml}}{2 \cancel{\text{hr}}} = \frac{500 \text{ ml} \times 1 \cancel{\text{hr}}}{2 \cancel{\text{hr}}}$$

$$X = \frac{500}{2}$$

$$X = 250 \text{ ml/hr}$$

The nurse should set the infusion rate at 250 ml/hr.

Take the shortcut

The doctor prescribes *1,000 ml of normal saline to be infused over 12 hours.* If your administration set delivers 15 gtt/ml, what's the drip rate?

- First, determine the flow rate *(X)* by dividing the number of milliliters to be delivered by the number of hours:

$$X = \frac{1{,}000 \text{ ml}}{12 \text{ hours}} = 83.3 \text{ ml/hour}$$

- Remember the rule: For sets that deliver 15 gtt/ml, divide the flow rate by 4 to determine the drip rate.
- Next, set up an equation to determine the drip rate, which now becomes X, and solve for X. Divide the flow rate by 4:

$$X = \frac{83.3}{4}$$

$$X = 20.8 \text{ gtt/minute}$$

The drip rate is 20.8 gtt/minute, rounded to 21 gtt/minute.

Follow the golden microdrip rule

See if you can solve the following problem without a pencil and paper or a calculator:

Your patient is to receive an I.V. infusion of 150 ml/hour using a 60 gtt/ml set. What's the drip rate?

First, determine the flow rate. Recall that the flow rate is the number of milliliters of fluid to administer over 1 hour. Simply from reading the problem, we see that the flow rate is 150 ml/hr.

Now remember the rule: With a microdrip set, the drip rate is the same as the flow rate. Thus, the drip rate is 150 gtt/minute. Just think: You're doing dosage calculations without any math!

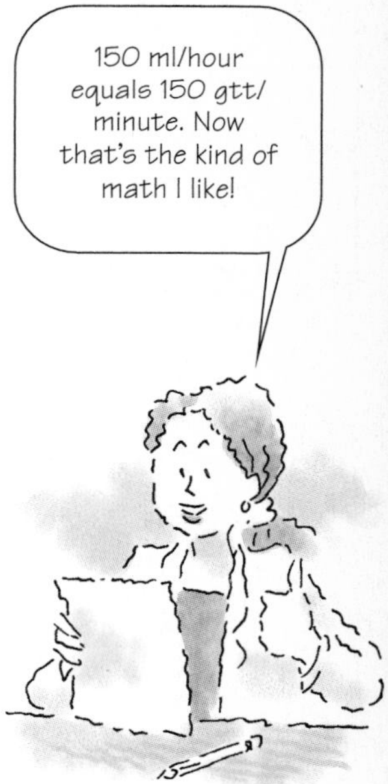

150 ml/hour equals 150 gtt/ minute. Now that's the kind of math I like!

Calculating infusion time

When you can calculate the flow rate and drip rate, you're ready to compute the time required for infusion of a specified volume of I.V. fluid. This calculation will help you keep the infusion on schedule and start the next infusion on time. It will also help you perform laboratory tests, such as the chemistry and electrolyte assessments that commonly accompany infusions, on time.

To calculate the infusion time, you must know the flow rate in milliliters per hour and the volume to be infused. Here's the formula:

$$\text{Infusion time} = \frac{\text{volume to be infused}}{\text{flow rate}}$$

The following examples show how to use this formula to calculate infusion times.

Be back in ______ minutes!

If you plan to infuse 1 L of D_5W at 50 ml/hour, what's the infusion time?

- First, convert 1 L to 1,000 ml to make units of measure that are equivalent.
- Then set up the fraction with the volume of the infusion as the numerator and the flow rate as the denominator:

$$\frac{1{,}000 \text{ ml}}{50 \text{ ml/hour}}$$

- Next, solve for X by dividing 1,000 by 50 and canceling units that appear in both the numerator and denominator:

$$X = \frac{1{,}000 \cancel{\text{ml}}}{50 \cancel{\text{ml}}\text{/hour}}$$

$$X = 20 \text{ hours}$$

The D_5W will infuse in 20 hours.

The bag will be empty at ______ o'clock

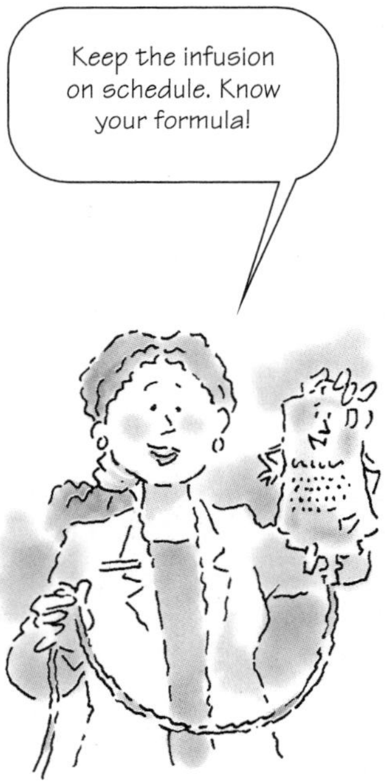
Keep the infusion on schedule. Know your formula!

Your patient requires 500 ml of normal saline solution at 80 ml/hour. What's the infusion time? If the normal saline solution is hung at 5 a.m., what time will the infusion end?

- Set up a fraction. Place the volume of the infusion as the numerator and the flow rate as the denominator:

$$X = \frac{500 \text{ ml}}{80 \text{ ml/hour}}$$

- Solve for X by dividing 500 by 80 and canceling units that appear in both the numerator and denominator:

$$X = \frac{500 \cancel{\text{ml}}}{80 \cancel{\text{ml}}\text{/hour}}$$

$$X = 6.25 \text{ hours}$$

The normal saline solution will infuse in 6.25 hours, which means that the bag will be empty at 11:15 a.m.

An alternative formula

Suppose all you know are the volume to be infused, the drip rate, and the drop factor. Then you would use the alternative formula shown here to calculate the infusion time:

$$\text{Infusion time in hours} = \frac{\text{volume to be infused}}{(\text{drip rate} \div \text{drop factor}) \times 60 \text{ minutes}}$$

Dosage drill

Test your math skills with this drill.

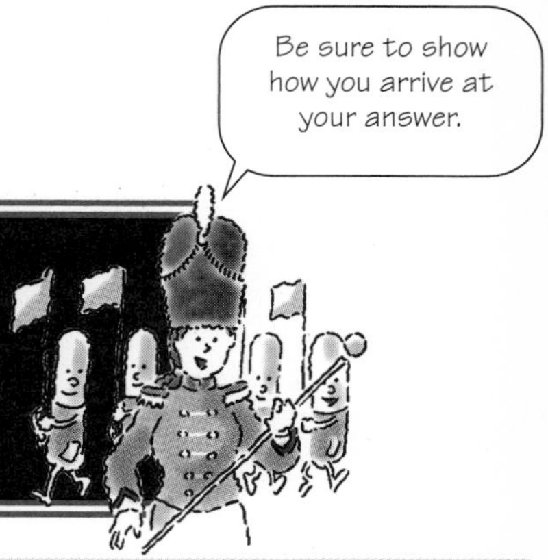
Be sure to show how you arrive at your answer.

At 6:00 a.m., a patient receives a preoperative infusion of 1,000 ml of dextrose 5% in half-normal saline solution at 125 ml/hr, followed by 1,000 ml of dextrose 5% in water at 100 ml/hr. What's the total infusion time?

Your answer: ______________________

First determine the infusion time of the first solution.

$$125 \text{ ml} : 1 \text{ hr} :: 1{,}000 \text{ ml} : X \text{ hr}$$

$$125 \text{ ml} \times X \text{ hr} = 1 \text{ hr} \times 1{,}000 \text{ ml}$$

$$\frac{\cancel{125 \text{ ml}} \times X \text{ hr}}{\cancel{125 \text{ ml}}} = \frac{1 \text{ hr} \times 1{,}000 \cancel{\text{ ml}}}{125 \cancel{\text{ ml}}}$$

$$X = \frac{1{,}000}{125}$$

$$X = 8 \text{ hr}$$

Next, determine the infusion time of the second solution.

$$100 \text{ ml} : 1 \text{ hr} :: 1{,}000 \text{ ml} : X \text{ hr}$$

$$100 \text{ ml} \times X \text{ hr} = 1 \text{ hr} \times 1{,}000 \text{ ml}$$

$$\frac{\cancel{100 \text{ ml}} \times X \text{ hr}}{\cancel{100 \text{ ml}}} = \frac{1 \text{ hr} \times 1{,}000 \cancel{\text{ ml}}}{100 \cancel{\text{ ml}}}$$

$$X = \frac{1{,}000}{100}$$

$$X = 10 \text{ hr}$$

Now add the times of both infusions together.

$$8 \text{ hr} + 10 \text{ hr} = 18 \text{ hr}$$

The total infusion time is 18 hours.

Another saline situation

A doctor prescribes *250 ml of normal saline I.V. at 32 gtt/minute*. The drop factor is 15 gtt/ml. What's the infusion time?

- Set up the formula with the known information:

$$\text{Infusion time} = \frac{250 \text{ ml}}{(32 \text{ gtt/minute} \div 15 \text{ gtt/ml}) \times 60 \text{ minutes}}$$

- Divide the drip rate by the drop factor. (Remember, to *divide* a complex fraction, multiply the dividend by the reciprocal of the divisor.) Cancel units that appear in both the numerator and denominator:

$$\frac{32 \cancel{\text{gtt}}}{1 \text{ min}} \times \frac{1 \text{ ml}}{15 \cancel{\text{gtt}}} = \frac{32 \text{ ml}}{15 \text{ min}} = 2.13 \text{ ml/min}$$

- Rewrite the equation (solve for *X*) with the result (2.13 ml/minute) placed in the denominator. Cancel units that appear in both the numerator and denominator:

$$X = \frac{250 \cancel{\text{ml}}}{\frac{2.13 \cancel{\text{ml}}}{1 \cancel{\text{min}}} \times \frac{60 \cancel{\text{min}}}{1 \text{ hour}}}$$

- To find the infusion time, solve for *X*:

$$X = \frac{250}{2.13 \times 60 \text{ hours}}$$

$$X = \frac{250}{127.8 \text{ hours}}$$

- Round off the denominator, and then divide it into the numerator:

$$X = \frac{250}{128 \text{ hours}}$$

$$X = 1.95 \text{ hours}$$

- The infusion time is 1.95 hours. Convert the decimal fraction portion of this time to minutes by multiplying by 60:

$$0.95 \text{ hour} \times 60 \text{ minutes} = 57 \text{ minutes}$$

The infusion time is 1 hour and 57 minutes.

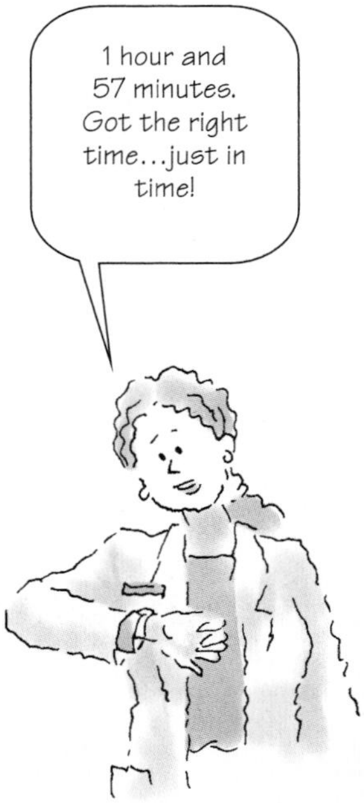
1 hour and 57 minutes. Got the right time...just in time!

Heads-up! Here comes Hespan...

If 500 ml of hetastarch (Hespan) are infusing at 40 gtt/minute with a set calibration of 20 gtt/ml, what's the infusion time?

- Use the information you know to set up a formula:

$$X = \frac{500 \text{ ml}}{(40 \text{ gtt/minute} \div 20 \text{ gtt/ml}) \times 60 \text{ minutes}}$$

- Divide the drip rate by the drop factor (remember to multiply the dividend by the reciprocal of the divisor). Cancel units that appear in both the numerator and denominator:

$$\frac{40 \cancel{\text{gtt}}}{1 \text{ min}} \times \frac{1 \text{ ml}}{20 \cancel{\text{gtt}}} = 2 \text{ ml/minute}$$

- Rewrite the equation (solving for X) with the new denominator (2 ml/minute). Cancel units that appear in both the numerator and denominator:

$$X = \frac{500 \cancel{\text{ml}}}{\frac{2 \cancel{\text{ml}}}{1 \cancel{\text{min}}} \times \frac{60 \cancel{\text{min}}}{1 \text{ hour}}}$$

- To find the infusion time, solve for X:

$$X = \frac{500}{2 \times 60 \text{ hours}}$$

$$X = \frac{500}{120 \text{ hours}}$$

- Divide the numerator by the denominator:

$$X = 4.166 = 4.17 \text{ hours}$$

- The infusion time is 4.166 hours, which rounds off to 4.17 hours. To convert the decimal fraction to minutes, multiply by 60 and then round off the number:

$$0.17 \text{ hour} \times 60 \text{ minutes} = 10.2 \text{ minutes} = 10 \text{ minutes}$$

The infusion time is 4 hours and 10 minutes.

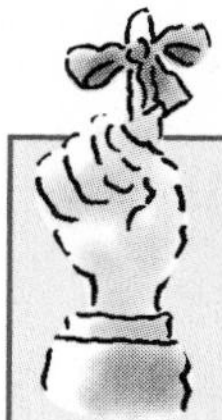

Memory jogger

When you need to divide a complex fraction, remember to multiply the *dividend* (the top number of the fraction) by the *reciprocal* (the inverse, or flipped, form) of the *divisor* (the bottom number).

In other words, change the division sign to a multiplication sign, and flip-flop the second fraction. Then proceed with the rest of the problem to solve for X.

Regulating infusions

After you start an infusion, you must be careful to regulate the I.V. flow. You can do this manually, using a pump, or using a patient-controlled analgesia (PCA) pump.

Regulating I.V. flow manually

To manually regulate the I.V. flow, count the number of drops going into the drip chamber. While counting the drops, adjust the flow with the roller clamp until the fluid is infusing at the appropriate number of drops per minute.

Save time. Calculate the drip rate for 15 seconds instead of a minute. Divide the prescribed rate by four.

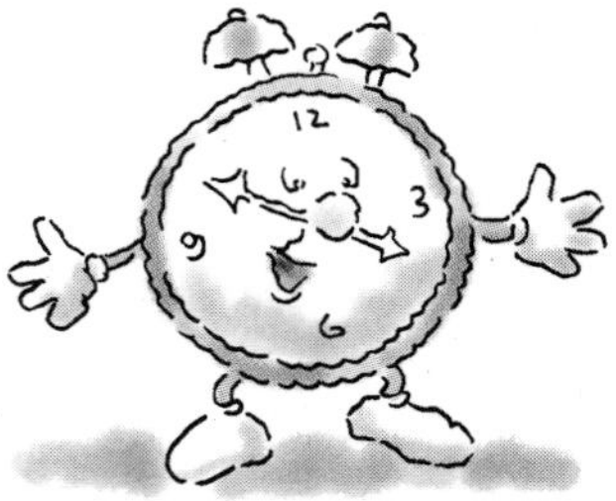

Fifteen seconds works fine

To save time, don't count for a full minute—calculate the drip rate for 15 seconds only. To do this, divide the prescribed drip rate by 4 (because 15 seconds is ¼ of a minute). For example, if the prescribed drip rate is 31 gtt/minute, divide 31 by 4 to get 8 (round 31 up to 32 first so it will divide evenly). Then adjust the roller clamp until the drip chamber shows 8 drops in 15 seconds.

Afterward, time-tape the I.V. bag to ensure that the solution is given at the prescribed rate and to make recording fluid intake easier. (See *Taped up and ready to drip*.)

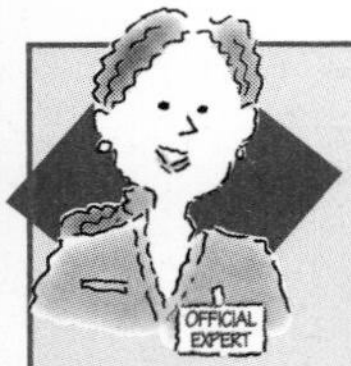

Advice from the experts

Taped up and ready to drip

Time-taping an I.V. bag helps ensure that an I.V. solution is administered at the prescribed rate. It also helps facilitate recording of fluid intake.

To time-tape an I.V. bag, place a strip of adhesive tape from the top to the bottom of the bag, next to the fluid level markings. (This illustration shows a bag time-taped for a rate of 100 ml/hour beginning at 10 a.m.)

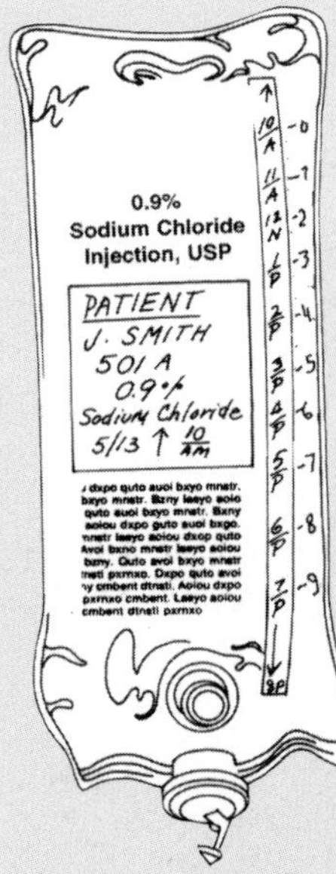

0 marks the spot.
Next to the "0" marking, record the time that you hung the bag. Then, knowing the hourly rate, mark each hour on the tape next to the corresponding fluid marking. At the bottom of the tape, mark the time at which the solution will be completely infused.

Ink alert
Don't write directly on the bag with a felt tip marker because the ink may seep into the fluid. Some manufacturers provide printed time-tapes for use with their solutions.

Electronic infusion pumps

Electronic infusion pumps facilitate I.V. administration. Pumps administer fluid under positive pressure and are calibrated by drip rate and volume.

Steady as she goes

When using a pump, set the device to deliver a constant amount of solution per hour, following the manufacturer's directions.

The electronic edge

Electronic infusion pumps offer many advantages, such as:

- allowing you easy control of the rate, or volume, by setting it on the machine
- shortening the time needed to calculate an infusion rate
- requiring less maintenance than standard devices that drip fluid by gravity
- providing greater accuracy than standard devices.

Special features

Most pumps keep track of the amount of fluid that has been infused, helping maintain accurate intake and output records. Many have alarms that signal when the fluid container is empty or when a mechanical problem occurs. Some devices have variable pressure limits that prevent them from pumping fluids into infiltrated sites.

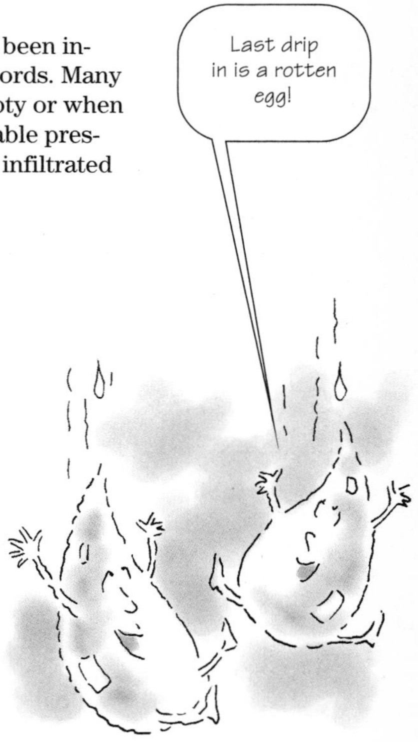
Last drip in is a rotten egg!

Regulating I.V. flow with pumps

When using a pump to regulate I.V. flow, program the device based on your calculation of the infusion rate. Remember that infusion pumps can make mistakes — they don't eliminate the need for careful calculations and assessment of infusion rates over time. So check the infusion by counting the drips in the chamber just as you would with manual regulation.

Programming the pump

To determine the pump settings, consider the volume of fluid to be given and the total infusion time. With most devices, you'll need to program both the amount of fluid to be infused and the hourly flow rate. However, some devices require you to program the flow rate per minute or the drip rate.

Patient-controlled analgesia pumps

One popular infusion device is the computerized PCA pump, which allows a patient to self-administer an analgesic by pushing a button. You program the pump to deliver a precise dose every time. The pump also can be programmed to deliver a basal dose of drug in addition to the patient-controlled dose. (See *Putting your patient in control.*)

No pain...all gains

The main advantage of using a PCA pump over the traditional approach — in which analgesics are injected intramuscularly every few hours — is that blood concentrations of analgesics remain consistent throughout the day. With the traditional approach, blood levels fluctuate, so patients have periods of heavy sedation alternating with periods of increasing pain.

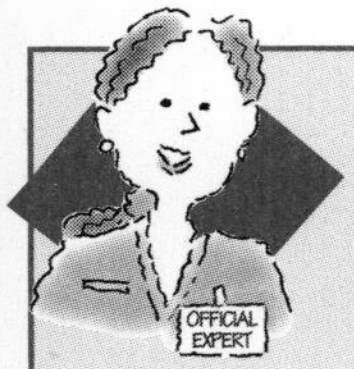

Advice from the experts

Putting your patient in control

A computerized patient-controlled analgesia (PCA) pump, such as the one shown here, allows your patient to give himself pain medication with the push of a button. With PCA pumps, patients tend to use less medication than they do with the traditional approach and they develop a greater feeling of control over their pain.

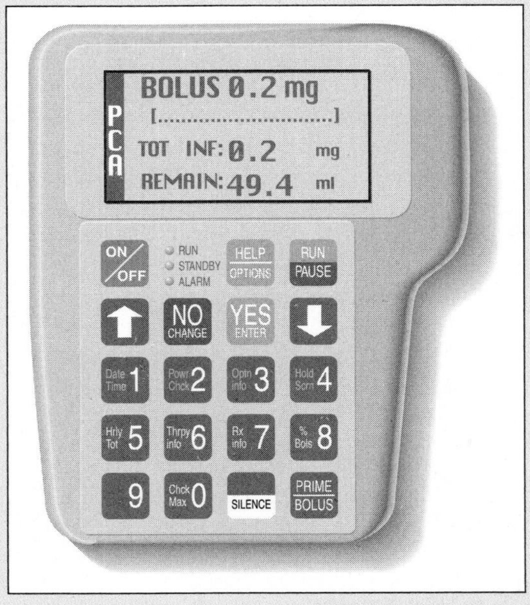

Two added benefits of PCA pumps are that patients tend to take less medication than they do with the traditional approach and that they develop a greater feeling of control over their pain.

Pump-provided protection

Several safety features are built into PCA pumps. Drug dose and administration frequency are programmed, preventing the patient from medicating himself too often. If the patient tries to overmedicate, the machine simply ignores the request. Also, some pumps record the number of requests and the number of times the patient actually receives medication, which helps you evaluate whether the doctor needs to increase or decrease the drug dose.

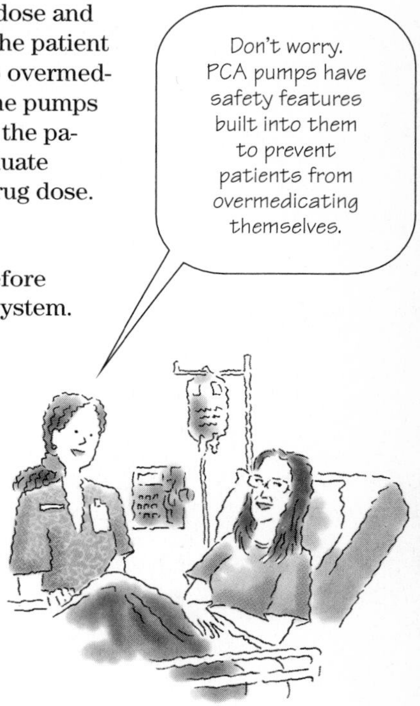

Don't worry. PCA pumps have safety features built into them to prevent patients from overmedicating themselves.

And the password is…

PCA pumps require you to use an access code or key before entering drug dose and frequency information into the system. This prevents unauthorized users from tampering with or accidentally resetting the pump. Some machines even record unauthorized entries.

PCA prep parameters

When preparing a PCA pump for a patient, follow these guidelines:

- Obtain the correct amount and concentration of drug — usually morphine — and insert it into the PCA pump. Prefilled cartridges are usually available.
- Program the pump according to the manufacturer's directions.
- Carefully read the PCA log, and then record the information based on your facility's policy. A typical order might state the following: *Start morphine sulfate PCA. Give 2 mg/hr basal rate and 1 mg/q15 min on demand, with a lock-out of 6 mg/4 hr.*

Recording drug dosage with a PCA

When interpreting the PCA log, note the strength (number of milligrams per milliliter) of drug solution in the container. You'll need this information to calculate the dose received by the patient.

Covering the basals

Also note the number of times the patient received the drug throughout the time covered by your assessment (usually over 4 hours). If your patient is receiving a basal dose, note that as well. By multiplying the number of injections by the volume of each injection and adding the basal dose, you can determine the amount of solution the patient received.

Multiply this amount by the solution strength to find the total amount of drug, as shown in this formula:

Fluid volume × solution strength = total medication received

Record this amount in milligrams in the patient's medication administration record.

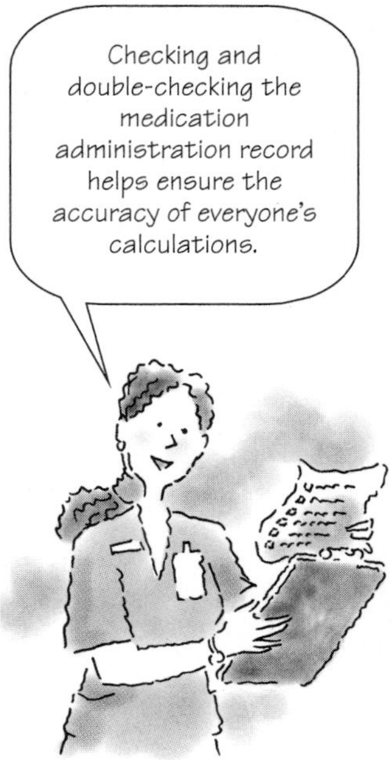

A double dose of accuracy

Most facilities require the nurse who prepares the infusion to record the amount of fluid and drug in the container. Each nurse who checks the PCA log double-checks and records this information. The record enables you to double-check the accuracy of everyone's calculations.

Adjusting the infusion rate

No matter how carefully you calculate the drip rate, and adjust the flow rate of an I.V. infusion, the rate still may change. Why? Perhaps the patient changed position, the I.V. tubing became kinked, or the drug infiltrated the patient's skin. Such factors cause the infusion to run ahead or behind schedule.

Don't hesitate to recalculate

When problems occur, notify the doctor and then recalculate the drip rate taking into account the remaining time and volume according to the doctor's order. If the fluid has infused too slowly, assess the patient to determine whether he can tolerate an increased rate. Look for a history of renal insufficiency, heart failure, pulmonary edema, or any other condition that increases the risk of fluid overload.

If I.V. fluid has infused too quickly, slow or stop the infusion and assess for signs of fluid overload, such as crackles and increased blood pressure. Call the doctor if these occur.

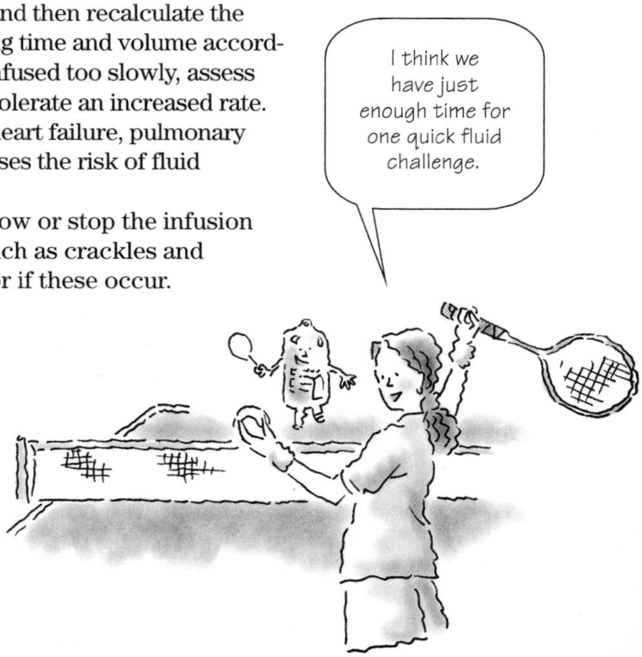

I think we have just enough time for one quick fluid challenge.

Are you up for a fluid challenge?

You may also need to adjust the infusion rate to administer a *fluid challenge*, if prescribed. A fluid challenge is prescribed when the patient needs fluid quickly. The fastest way to do a fluid challenge is by increasing the I.V. flow rate for a specified time and then reducing it to a maintenance rate. *However, be sure to use a fluid bolus cautiously in pediatric and elderly patients.*

Heparin and insulin infusions

The doctor may prescribe a heparin or insulin infusion. These drugs may be ordered in milliliters per hour, or units per hour. To administer them safely, you must calculate the drug dose so that it falls within therapeutic limits. (See chapter 12, Calculating parenteral injections, for more information on heparin and insulin.)

Calculating heparin doses

A common anticoagulant, heparin prevents the formation of new clots and slows the development of preexisting clots. It's usually given by the I.V. route and ordered in doses of units per hour or milliliters per hour. Each dose is individualized based on the patient's coagulation status, which is measured by the partial thromboplastin time.

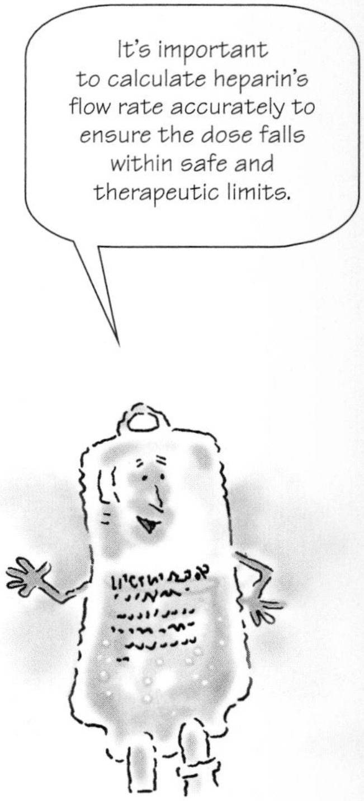
It's important to calculate heparin's flow rate accurately to ensure the dose falls within safe and therapeutic limits.

Flow rate

Accurately calculating the flow rate ensures that the heparin dose falls within safe and therapeutic limits. This type of calculation differs from the flow rate calculations discussed earlier because it's used to administer a drug, not just a fluid.

To calculate the hourly heparin flow rate, first determine the solution's concentration by dividing the units of drug added to the bag by the number of milliliters of solution. Then write a fraction stating the desired dose of heparin over the unknown flow rate. Then simply cross-multiply to find the unknown flow rate.

Here are some examples using simple proportions to find the solution.

Go with the flow!

An order states *heparin 40,000 units in 1 L of* D_5W *I.V. Infuse at 1,000 units/hr*. What's the flow rate in milliliters per hour?

- First, convert 1 L to 1,000 ml. Then write a fraction to express the known solution strength (units of drug divided by milliliters of solution):

$$\frac{40{,}000 \text{ units}}{1{,}000 \text{ ml}}$$

- Write a second fraction with the desired dose of heparin in the numerator and the unknown flow rate in the denominator:

$$\frac{1{,}000 \text{ units/hour}}{X}$$

- Put these fractions into a proportion:

$$\frac{40{,}000 \text{ units}}{1{,}000 \text{ ml}} = \frac{1{,}000 \text{ units/hour}}{X}$$

• To find the flow rate, solve for X by cross-multiplying:

$$40{,}000 \text{ units} \times X = 1{,}000 \text{ units/hour} \times 1{,}000 \text{ ml}$$

• Divide each side of the equation by 40,000 units and cancel units that appear in both the numerator and denominator:

$$\frac{\cancel{40{,}000 \text{ units}} \times X}{\cancel{40{,}000 \text{ units}}} = \frac{1{,}000 \ \cancel{\text{units}}\text{/hour} \times 1{,}000 \text{ ml}}{40{,}000 \ \cancel{\text{units}}}$$

$$X = \frac{1{,}000{,}000 \text{ ml/hour}}{40{,}000}$$

$$X = 25 \text{ ml/hour}$$

To administer heparin at 1,000 units/hour, you should set the flow rate at 25 ml/hour.

Know this flow?

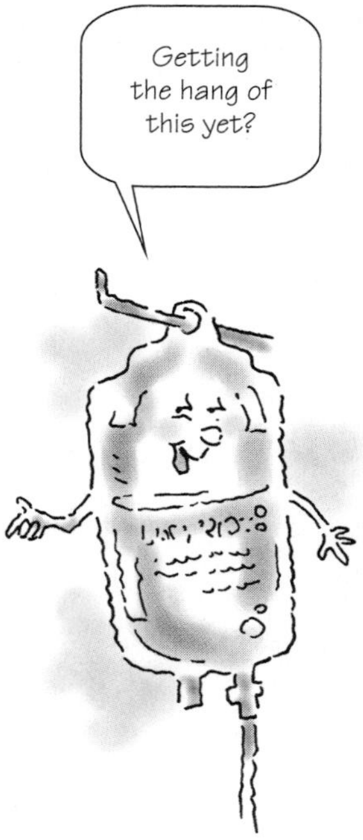
Getting the hang of this yet?

You're about to administer a continuous infusion of 25,000 units of heparin in 250 ml of D_5W. If the patient is to receive 600 units/hour, what's the flow rate?

• Write a ratio to express the known solution strength (units of drug to milliliters of solution):

$$25{,}000 \text{ units} : 250 \text{ ml}$$

• Write a second ratio to describe the desired dose of heparin in relation to the unknown flow rate:

$$600 \text{ units/hour} : X$$

• Put these ratios into a proportion:

$$25{,}000 \text{ units} : 250 \text{ ml} :: 600 \text{ units/hour} : X$$

• Solve for X by multiplying the extremes and the means:

$$25{,}000 \text{ units} \times X = 600 \text{ units/hour} \times 250 \text{ ml}$$

• Divide each side of the equation by 25,000 units and cancel units that appear in both the numerator and denominator:

$$\frac{\cancel{25{,}000 \text{ units}} \times X}{\cancel{25{,}000 \text{ units}}} = \frac{600 \ \cancel{\text{units}}\text{/hour} \times 250 \text{ ml}}{25{,}000 \ \cancel{\text{units}}}$$

$$X = \frac{600 \times 250 \text{ ml/hour}}{25{,}000}$$

$$X = \frac{150{,}000 \text{ ml/hour}}{25{,}000}$$

$$X = 6 \text{ ml/hour}$$

To administer 600 units/hour, you should set the flow rate at 6 ml/hour.

Dosage drill

Test your math skills with this drill.

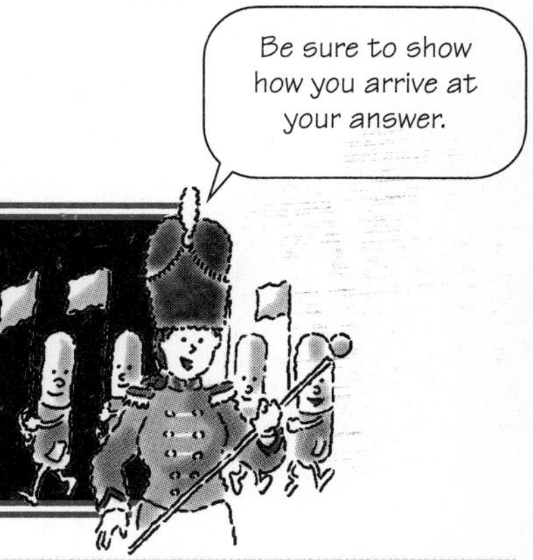
Be sure to show how you arrive at your answer.

A doctor's order reads Heparin I.V. at 1,400 units/hr. The pharmacy sends heparin in a bag containing 25,000 units of dextrose 5% in water. What infusion rate should be set on the I.V. pump?

Your answer: ______________________

To find the answer, begin by setting up ratios and a proportion.

$$25{,}000 \text{ units} : 250 \text{ ml} :: 1{,}400 \text{ units} \times X \text{ ml}$$

$$25{,}000 \text{ units} \times X \text{ ml} = 250 \text{ ml} \times 1{,}400 \text{ units}$$

Solve for *X*.

$$\frac{\cancel{25{,}000 \text{ units}} \times X \text{ ml}}{\cancel{25{,}000 \text{ units}}} = \frac{250 \text{ ml} \times 1{,}400 \cancel{\text{ units}}}{25{,}000 \cancel{\text{ units}}}$$

$$X = \frac{350{,}000}{25{,}000}$$

$$X = 14 \text{ ml/hr}$$

The infusion pump should be set to run at 14 ml/hour.

Units per hour

If a heparin infusion is ordered in milliliters per hour, you may want to calculate it in units per hour, too. This determines the patient's drug dose so you can be sure it falls within a safe and therapeutic range.

Here's an example calculating units per hour.

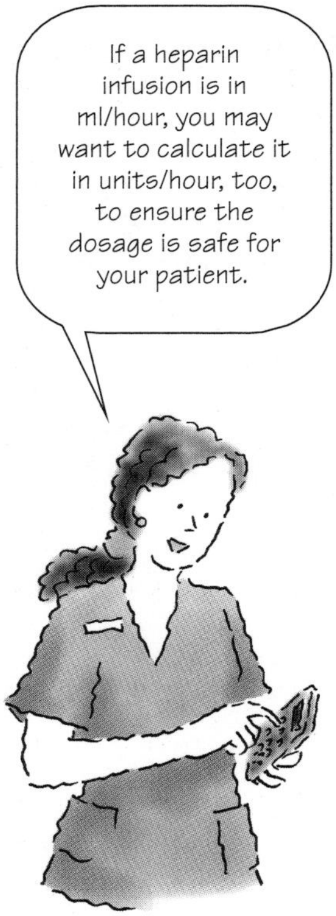
If a heparin infusion is in ml/hour, you may want to calculate it in units/hour, too, to ensure the dosage is safe for your patient.

Knowing your therapeutic range

A patient is receiving 20,000 units of heparin in 1,000 ml of D_5W I.V. at 30 ml/hour. What heparin dose is he receiving?

- Write a fraction to describe the known solution strength (units of drug divided by milliliters of solution):

$$\frac{20{,}000 \text{ units}}{1{,}000 \text{ ml}}$$

- Set up the second fraction with the flow rate in the denominator and the unknown dose of heparin in the numerator:

$$\frac{X}{30 \text{ ml/hour}}$$

- Write these fractions into a proportion:

$$\frac{20{,}000 \text{ units}}{1{,}000 \text{ ml}} = \frac{X}{30 \text{ ml/hour}}$$

- Solve for X by cross-multiplying:

$$1{,}000 \text{ ml} \times X = 30 \text{ ml/hour} \times 20{,}000 \text{ units}$$

- Divide each side of the equation by 1,000 ml and cancel units that appear in both the numerator and denominator:

$$\frac{\cancel{1{,}000 \text{ ml}} \times X}{\cancel{1{,}000 \text{ ml}}} = \frac{30 \cancel{\text{ ml}}\text{/hour} \times 20{,}000 \text{ units}}{1{,}000 \cancel{\text{ ml}}}$$

$$X = \frac{30 \times 20{,}000 \text{ units/hour}}{1{,}000}$$

$$X = \frac{600{,}000 \text{ units/hour}}{1{,}000}$$

$$X = 600 \text{ units/hour}$$

With the flow rate set at 30 ml/hour, the patient is receiving 600 units/hour of heparin.

Calculating continuous insulin infusions

An acutely ill diabetic patient may need to receive insulin by continuous infusion. Continuous infusion allows close control of insulin administration based on serial measurements of blood glucose levels.

You'll use an infusion pump to administer I.V. insulin. Regular insulin is the only type that can be administered by the I.V. route because it has a shorter duration of action than other insulins.

Insulin is usually prescribed in units per hour, but it may be ordered in milliliters per hour. In either case, the infusion should be in a concentration of 1 unit/ml to avoid calculation errors that may have serious consequences. The examples here are based on common patient situations.

Insulin inquiry #1

Your patient needs a continuous infusion of 150 units of regular insulin in 150 ml of normal saline at 6 units/hour. What's the flow rate?

- Write a fraction to describe the known solution strength (units of drug over milliliters of solution):

$$\frac{150 \text{ units}}{150 \text{ ml}}$$

- Write a second fraction with the infusion rate in the numerator and the unknown flow rate in the denominator:

$$\frac{6 \text{ units/hour}}{X}$$

- Write the two fractions as a proportion:

$$\frac{150 \text{ units}}{150 \text{ ml}} = \frac{6 \text{ units/hour}}{X}$$

- Solve for X by cross-multiplying:

$$150 \text{ units} \times X = 6 \text{ units/hour} \times 150 \text{ ml}$$

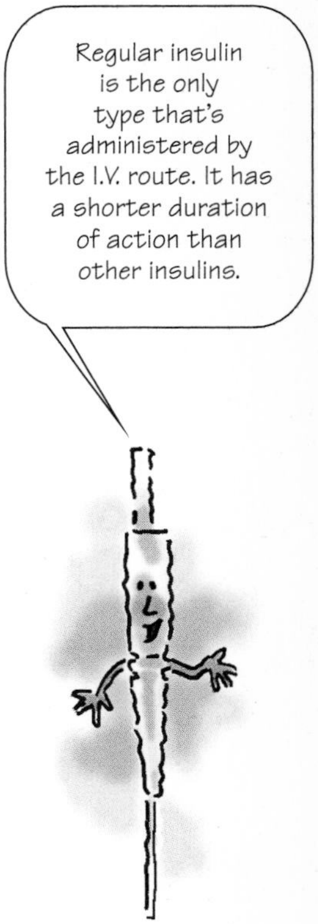
Regular insulin is the only type that's administered by the I.V. route. It has a shorter duration of action than other insulins.

Dosage drill

Test your math skills with this drill.

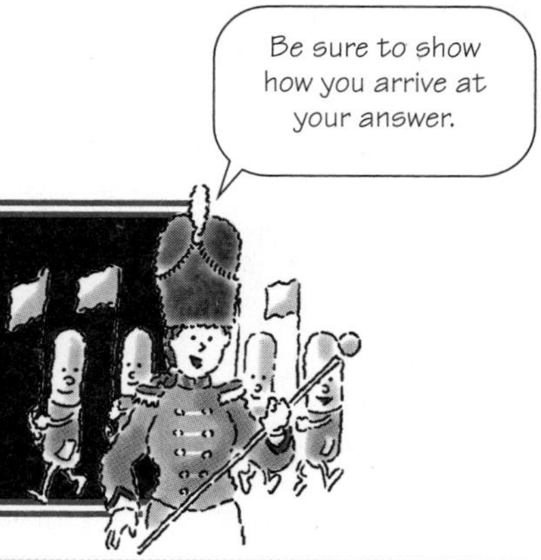
Be sure to show how you arrive at your answer.

A 25-year-old patient is admitted to your unit with diabetic ketoacidosis. The doctor orders a continuous infusion of 100 units of regular insulin in 100 ml normal saline at 12 units/hour. What's the infusion rate?

Your answer: ____________________

To find the answer, first write a fraction to describe the solution strength.

$$\frac{100 \text{ units}}{100 \text{ ml}}$$

Write a second fraction with the infusion rate and the unknown flow rate.

$$\frac{12 \text{ units/hr}}{X}$$

Write the two fractions as a proportion.

$$\frac{100 \text{ units}}{100 \text{ ml}} = \frac{12 \text{ units/hr}}{X}$$

Solve for X by cross-multiplying.

$$100 \text{ units} \times X = 12 \text{ units/hour} \times 100 \text{ ml}$$

$$\frac{\cancel{100 \text{ units}} \times X}{\cancel{100 \text{ units}}} = \frac{12 \cancel{\text{ units}}\text{/hour} \times 100 \text{ ml}}{100 \cancel{\text{ units}}}$$

$$X = 12 \text{ ml/hr}$$

The infusion rate is 12 ml/hour.

• Divide each side of the equation by 150 units and cancel units that appear in both the numerator and denominator:

$$\frac{\cancel{150\ \text{units}} \times X}{\cancel{150\ \text{units}}} = \frac{6\ \cancel{\text{units}}/\text{hour} \times 150\ \text{ml}}{150\ \cancel{\text{units}}}$$

$$X = 6\ \text{ml/hour}$$

To administer 6 units/hour of the prescribed insulin, you set the infusion pump's flow rate at 6 ml/hour.

Insulin inquiry #2

Your patient is receiving a continuous infusion of 100 units of regular insulin in 100 ml of normal saline at 10 ml/hour. How many units per hour is your patient receiving?

• Write a ratio to describe the known solution strength (units of insulin to milliliters of solution):

$$100\ \text{units} : 100\ \text{ml}$$

• Set up a second ratio comparing the unknown amount of insulin to the prescribed infusion rate:

$$X : 10\ \text{ml/hour}$$

• Put these ratios into a proportion:

$$100\ \text{units} : 100\ \text{ml} :: X : 10\ \text{ml/hour}$$

• Solve for X by multiplying the means and the extremes:

$$X \times 100\ \text{ml} = 100\ \text{units} \times 10\ \text{ml/hour}$$

• Divide each side of the equation by 100 ml and cancel units that appear in both the numerator and denominator:

$$\frac{X \times \cancel{100\ \text{ml}}}{\cancel{100\ \text{ml}}} = \frac{100\ \text{units} \times 10\ \cancel{\text{ml}}/\text{hour}}{100\ \cancel{\text{ml}}}$$

$$X = 10\ \text{units/hour}$$

When the insulin infusion runs at 10 ml/hour, the patient receives 10 units/hour.

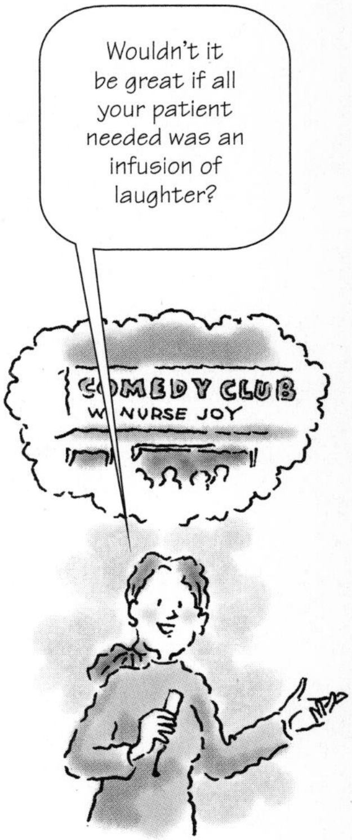
Wouldn't it be great if all your patient needed was an infusion of laughter?
COMEDY CLUB
NURSE JOY

Electrolyte and nutrient infusions

I.V. fluids can be used to deliver electrolytes and nutrients directly into the patient's bloodstream.

Adding up the additives

Large-volume infusions with additives maintain or restore hydration or electrolyte status or supply additional electrolytes, vitamins, or other nutrients. Common additives include potassium chloride, vitamins B and C, and trace elements.

Piggyback ride

Electrolytes may also be given in small-volume, intermittent infusions piggybacked into existing I.V. lines. (See *Calculating piggyback infusions.*)

Prepare to prepare

Additives are commonly prepackaged in solution, either by the manufacturer or by the pharmacy. You must calculate the flow rate and the drip rate. In a rare occasion, if you must add the additive yourself, use the proportion method as you would for any prepared liquid drug to calculate the amount of additive. Here's an example.

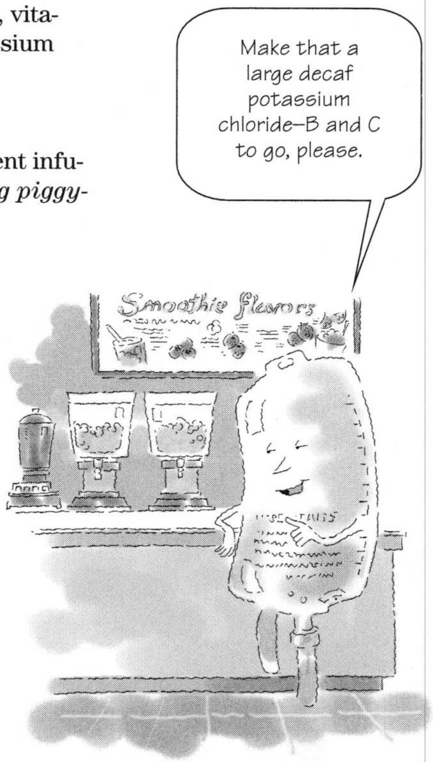
Make that a large decaf potassium chloride—B and C to go, please.
Smoothie flavors

Thinking about thiamine

Your patient requires 1,000 ml of D_5W with 150 mg of thiamine/L infused over 12 hours. The thiamine is available in a prepared syringe of 100 mg/ml. How many milliliters of thiamine must be added to the solution? What's the flow rate?

- Write the first ratio to describe the known solution strength (amount of drug per 1 ml):

$$100 \text{ mg} : 1 \text{ ml}$$

- Set up the second ratio. Write the amount of thiamine ordered on one side and the unknown amount to be added to the solution on the other side:

$$150 \text{ mg} : X$$

Calculating piggyback infusions

An I.V. piggyback is a small-volume, intermittent infusion that's connected to an existing I.V. line containing maintenance fluid. Most piggybacks contain antibiotics or electrolytes. To calculate piggyback infusions, use proportions.

Piggyback problem

You receive an order for 500 mg of imipenem in 100 ml of normal saline solution to be infused over 1 hour. The imipenem vial contains 1,000 mg (1 g). The insert says to reconstitute the powder with 5 ml of normal saline solution. How much solution should you draw? What's the flow rate?

Solution solution

- Write the first ratio to describe the known solution strength (amount of drug compared to the known amount of solution):

$$1{,}000 \text{ mg} : 5 \text{ ml}$$

- Write the second ratio, which compares the desired dose of imipenem and the unknown amount of solution:

$$500 \text{ mg} : X$$

- Put these ratios into a proportion:

$$1{,}000 \text{ mg} : 5 \text{ ml} :: 500 \text{ mg} : X$$

- Multiply the extremes and the means:

$$1{,}000 \text{ mg} \times X = 500 \text{ mg} \times 5 \text{ ml}$$

- Solve for X by dividing each side of the equation by 1,000 mg and canceling units that appear in both the numerator and denominator:

$$\frac{\cancel{1{,}000 \text{ mg}} \times X}{\cancel{1{,}000 \text{ mg}}} = \frac{500 \cancel{\text{mg}} \times 5 \text{ ml}}{1{,}000 \cancel{\text{mg}}}$$

$$X = \frac{500 \times 5 \text{ ml}}{1{,}000}$$

$$X = \frac{2{,}500 \text{ ml}}{1{,}000}$$

$$X = 2.5 \text{ ml}$$

You should draw 2.5 ml of solution to get 500 mg of imipenem.

Flow rate

Recall that the flow rate is the number of milliliters of fluid to administer over 1 hour. So, in this case, the flow rate is 100 ml/hour.

Compatibility counts

After you've calculated an I.V. piggyback dose, make sure that the drugs to be infused together are compatible. The same goes for drugs mixed in the same syringe or I.V. bag. Drug compatibility charts can be time-savers—you should have one hanging in your unit's medication room. If not, use a drug handbook that includes a compatibility chart.

- Put these ratios into a proportion:

$$100 \text{ mg} : 1 \text{ ml} :: 150 \text{ mg} : X$$

- Solve for X by multiplying the extremes and the means:

$$X \times 100 \text{ mg} = 150 \text{ mg} \times 1 \text{ ml}$$

• Divide each side of the equation by 100 mg and cancel units that appear in both the numerator and denominator:

$$\frac{X \times \cancel{100\text{ mg}}}{\cancel{100\text{ mg}}} = \frac{150\ \cancel{\text{mg}} \times 1\text{ ml}}{100\ \cancel{\text{mg}}}$$

$$X = \frac{150\text{ ml}}{100}$$

$$X = 1.5\text{ ml}$$

• You must add 1.5 ml of thiamine to the solution. If the flow rate is 1,000 ml over 12 hours, divide 1,000 by 12 to find the flow rate for 1 hour:

$$\frac{1{,}000\text{ ml}}{12\text{ hr}} = 83.3\text{ ml/hr}$$

The flow rate is 83 ml/hour.

Blood and blood product infusions

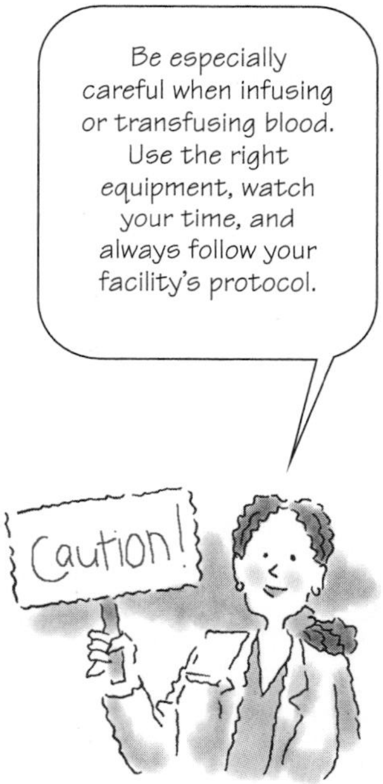

Be especially careful when infusing or transfusing blood. Use the right equipment, watch your time, and always follow your facility's protocol.
Caution!

The volume of fluid to be infused and the drop factor can be used to calculate transfusions of blood and blood products. During such transfusions, take care to prevent cell damage and ensure an adequate blood flow by using a special administration set that contains filters to remove agglutinated cells. The drop factor for these sets is usually 10 to 15 gtt/ml.

Generally, you'll use a 20G or larger I.V. catheter for administration. However, you may need a smaller catheter for elderly or pediatric patients, those with chronic illnesses who are hospitalized frequently, or severely dehydrated patients.

Written in blood

Your facility probably has specific protocols for infusing blood and blood products. For example, a unit of whole blood—about 500 ml—or packed red blood cells (PRBCs)—about 250 ml—should infuse for no longer than 4 hours because the blood can deteriorate and become contaminated with bacteria after this time. Many facilities recommend completing a transfusion in about 2 hours. However, this rate may be too fast for pediatric and elderly patients.

Product precautions

You'll also need to take special precautions when transfusing blood products, such as platelets, cryoprecipitate, and granulocytes. Consult your facility's procedure manual to find out the type of tubing to use and the rate and duration of the transfusion.

In addition, some medical conditions require the use of special tubing. For example, cancer patients may need to use a leukocyte filter with blood products to prevent complications.

Blood cell brain teaser

Here's an example of a dosage calculation problem that involves PRBCs: Your patient is to receive 250 ml of PRBCs over 4 hours. The drop factor of the tubing is 10 gtt/ml. What's the drip rate in drops per minute?

- First, find the flow rate in milliliters per minute:

$$\frac{250 \text{ ml PRBC}}{4 \text{ hours}} = \frac{62.5 \text{ ml}}{1 \text{ hour}}$$

Use the flow rate in milliliters per hour...

$$\frac{62.5 \text{ ml}}{\cancel{1 \text{ hour}}} \times \frac{\cancel{1 \text{ hour}}}{60 \text{ minutes}} = 1.04 \text{ ml/minute} = \text{flow rate}$$

- Multiply the flow rate by the drop factor to find the drip rate in drops per minute:

$$\frac{1.04 \cancel{\text{ ml}}}{1 \text{ minute}} \times \frac{10 \text{ gtt}}{\cancel{\text{ml}}} = 10.4 \text{ gtt/minute}$$

...to find the drip rate in drops per minute.

The drip rate is 10.4 gtt/minute, or approximately 10 gtt/minute.

Total parenteral nutrition

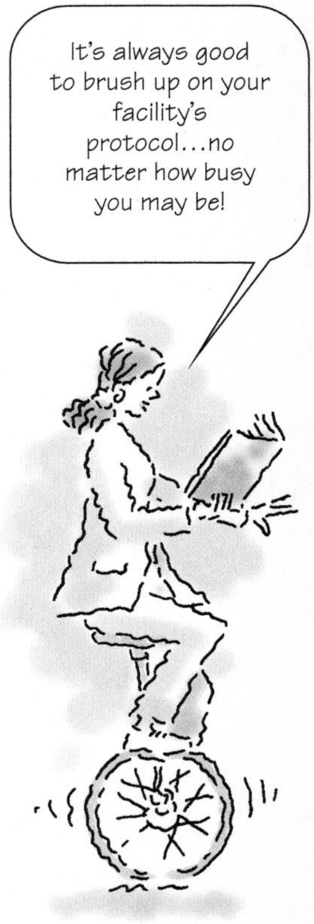

It's always good to brush up on your facility's protocol...no matter how busy you may be!

A patient receives parenteral nutrition when his nutritional needs can't be met enterally because of elevated requirements or impaired digestion or absorption in the GI tract. *Total parenteral nutrition* (TPN) refers to any nutrient solution, including lipids, given through a central venous line.

TPN can be administered through a central vein, such as the subclavian vein or internal jugular vein. *Peripheral parenteral nutrition* (PPN), which is administered through the veins of the arms, legs, or scalp, supplies full caloric needs while avoiding the risks that accompany a central line. Most facilities have a written protocol regarding insertion sites and recommended solutions for both TPN and PPN.

TPN is available as commercially prepared products or individually formulated solutions from the pharmacy. Solutions are prepared under sterile conditions to guard against patient infection. Very rarely are nurses responsible for preparing TPN solutions on the unit.

Added attractions

TPN solutions contain a 10% or greater dextrose concentration. Amino acids are added to maintain or restore nitrogen balance, and vitamins, electrolytes, and trace minerals are added to meet individual patient needs.

Lipids also may be added, but they're commonly given separately to prevent their destruction by the other nutrients. Remember that additives increase a solution's total volume, so they affect intake measurements.

For example, when assessing the amount of fluid remaining in the TPN bottle, don't be surprised to find 20 to 50 ml more than you expected. If this happens, find out whether the volume of additives explains the discrepancy.

What goes up...must come down

Initially, TPN is infused at a slow rate — usually 40 ml/hour — which is gradually increased to a maintenance level. The rate is gradually decreased before discontinuing TPN. Solutions are administered through an infusion pump.

For example, a patient's TPN may be increased to a maintenance level of 2,000 ml in 24 hours. To set the maintenance flow rate of the infusion pump, you need to find the hourly flow rate. To do this, simply divide the amount to be infused daily — 2,000 ml — by 24 hours. You find that you should set the infusion pump at 83 ml/hour.

Infusion calculations

These problems are typical of the infusion calculations you're likely to encounter.

Real world problems

Your patient needs 15 ml of erythromycin, which is equal to 500 mg. The infusion is to be completed in 30 minutes using a tubing set calibrated to 20 gtt/ml. What's the drip rate?

Here's how to determine the answer.

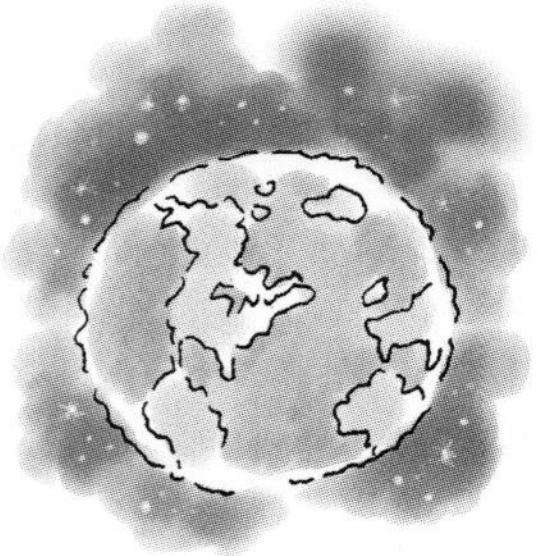

Erythromycin drip rate drill

• Set up a fraction. Place the volume of the infusion in the numerator. Place the number of minutes in which the volume is to be infused in the denominator:

$$\frac{15 \text{ ml}}{30 \text{ minutes}}$$

• Multiply the fraction by the drop factor to determine the number of drops per minute to be infused (solve for X). Cancel units that appear in both the numerator and denominator:

$$X = \frac{15\ \cancel{ml}}{30\ \text{minutes}} \times \frac{20\ \text{gtt}}{\cancel{ml}}$$

- Solve for X by dividing the numerator by the denominator:

$$X = \frac{15 \times 20\ \text{gtt}}{30\ \text{minutes}}$$

$$X = \frac{300\ \text{gtt}}{30\ \text{minutes}}$$

$$X = 10\ \text{gtt/minute}$$

The drip rate is 10 gtt/minute.

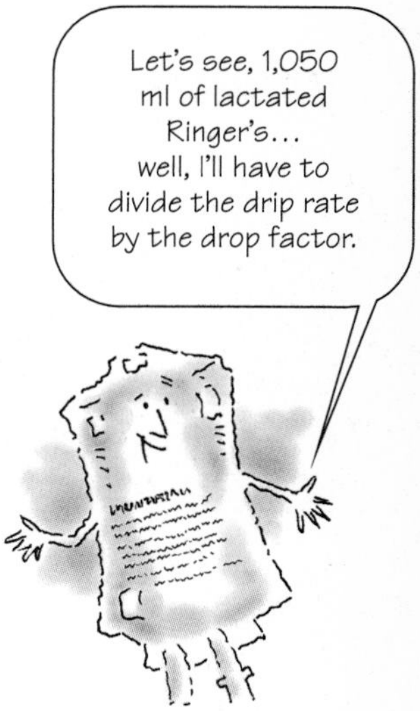
Let's see, 1,050 ml of lactated Ringer's... well, I'll have to divide the drip rate by the drop factor.

This should ring 'er bell

If you infuse 1,050 ml of lactated Ringer's solution at 25 gtt/minute using a set calibration of 10 gtt/ml, what's the infusion time?

- Use the information you know to set up the formula:

$$X = \frac{1{,}050\ \text{ml}}{(25\ \text{gtt/minute} \div 10\ \text{gtt/ml}) \times 60\ \text{minutes}}$$

- Divide the drip rate by the drop factor. (Remember to multiply the dividend by the reciprocal of the divisor.) Cancel units that appear in both the numerator and denominator:

$$\frac{25\ \cancel{gtt}}{1\ \text{min}} \times \frac{1\ \text{ml}}{10\ \cancel{gtt}} = 2.5\ \text{ml/minute}$$

- Rewrite the equation (solving for X) using the result (2.5 ml/minute) in the denominator. Cancel units that appear in both the numerator and denominator:

$$X = \frac{1{,}050\ \cancel{ml}}{\frac{2.5\ \cancel{ml}}{1\ \cancel{min}} \times \frac{60\ \cancel{min}}{1\ \text{hour}}}$$

- To find the infusion time, solve for X:

$$X = \frac{1{,}050}{2.5 \times 60\ \text{hours}}$$

$$X = \frac{1{,}050}{150\ \text{hours}}$$

- Divide the numerator by the denominator:

$$X = 7\ \text{hours}$$

The infusion time is 7 hours.

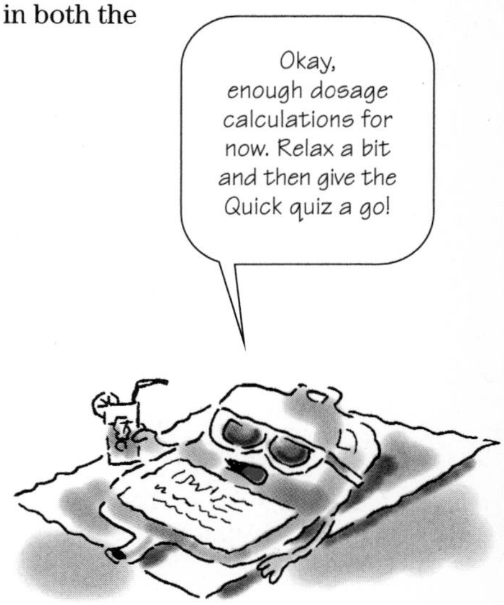

Dosage drill

Test your math skills with this drill.

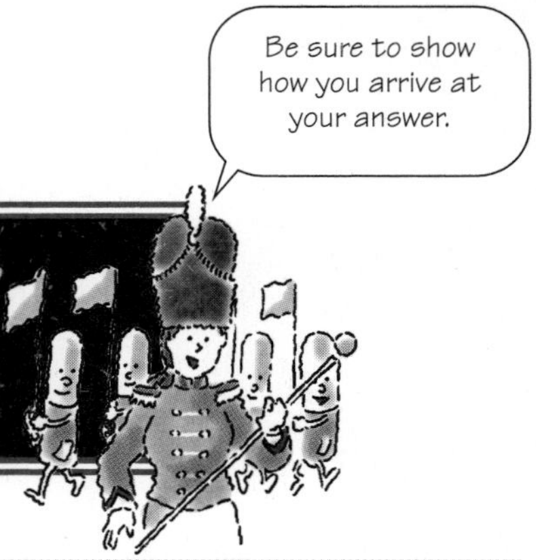
Be sure to show how you arrive at your answer.

The order for a patient reads 250 ml hypertonic saline solution to run over 4 hours. What should the infusion rate be for the solution?

Your answer: ______________________

To find the answer, first set up your ratios and a proportion.

$$4 \text{ hr} : 250 \text{ ml} :: 1 \text{ hr} : X \text{ ml}$$

Now, solve for *X*.

$$\frac{\cancel{4 \text{ hr}} \times X \text{ ml}}{\cancel{4 \text{ hr}}} = \frac{250 \text{ ml} \times 1 \cancel{\text{hr}}}{4 \cancel{\text{hr}}}$$

$$X = \frac{250}{4}$$

$$X = 62.5 \text{ ml/hr}$$

Rounding this off, the infusion rate would be 63 ml/hour.

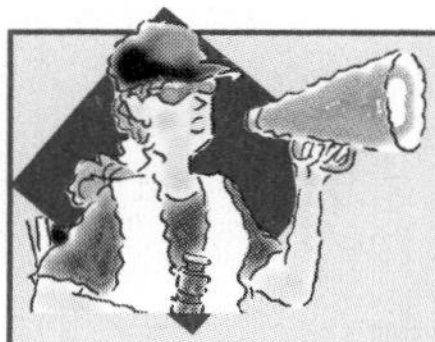

That's a wrap!

Calculating I.V. infusions review

Some important information about calculating I.V. infusions is highlighted below.

Drip rate

- Represents the number of drops infused per minute
- Formula to use:

total milliliters ÷ total minutes × drop factor in drops (gtt)/milliliter

- Drop factor represents the number of drops per milliliter of solution that the I.V. tubing is designed to deliver

Flow rate

- Represents the number of milliliters of fluid administered over 1 hour
- Formula to use:

total volume ordered ÷ number of hours

Drip rate shortcut

Macrodrips

- For 10 gtt/ml sets, divide hourly flow rate by 6
- For 15 gtt/ml sets, divide hourly flow rate by 4
- For 20 gtt/ml sets, divide hourly flow rate by 3

Microdrips

- Drip rate = flow rate

Infusion time

- The amount of time required for infusion of a specified volume of I.V. fluid
- Method #1:

infusion time = infused volume ÷ flow rate

- Method #2:

infusion time = infused volume ÷ drip rate/drop factor × 60 minutes

Regulating I.V. flow manually

- Count the number of drops going into the drip chamber.
- Adjust the flow with the roller clamp to the appropriate drip rate.
- Time-tape the I.V. bag.

Regulating I.V. flow with electronic infusion pumps

- Program the device based on the infusion rate.
- Count drips in the chamber to check the infusion.

PCA pump

- Allows the patient to self-administer an analgesic
- Also can be programmed to deliver a basal dose of drug
- Requires use of an access code or key to prevent unauthorized use of the device

Using a PCA pump

- Program the pump according to manufacturer's directions
- Read the PCA log; then record information per facility policy

PCA log notes

- Strength of drug solution in the container
- Number of drug administrations during assessment period
- Basal dose patient received, if any
- Amount of solution received (equals the number of injections × volume of injections + basal doses)
- Total amount of drug received (equals total amount of solution × solution strength)

(continued)

Calculating I.V. infusions review *(continued)*

Heparin flow rate formula
- First determine the solution's concentration: Divide units of drug added by the amount of solution in milliliters.
- Then state as a fraction (the desired dose over the unknown flow rate).
- Lastly, cross-multiply and solve for *X*.

Insulin infusions
- Regular insulin is the only type administered by I.V. route.
- Use an infusion pump.
- Use concentrations of 1 unit/ml.

Electrolyte and nutrient infusions
- Make sure that drugs to be infused together are compatible.
- Calculate the amount of additive using the proportion method as you would for any prepared liquid drug.
- Calculate the flow rate and the drip rate.

Blood infusions
- Filter out agglutinated cells with special administration sets.
- Drop factor is 10 to 15 gtt/ml.
- Use at least a 20G I.V. catheter.

TPN administration
- Can be given centrally or peripherally
- Initially infused at 40 ml/hour, then increased to maintenance
- Administered with an infusion pump

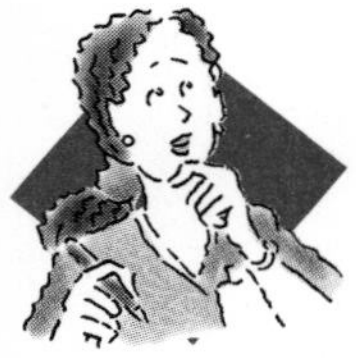

Quick quiz

1. To calculate the drip rate of an I.V. solution, you must first determine the:

A. drop factor.
B. flow rate.
C. size of the tubing.
D. total volume of the I.V. solution.

Answer: A. The drop factor, or number of drops/milliliter of solution, depends on the administration set you're using and is listed on the set's label.

2. The doctor orders 1,000 ml of a drug to infuse over 10 hours at 25 gtt/minute. The set calibration is 15 gtt/ml. After 5 hours, 650 ml have infused instead of 500. To recalculate the drip rate for the remaining solution, you would:

A. increase the rate to 18 gtt/minute.
B. increase the rate to 35 gtt/minute.
C. slow the rate to 10 gtt/minute.
D. slow the rate to 18 gtt/minute.

Answer: D. To solve this problem, determine the amount of fluid remaining by subtracting 650 ml from 1,000 ml. Convert the time remaining to minutes. Set up the equation using this formula:

$$\frac{\text{total ml}}{\text{total minutes}} \times \text{drop factor in gtt/ml} = \text{drip rate in gtt/minute}$$

3. Which test determines the therapeutic range for heparin?

A. Activated partial thrombin test
B. Partial thromboplastin time (PTT)
C. Partial thrombin activation test
D. Clotting test

Answer: B. Heparin doses are individualized based on the patient's coagulation status, which is measured by PTT.

4. For a microdrip set with a drop factor of 60 gtt/ml, the drip rate is:

A. half the hourly flow rate.
B. 10 times greater than the hourly flow rate.
C. the same as the hourly flow rate.
D. 4 times greater than the hourly flow rate.

Answer: C. The drip rate is the same as the hourly flow rate because the number of minutes in an hour—60—is the same as the drop factor.

5. You start a continuous infusion of 150 units of regular insulin in 150 ml of normal saline solution. If the prescribed dose is 8 units/hour, what's the hourly flow rate?

A. 8 ml/hour
B. 10 ml/hour
C. 18 ml/hour
D. 80 ml/hour

Answer: A. Solve this problem by setting up the first fraction with the known solution strength and the second fraction with the desired dose and the unknown volume, putting these fractions into a proportion, cross-multiplying, and then dividing and canceling the units of measure that appear in both the numerator and denominator.

6. The PCA pump can provide a dose of medication on demand or at a:

A. dropped rate.
B. basal rate.
C. ratio rate.
D. lock-out rate.

Answer: B. The basal rate is a continuous infusion administered by the PCA.

7. You need to infuse 1,500 ml of D_5W over 10 hours. What's the flow rate?

A. 50 ml/hour
B. 100 ml/hour
C. 150 ml/hour
D. 250 ml/hour

Answer: C. Set up the equation using this formula:

$$\frac{\text{total volume ordered}}{\text{number of hours}}$$

8. Your patient needs an infusion of D_5W at 75 ml/hour. If the tubing set is calibrated at 20 gtt/ml, what's the drip rate?

A. 20 gtt/minute
B. 25 gtt/minute
C. 50 gtt/minute
D. 75 gtt/minute

Answer: B. Set up the equation using this formula:

$$\frac{\text{total ml}}{\text{total minutes}} \times \text{drop factor in gtt/ml} = \text{drip rate in gtt/minute}$$

Scoring

☆☆☆ If you answered all eight items correctly, excellent! Enjoy every gtt of success.

☆☆ If you answered five to seven items correctly, great job! Your drop factor is beyond measure. (All right, if you insist, we'll give you 15 gtt/ml.)

☆ If you answered fewer than five items correctly, no problem! Go with the flow, keep calculatin', and infuse in peace and joy.

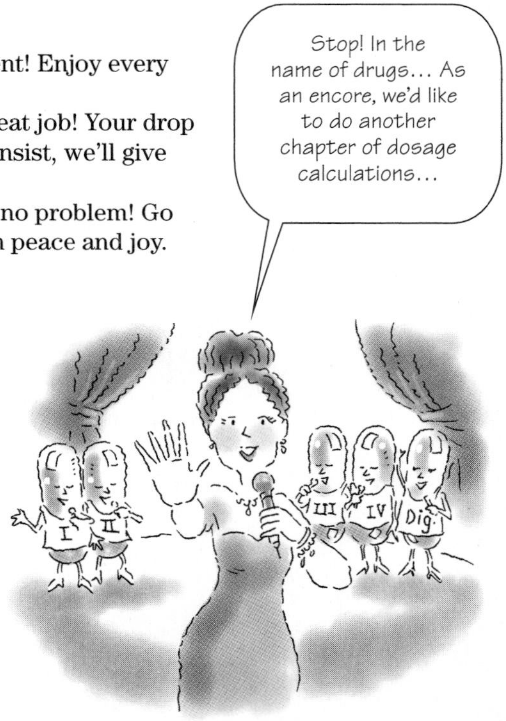

Stop! In the name of drugs... As an encore, we'd like to do another chapter of dosage calculations...
I
II
III
IV
Dig

Part VI Special calculations

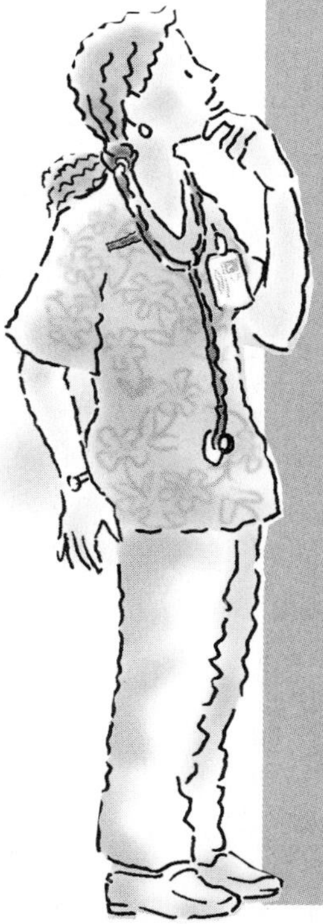

14

Calculating pediatric dosages

Just the facts

In this chapter, you'll learn:

- how to prepare drugs and administer them to infants and children by the four major routes
- methods for calculating safe pediatric drug dosages according to body weight and body surface area
- recommended pediatric infusion guidelines and protocols
- how to calculate pediatric fluid needs based on body weight, calories of metabolism, and body surface area.

A look at calculating pediatric dosages

When calculating drug dosages for pediatric patients, remember that children aren't just small adults. Because of their size, metabolism, and other factors, children have special medication needs and require special care. Also, an incorrect dose is more likely to harm a child than an adult.

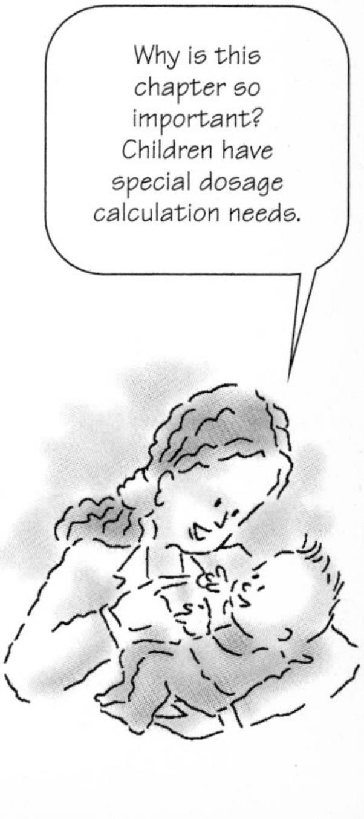

Why is this chapter so important? Children have special dosage calculation needs.

Same routes, different needs

Although children and adults receive drugs by the oral (P.O.), subcutaneous (subQ), intramuscular (I.M.), intravenous (I.V.), and topical routes, the similarity ends there. The pharmacokinetics, pharmacodynamics, and pharmacotherapeutics of drugs differ greatly between children and adults.

For example, a child's immature body systems may be unable to handle certain drugs. Also, a child's total volume of body water is much greater proportionally than an adult's, so drug distribution is altered. Because of these differences, you must be especially careful when calculating dosages for children. (See *A trio of time-saving tips*, page 286.)

Administering pediatric drugs

The methods used to prepare drugs and administer them to pediatric patients also differ from the methods used for adults, depending on which route is used. There are specific administration guidelines and precautions for each route as well. However, there is one step that is always the same no matter what age the patient is. Always verify the child's identity using two patient identifiers. Involve the parent and the patient in the identification process, when possible. (See *Giving medications to children.*)

Oral route

Infants and young children who can't swallow tablets or capsules are given oral drugs in liquid form. When a liquid preparation isn't available, you may generally crush a tablet and mix it with a small amount of liquid. Don't use essential fluids, such as breast milk and infant formula, because this could lead to feeding refusal. Additionally, mix it in only a small amount of liquid. If the medication is mixed in a large amount of liquid, such as a full bottle, the child won't receive the entire dose if he doesn't finish the bottle.

Remember: Never crush timed-release capsules or tablets or enteric-coated drugs. Crushing destroys the coating that causes drugs to release at the right time and prevent stomach irritation.

Measuring device advice

If a child can drink from a cup, measure and give liquid medications in a cup that's calibrated in metric and household units. If the child is very young or can't drink from a cup, use a medication dropper, syringe, or hollow-handle spoon. These devices are sold individually and also come prepackaged with some drugs.

Advice from the experts

A trio of time-saving tips

When calculating safe pediatric dosages, save time and avoid errors by following these suggestions:

- Carry a calculator for use in solving equations.
- Consult a formulary or drug handbook to verify a drug dose. When in doubt, call the pharmacist.
- Keep your patient's weight in kilograms at his bedside so you don't have to estimate it or weigh him in a rush.

Advice from the experts

Giving medications to children

When giving oral and parenteral medications to children, safety is essential. Keep these points in mind:

- Check the child's mouth to make sure he has swallowed the oral drug.
- Carefully mix oral drugs that come in suspension form.
- Give intramuscular (I.M.) injections in the vastus lateralis muscle or ventrogluteal muscle.
- Don't inject more than 1 ml into I.M. or subcutaneous sites.
- Rotate injection sites.

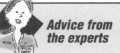

I.M. injections for infants

When giving intramuscular (I.M.) injections to infants, use the vastus lateralis muscle. Don't inject into the gluteus muscle until it's fully developed, which occurs when the child learns to walk. Use a 23G to 25G needle that's ⅝″ to 1″ in length. These illustrations show how to give an I.M. injection using one- and two-person methods.

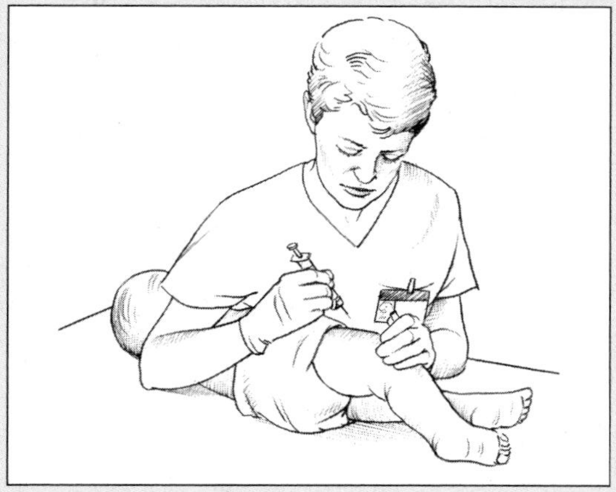

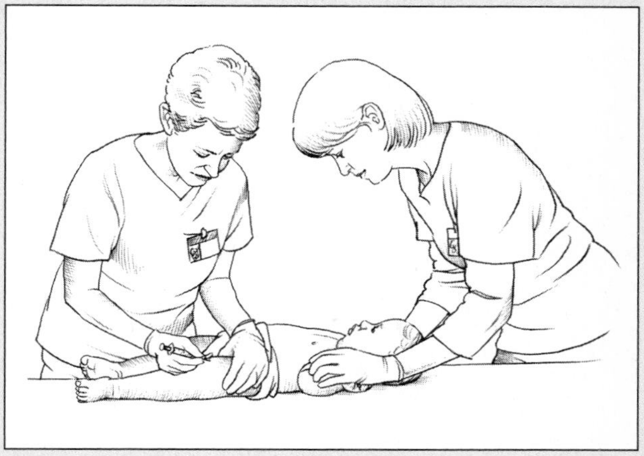

Mix it up

If the liquid drug is prepared as a suspension or as an insoluble drug in a liquid base, mix it thoroughly before you measure and administer it. This ensures that none of the drug remains settled out of the solution. Whenever you give an oral drug, check the child's mouth to make sure that all of the drug was swallowed.

Subcutaneous route

Pediatric patients also may receive childhood immunizations (such as the measles, mumps, and rubella vaccine and other virus vaccines) and drugs such as insulin by the subQ route. When giving subQ injections, make sure each injection contains no more than 1 ml of solution. Any area with sufficient subcutaneous tissue may be used—the upper arm, abdomen, and thigh are the most common.

I.M. route

Vaccines, such as that against diphtheria, pertussis, and tetanus, are commonly administered by the I.M. route. (See *I.M. injections for infants.*)When giving I.M. injections, make sure each injection contains no more than 1 ml of solution. Give I.M. injections in the vastus lateralis (outer thigh) or the ventrogluteal muscle.

Finding the nerve

Be aware of the risk of nerve damage when selecting the site, needle length, and injection technique.

I.V. route

Fluids and drugs may also be administered by the I.V. route. I.V. site placement may be in a peripheral or central vein. Because pediatric patients can tolerate only a limited amount of fluid, dilute I.V. drugs and administer I.V. fluids cautiously. Always use an infusion pump with infants and small children.

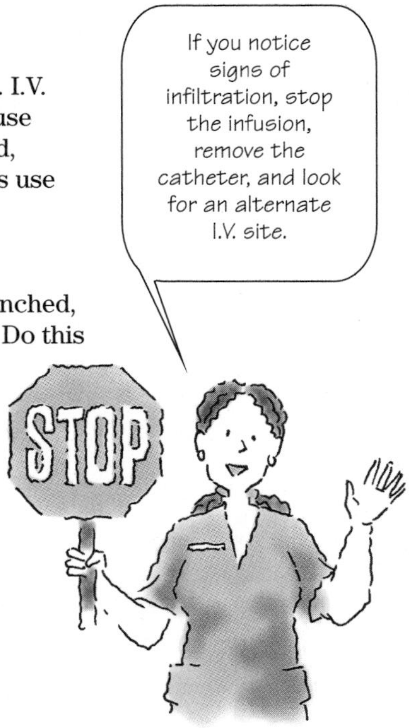
If you notice signs of infiltration, stop the infusion, remove the catheter, and look for an alternate I.V. site.
STOP

Infiltration and inflammation alert!

Inspect I.V. sites frequently for signs of infiltration (cool, blanched, and puffy skin) or inflammation (warm and reddened skin). Do this before, during, and after the infusion because children's vessels are immature and easily damaged by drugs. If infiltration occurs, stop the infusion, remove the catheter, and consider placement for a new I.V. site.

Topical route

Medications may be administered topically in children as in adults. However, in infants and small children, the absorption of topical medications is greater because these children have:

- a thinner stratum corneum
- increased skin hydration
- a greater ratio of total body surface area to weight.

Also, the use of disposable diapers with a plastic-coated layer can increase topical drug absorption in the diaper area because the plastic coating can act like an occlusive dressing.

Baby wipes

When applying topical drugs on pediatric patients, wipe off any drug that remains on the skin from the previous application, and apply the new drug according to the doctor's order and the drug manufacturer's recommendations.

Calculation methods

To calculate and verify the safety of pediatric drug dosages, use the dosage-per-kilogram-of-body-weight method or the body-surface-area (BSA) method. Other methods, such as those based on age or the standard dosing used for adults, are less accurate and typically aren't used.

Whichever method you use, remember that you're professionally and legally responsible for checking the safety of a prescribed dose prior to administration.

Dosage per kilogram of body weight

Many pharmaceutical companies provide information about safe drug dosages for pediatric patients in milligrams per kilogram of body weight. This is the most accurate and common way to calculate pediatric dosages. Pediatric dosages are usually expressed as *mg/kg/day* or *mg/kg/dose*. Based on this information, you can determine the pediatric dose by multiplying the child's weight in kilograms by the required number of milligrams of drug per kilogram.

Shifting weight: From pounds to kilograms

Because most patients' weights are measured in pounds (lb), you must convert from pounds to kilograms before calculating the dosage per kilogram of body weight. Remember that 1 kg equals 2.2 lb.

Real world problems

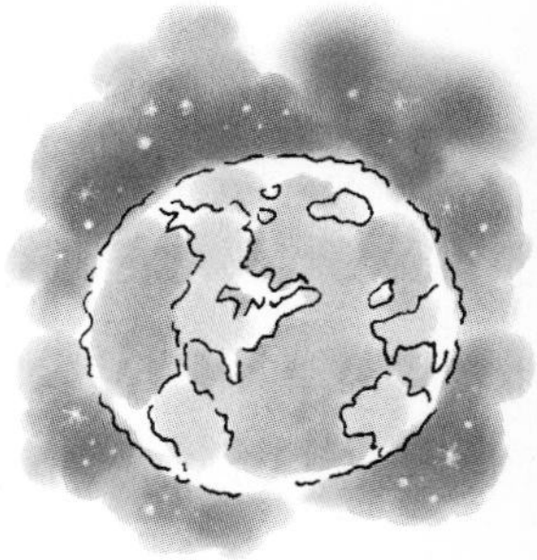

The following examples show how to use proportions to convert pounds to kilograms, how to calculate mg/kg/dose for one-time or as-needed (p.r.n.) medications, and how to calculate mg/kg/day for doses given around-the-clock to maintain a continuous drug effect.

A weighty problem

If your 6-year-old patient weighs 41.5 lb, how much does he weigh in kilograms?

Here's how to solve this problem using ratios.

- Set up the proportion, remembering that 2.2 lb equals 1 kg:

$$X : 41.5 \text{ lb} :: 1 \text{ kg} : 2.2 \text{ lb}$$

• Multiply the extremes and the means:

$$X \times 2.2 \text{ lb} = 1 \text{ kg} \times 41.5 \text{ lb}$$

• Solve for X by dividing each side of the equation by 2.2 lb and canceling units that appear in both the numerator and denominator:

$$\frac{X \times 2.2 \cancel{\text{lb}}}{2.2 \cancel{\text{lb}}} = \frac{1 \text{ kg} \times 41.5 \cancel{\text{lb}}}{2.2 \cancel{\text{lb}}}$$

$$X = \frac{41.5 \text{ kg}}{2.2}$$

$$X = 18.9 \text{ kg}$$

The child weighs 18.9 kg, rounded off to 19 kg.

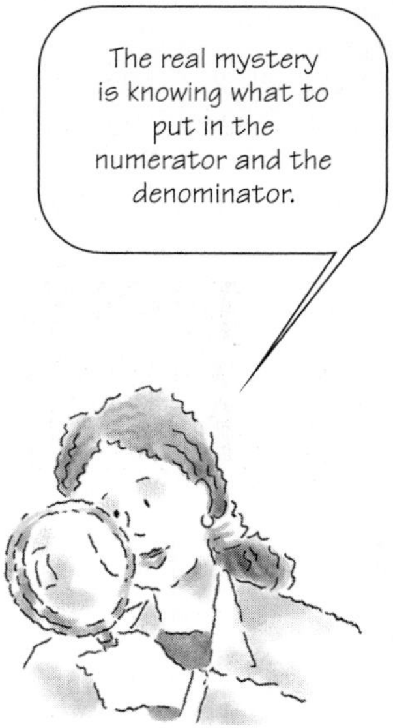

The real mystery is knowing what to put in the numerator and the denominator.

Milligram mystery

The doctor orders a single dose of 20 mg/kg/dose of amoxicillin oral suspension for a toddler who weighs 20 lb (9.1 kg). What's the dose in milligrams?

Here's how to solve this problem using fractions.

• Set up the proportion with the ordered dosage in one fraction and the unknown dosage and the patient's weight in the other fraction:

$$\frac{20 \text{ mg}}{1 \text{ kg/dose}} = \frac{X}{9 \text{ kg/dose}}$$

• Cross-multiply the fractions:

$$X \times 1 \text{ kg/dose} = 20 \text{ mg} \times 9 \text{ kg/dose}$$

• Solve for X by dividing each side of the equation by 1 kg/dose and canceling units that appear in both the numerator and denominator:

$$\frac{X \times \cancel{1 \text{ kg/dose}}}{\cancel{1 \text{ kg/dose}}} = \frac{20 \text{ mg} \times 9 \cancel{\text{kg/dose}}}{1 \cancel{\text{kg/dose}}}$$

$$X = 180 \text{ mg}$$

The patient needs 180 mg of amoxicillin.

Dosage drill

Test your math skills with this drill.

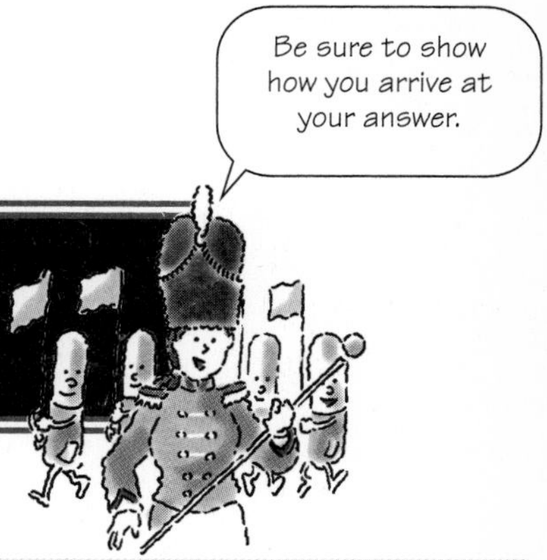
Be sure to show how you arrive at your answer.

How many milligrams of a medication will a nurse give to a 32-lb child if the order calls for 25 mg/kg?

Your answer: ______________________

First find the child's weight in kilograms by setting up ratios and a proportion and solving for *X*.

$$2.2 \text{ lb} : 1 \text{ kg} :: 32 \text{ lb} : X \text{ kg}$$

$$2.2 \text{ lb} \times X \text{ kg} = 1 \text{ kg} \times 32 \text{ lb}$$

$$\frac{\cancel{2.2 \text{ lb}} \times X \text{ kg}}{\cancel{2.2 \text{ lb}}} = \frac{1 \text{ kg} \times 32 \cancel{\text{ lb}}}{2.2 \cancel{\text{ lb}}}$$

$$X = \frac{32}{2.2}$$

$$X = 14.5454 \text{ kg}$$

Now, find the total number of milligrams to give based on the child's weight.

$$1 \text{ kg} : 25 \text{ mg} :: 14.5454 \text{ kg} : X \text{ mg}$$

$$1 \text{ kg} \times X \text{ mg} = 25 \text{ mg} \times 14.5454 \text{ kg}$$

$$\frac{\cancel{1 \text{ kg}} \times X \text{ mg}}{\cancel{1 \text{ kg}}} = \frac{25 \text{ mg} \times 14.5454 \cancel{\text{ kg}}}{1 \cancel{\text{ kg}}}$$

$$X = 25 \times 14.5454$$

$$X = 363.6 \text{ mg}$$

The nurse would give 363.6 mg of medication.

A perplexing penicillin problem

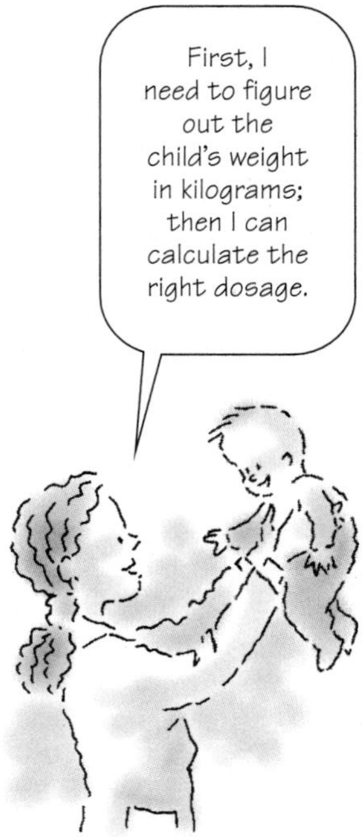
First, I need to figure out the child's weight in kilograms; then I can calculate the right dosage.

The doctor orders *penicillin V potassium oral suspension 56 mg/kg/day in four divided doses* for a patient who weighs 55 lb. The suspension that's available is penicillin V potassium 125 mg/5 ml. What volume should you administer for each dose?

Here's how to solve this problem using ratios and fractions.

- First, convert the child's weight from pounds to kilograms by setting up the following proportion:

$$X : 55\text{ lb} :: 1\text{ kg} : 2.2\text{ lb}$$

- Multiply the extremes and the means:

$$X \times 2.2\text{ lb} = 1\text{ kg} \times 55\text{ lb}$$

- Solve for X by dividing each side of the equation by 2.2 lb and canceling units that appear in both the numerator and denominator:

$$\frac{X \times \cancel{2.2\text{ lb}}}{\cancel{2.2\text{ lb}}} = \frac{1\text{ kg} \times 55\,\cancel{\text{lb}}}{2.2\,\cancel{\text{lb}}}$$

$$X = \frac{55\text{ kg}}{2.2}$$

$$X = 25\text{ kg}$$

- The child weighs 25 kg. Next, determine the total daily dosage by setting up a proportion with the patient's weight and the unknown dosage on one side and the ordered dosage on the other side:

$$\frac{25\text{ kg}}{X} = \frac{1\text{ kg}}{56\text{ mg}}$$

- Cross-multiply the fractions:

$$X \times 1\text{ kg} = 56\text{ mg} \times 25\text{ kg}$$

- Solve for X by dividing each side of the equation by 1 kg and canceling units that appear in both the numerator and denominator:

$$\frac{X \times \cancel{1\text{ kg}}}{\cancel{1\text{ kg}}} = \frac{56\text{ mg} \times 25\,\cancel{\text{kg}}}{1\,\cancel{\text{kg}}}$$

$$X = \frac{56\text{ mg} \times 25}{1}$$

$$X = 1{,}400\text{ mg}$$

• The child's daily dosage is 1,400 mg. Now, divide the daily dosage by 4 doses to determine the dose to administer every 6 hours:

$$X = \frac{1{,}400 \text{ mg}}{4 \text{ doses}}$$

$$X = 350 \text{ mg/dose}$$

The child should receive 350 mg every 6 hours.

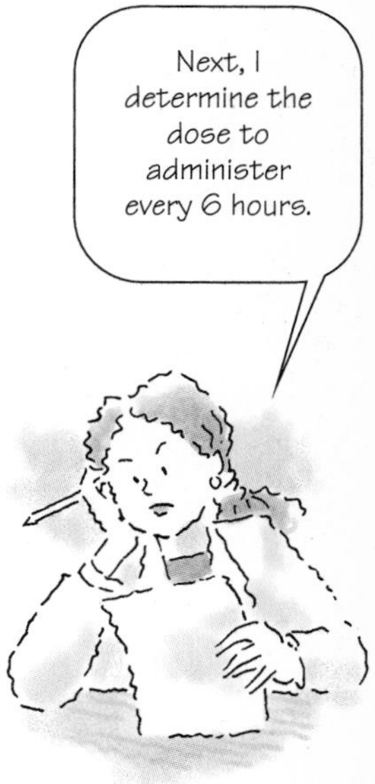
Next, I determine the dose to administer every 6 hours.

• Lastly, calculate the volume to give for each dose by setting up a proportion with the unknown volume and the amount in one dose on one side and the available dose on the other side:

$$\frac{X}{350 \text{ mg}} = \frac{5 \text{ ml}}{125 \text{ mg}}$$

• Cross-multiply the fractions:

$$X \times 125 \text{ mg} = 5 \text{ ml} \times 350 \text{ mg}$$

• Solve for *X* by dividing each side of the equation by 125 mg and canceling units that appear in both the numerator and denominator:

$$\frac{X \times \cancel{125 \text{ mg}}}{\cancel{125 \text{ mg}}} = \frac{5 \text{ ml} \times 350 \cancel{\text{ mg}}}{125 \cancel{\text{ mg}}}$$

$$X = \frac{5 \text{ ml} \times 350}{125}$$

$$X = \frac{1{,}750 \text{ ml}}{125}$$

$$X = 14 \text{ ml}$$

You should administer 14 ml of the drug at each dose.

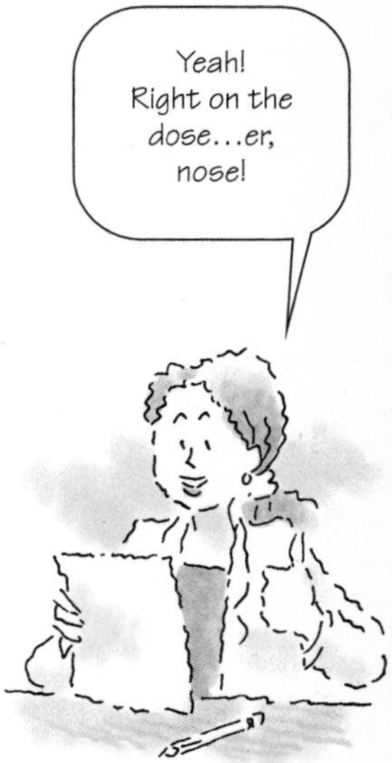
Yeah! Right on the dose…er, nose!

Dosage by BSA

The BSA method is used to calculate safe pediatric dosages for a limited number of drugs, such as antineoplastic or chemotherapeutic agents. (It's also used to calculate safe dosages for adult patients receiving these extremely potent drugs or drugs requiring great precision.)

Dosage drill

Test your math skills with this drill.

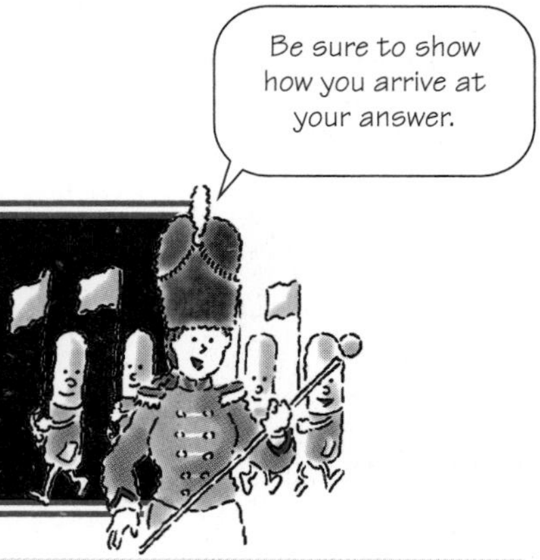
Be sure to show how you arrive at your answer.

A 52-lb (23.6-kg) child receives 5 mg/kg of phenytoin (Dilantin) for seizure control in two divided doses. The bottle contains a concentration of 125 mg/5 ml. How many milliliters per dose should the nurse instruct the parents to administer?

Your answer: ______________________

First calculate the required milligrams.

$$1 \text{ kg} : 5 \text{ mg} :: 23.6 \text{ kg} : X \text{ mg}$$

$$1 \text{ kg} \times X \text{ mg} = 5 \text{ mg} \times 23.6 \text{ kg}$$

$$\frac{\cancel{1 \text{ kg}} \times X \text{ mg}}{\cancel{1 \text{ kg}}} = \frac{5 \text{ mg} \times 23.6 \cancel{\text{ kg}}}{1 \cancel{\text{ kg}}}$$

$$X = 118 \text{ mg}$$

Then calculate the required milliliters.

$$125 \text{ mg} : 5 \text{ ml} :: 118 \text{ mg} : X \text{ ml}$$

$$125 \text{ mg} \times X \text{ ml} = 5 \text{ ml} \times 118 \cancel{\text{ mg}}$$

$$\frac{\cancel{125 \text{ mg}} \times X \text{ ml}}{\cancel{125 \text{ mg}}} = \frac{5 \text{ ml} \times 118 \cancel{\text{ mg}}}{125 \text{ mg}}$$

$$X = \frac{590}{125}$$

$$X = 4.7 \text{ ml}$$

Finally, determine the amount per dose.

$$4.7 \text{ ml} : 2 \text{ doses} :: X \text{ ml} : 1 \text{ dose}$$

$$4.7 \text{ ml} \times 1 \text{ dose} = 2 \text{ doses} \times X \text{ ml}$$

$$\frac{4.7 \text{ ml} \times 1 \cancel{\text{ dose}}}{2 \cancel{\text{ doses}}} = \frac{\cancel{2 \text{ doses}} \times X \text{ ml}}{\cancel{2 \text{ doses}}}$$

$$X = \frac{4.7}{2}$$

$$X = 2.35 \text{ ml/dose}$$

The parents should give 2.35 ml with each dose.

BSA plot thickens

Calculating dosages by BSA involves two steps:

Plot the patient's height and weight on a chart called a *nomogram* to determine the BSA in square meters (m^2). (See *What's in a nomogram?*, page 296.)

Multiply the BSA by the prescribed pediatric dose in $mg/m^2/day$.

Here's the formula:

$$\text{child's dose in mg} = \text{child's BSA in m}^2 \times \frac{\text{pediatric dose in mg}}{\text{m}^2\text{/day}}$$

The BSA method can also be used to calculate a child's dose based on the average adult BSA—1.73 m^2—and an average adult dose.

The formula looks like this:

$$\text{child's dose in mg} = \frac{\text{child's BSA in m}^2}{\text{average adult BSA (1.73 m}^2\text{)}} \times \text{average adult dose}$$

Real world problems

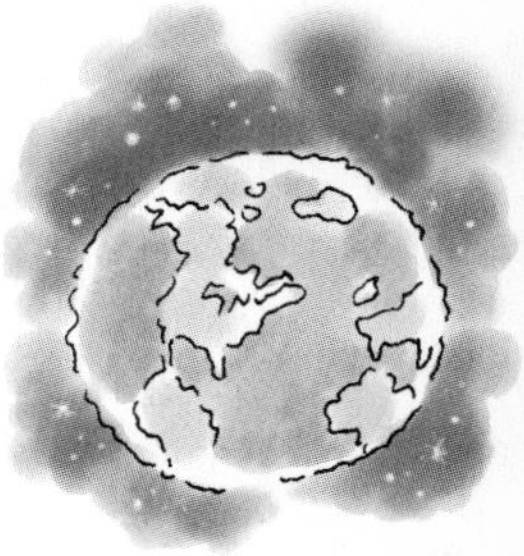

The following problems show how these two formulas are used in the BSA method of dosage calculation.

An engrossing ephedrine equation

The doctor orders *ephedrine 100 mg/m²/day* for a child who's 40″ tall and weighs 64 lb. How much ephedrine should the child receive daily?

- Use the nomogram to determine that the child's BSA is 0.96 m^2.
- Using the appropriate formula, determine the daily dosage:

$$X = 0.96\ \text{m}^2 \times \frac{100\ \text{mg}}{1\ \text{m}^2\text{/day}}$$

- Solve for X:

$$X = 0.96\ \cancel{\text{m}^2} \times \frac{100\ \text{mg}}{1\ \cancel{\text{m}^2}\text{/day}}$$

$$X = 96\ \text{mg/day}$$

The child needs 96 mg of ephedrine per day.

A captivating chemotherapy question

A child who needs chemotherapy is 36″ tall and weighs 40 lb. What's the safe drug dose if the average adult dose is 1,000 mg?

- Use the nomogram to determine that the child's BSA is 0.72 m^2.

What's in a nomogram?

Body surface area (BSA) is critical when calculating dosages for pediatric patients or for drugs that are extremely potent and need to be given in precise amounts. The nomogram shown here lets you plot the patient's height and weight to determine the BSA. Here's how it works:

- Locate the patient's height in the left column of the nomogram and his weight in the right column.
- Use a ruler to draw a straight line connecting the two points. The point where the line intersects the surface area column indicates the patient's BSA in square meters.
- For an average-sized child, use the simplified nomogram in the box. Just find the child's weight in pounds on the left side of the scale, and then read the corresponding BSA on the right side.

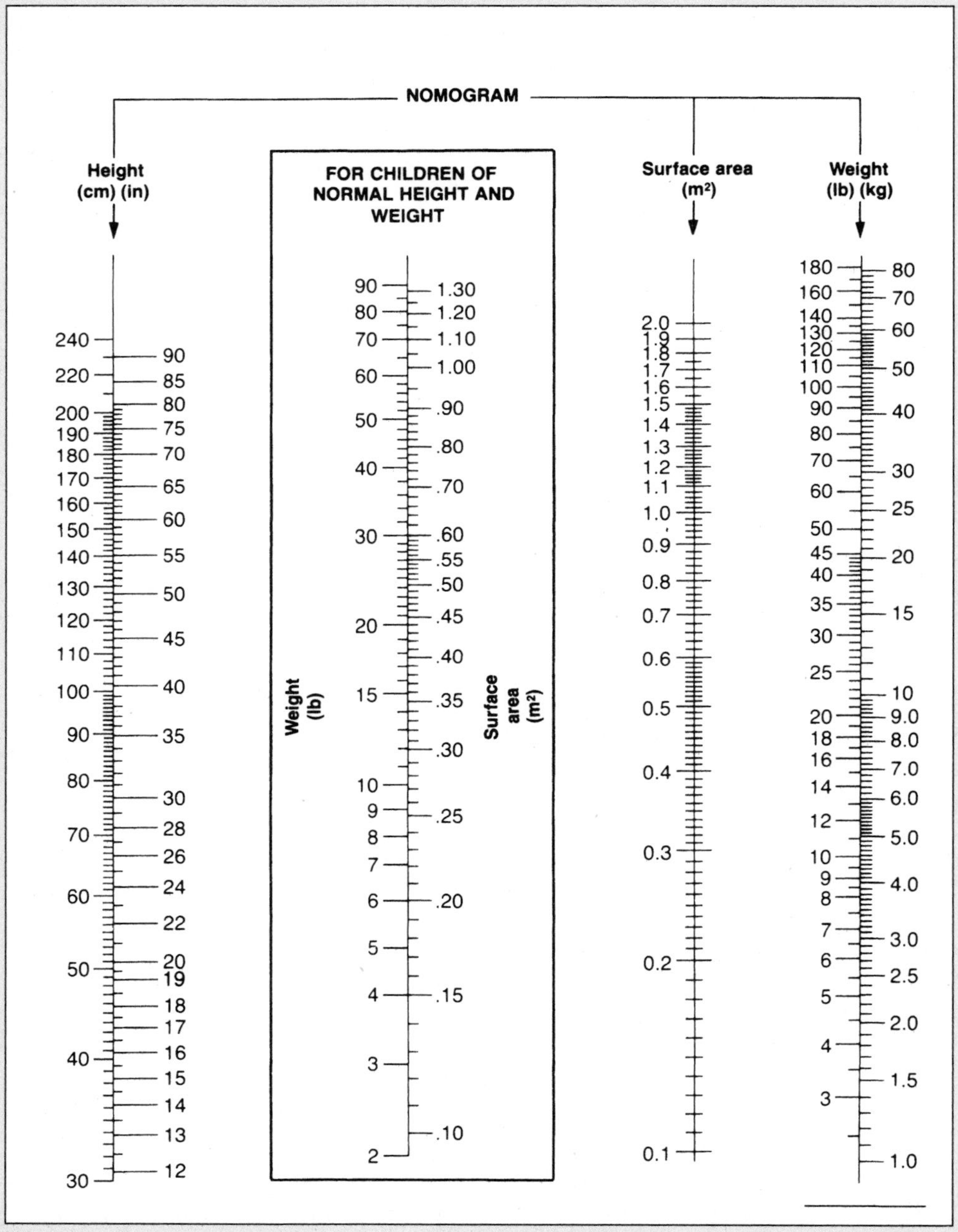

- Then set up an equation using the appropriate formula. Divide the child's BSA by 1.73 m^2 (the average adult BSA), and multiply by the average adult dose, 1,000 mg:

$$X = \frac{0.72 \text{ m}^2}{1.73 \text{ m}^2} \times 1{,}000 \text{ mg}$$

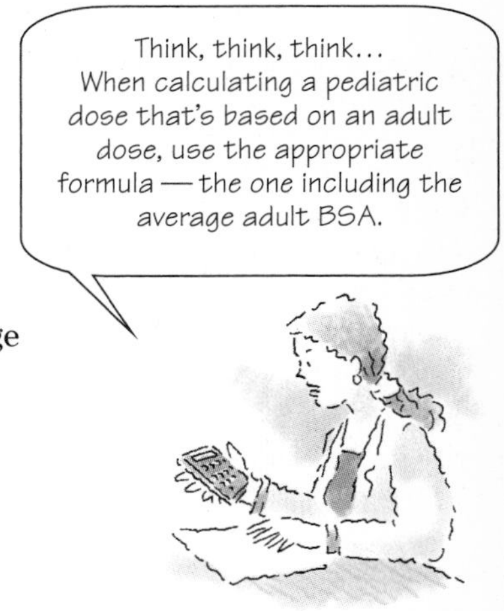
Think, think, think...
When calculating a pediatric dose that's based on an adult dose, use the appropriate formula — the one including the average adult BSA.

- Solve for X by canceling units that appear in both the numerator and denominator, multiplying the child's BSA by the average adult dose, and dividing the result by the average adult BSA:

$$X = \frac{0.72 \cancel{\text{m}^2} \times 1{,}000 \text{ mg}}{1.73 \cancel{\text{m}^2}}$$

$$X = 416 \text{ mg}$$

The safe dose for this child is 416 mg.

Verifying calculations

Although the doctor determines the medication dosage, the nurse is an important "last line of defense" who verifies that the ordered dosage is safe. Depending on your facility, you may have access to several reliable sources of information, including on-line computer services, drug references, and other staff.

Look it up

Some nursing drug handbooks contain usual (recommended) pediatric dosages for commonly prescribed drugs (pediatric drug handbooks specifically developed for the special needs of infants and children are also available). The pharmacist is another excellent resource for verifying drug safety. And remember, you should always double-check complex calculations with another nurse.

Real world problems

Here are some real world examples of verifying calculations.

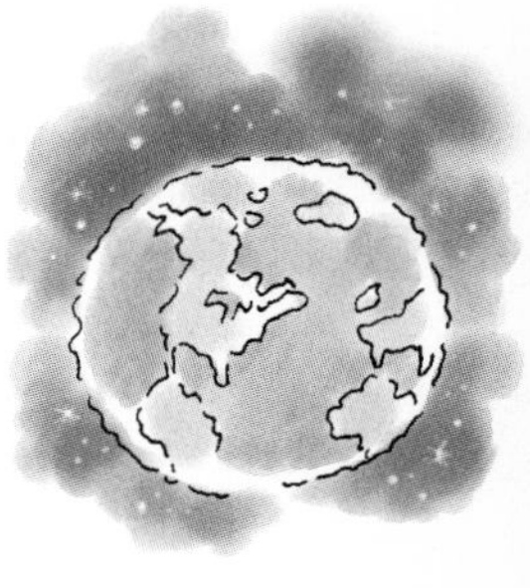

Clearing the way for chloral hydrate

The doctor orders *chloral hydrate 75 mg P.O.* to sedate a 3-kg neonate for an electroencephalogram. The drug resource states that the usual (recommended) dosage of chloral hydrate for a neonate is 25 mg/kg/dose for sedation prior to a procedure. Did the doctor order the correct dosage? Here's how to solve this problem using fractions.

Dosage drill

Test your math skills with this drill.

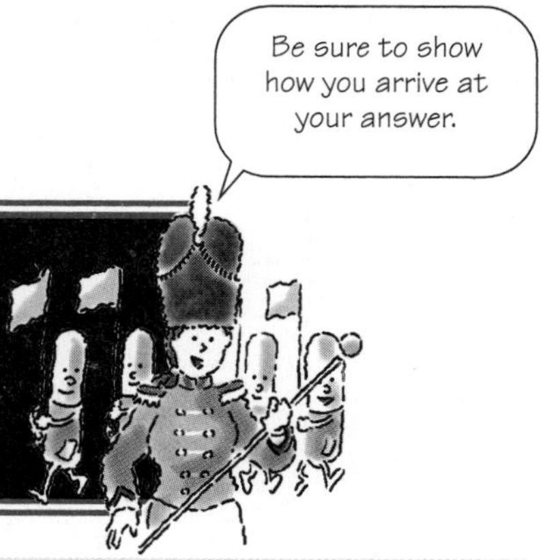
Be sure to show how you arrive at your answer.

The average adult dose of codeine phosphate for pain is 60 mg P.O. every 4 hours. How much should a nurse administer in a single dose to a child with a body surface area of 0.55 m²?

Your answer: ______________________

Set up ratios and a proportion, then solve for *X* to find the answer.

$$1.73\ m^2 : 60\ mg :: 0.55\ m^2 : X\ mg$$

$$1.73\ m^2 \times X\ mg = 60\ mg \times 0.55\ m^2$$

$$\frac{\cancel{1.73\ m^2} \times X\ mg}{\cancel{1.73\ m^2}} = \frac{60\ mg \times 0.55\ \cancel{m^2}}{1.73\ \cancel{m^2}}$$

$$X = \frac{33}{1.73}$$

$$X = 19.1\ mg$$

The nurse should administer 19.1 mg of the codeine phosphate in a single dose.

- Set up the proportion with the usual dosage in one fraction and the unknown dosage and the patient's weight in the other fraction:

$$\frac{25 \text{ mg}}{1 \text{ kg/dose}} = \frac{X}{3 \text{ kg/dose}}$$

- Cross-multiply the fractions:

$$X \times 1 \text{ kg/dose} = 25 \text{ mg} \times 3 \text{ kg/dose}$$

- Solve for X by dividing each side of the equation by 1 kg/dose and canceling units that appear in both the numerator and denominator:

$$\frac{X \times \cancel{1 \text{ kg/dose}}}{\cancel{1 \text{ kg/dose}}} = \frac{25 \text{ mg} \times 3 \cancel{\text{ kg/dose}}}{1 \cancel{\text{ kg/dose}}}$$

$$X = 75 \text{ mg}$$

The patient needs 75 mg of chloral hydrate. That's what the doctor ordered and, therefore, the dose is safe to administer.

Penicillin puzzler

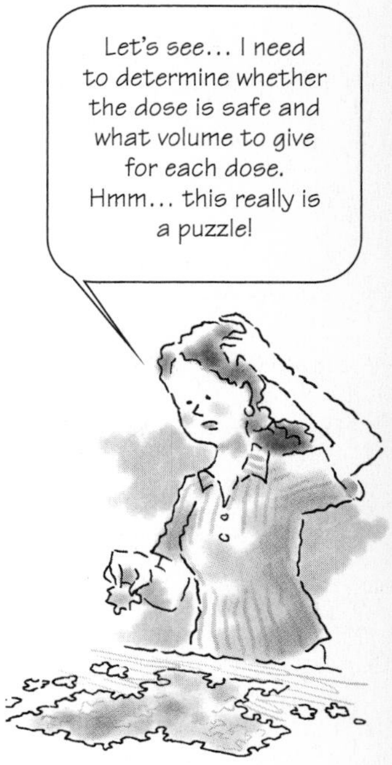

Let's see... I need to determine whether the dose is safe and what volume to give for each dose. Hmm... this really is a puzzle!

The doctor orders *penicillin V potassium oral suspension 250 mg P.O. q6h* for a patient who weighs 55 lb. Is the dose safe? The suspension that's available is penicillin V potassium 125 mg/5 ml. What volume should you administer for each dose?

Here's how to answer these questions using ratios and fractions:

- First, convert the child's weight from pounds to kilograms by setting up the following proportion:

$$X : 55 \text{ lb} :: 1 \text{ kg} : 2.2 \text{ lb}$$

- Multiply the extremes and the means:

$$X \times 2.2 \text{ lb} = 1 \text{ kg} \times 55 \text{ lb}$$

- Solve for X by dividing each side of the equation by 2.2. lb and canceling units that appear in both the numerator and denominator:

$$\frac{X \times \cancel{2.2 \text{ lb}}}{\cancel{2.2 \text{ lb}}} = \frac{1 \text{ kg} \times 55 \cancel{\text{ lb}}}{2.2 \cancel{\text{ lb}}}$$

$$X = \frac{55 \text{ kg}}{2.2}$$

$$X = 25 \text{ kg}$$

The child weighs 25 kg.

- Now verify the usual (recommended) dosage. The drug reference states to give penicillin V potassium 25 to 50 mg/kg/day orally in divided doses every 6 to 8 hours. This indicates a safe daily dosage range — a low dosage (25 mg/kg/day) and a high dosage

Dosage drill

Test your math skills with this drill.

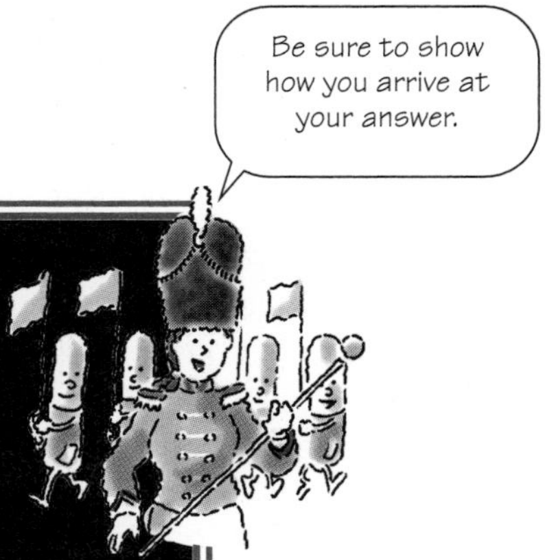
Be sure to show how you arrive at your answer.

The doctor orders furosemide (Lasix) 12 mg P.O. daily for a 6-kg infant diagnosed with heart failure. The drug reference on your unit states that the recommended dosage of furosemide for a child is 2 mg/kg/dose. Did the doctor order the correct dosage?

Your answer: ______________________

To find the answer, first set up a proportion with the recommended dosage in one fraction and the unknown dosage and the patient's weight in the other fraction.

$$\frac{2\text{ mg}}{1\text{ kg/dose}} = \frac{X}{6\text{ kg/dose}}$$

Next, cross-multiply the fractions.

$$2\text{ mg} \times 6\text{ kg/dose} = X \times 1\text{ kg/dose}$$

Finally, solve for X by dividing each side of the equation by 1 kg/dose and canceling units that appear in both the numerator and denominator.

$$\frac{2\text{ mg} \times 6\ \cancel{\text{kg/dose}}}{1\ \cancel{\text{kg/dose}}} = \frac{X \times \cancel{1\text{ kg/dose}}}{\cancel{1\text{ kg/dose}}}$$

$$X = 12\text{ mg}$$

The patient needs 12 mg of furosemide, which is exactly what the doctor ordered. The dose is safe to administer.

(50 mg/kg/day). These are also the minimum (low) dosage and the maximum (high) dosage for the day.

- Next, determine the usual total daily dosage range by setting up two proportions with the patient's weight on one side and the usual dosage (either the low dosage and or the high dosage) on the other side. Let's look at the high dose first:

$$\frac{25\text{ kg}}{X} = \frac{1\text{ kg}}{50\text{ mg}}$$

- Cross-multiply the fractions:

$$X \times 1\text{ kg} = 50\text{ mg} \times 25\text{ kg}$$

- Solve for X by dividing each side of the equation by 1 kg and canceling units that appear in both the numerator and denominator:

$$\frac{X \times \cancel{1\text{ kg}}}{\cancel{1\text{ kg}}} = \frac{50\text{ mg} \times 25\ \cancel{\text{kg}}}{1\ \cancel{\text{kg}}}$$

$$X = \frac{50\text{ mg} \times 25}{1}$$

$$X = 1{,}250\text{ mg}$$

- The child's maximum daily dosage is 1,250 mg. Now divide the daily dosage by four doses, to determine the maximum safe dose to administer every 6 hours:

$$X = \frac{1{,}250\text{ mg}}{4\text{ doses}}$$

$$X = 312.5\text{ mg/dose or } 313\text{ mg/dose}$$

- Now repeat the same steps to determine the low or minimum dose:

$$\frac{25\text{ kg}}{X} = \frac{1\text{ kg}}{25\text{ mg}}$$

- Cross-multiply the fractions:

$$X \times 1\text{ kg} = 25\text{ mg} \times 25\text{ kg}$$

- Solve for X by dividing each side of the equation by 1 kg and canceling like units:

$$\frac{X \times \cancel{1\text{ kg}}}{\cancel{1\text{ kg}}} = \frac{25\text{ mg} \times 25\ \cancel{\text{kg}}}{1\ \cancel{\text{kg}}}$$

$$X = \frac{25\text{ mg} \times 25}{1}$$

$$X = 625\text{ mg}$$

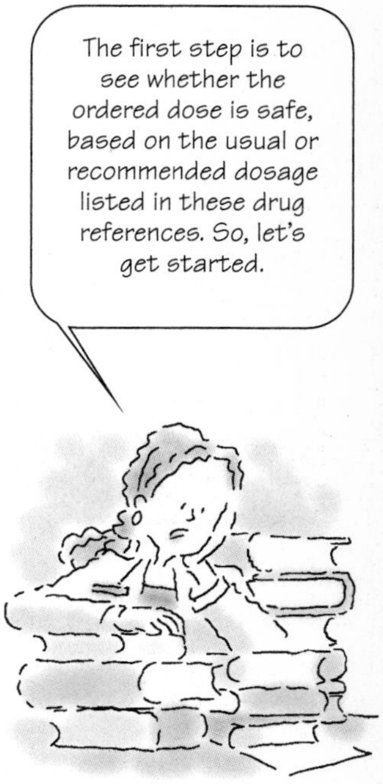

The first step is to see whether the ordered dose is safe, based on the usual or recommended dosage listed in these drug references. So, let's get started.

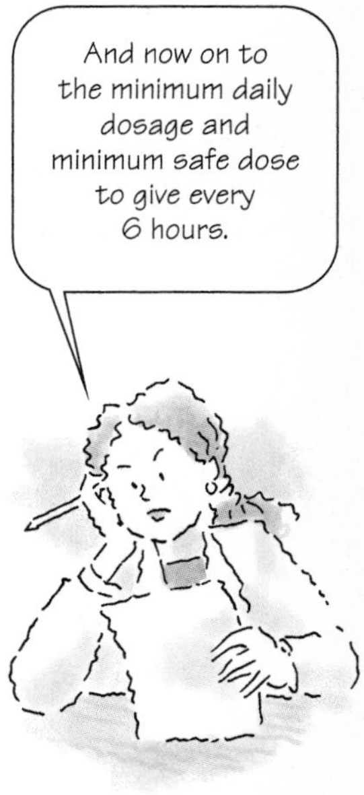

And now on to the minimum daily dosage and minimum safe dose to give every 6 hours.

• The child's minimum daily dosage is 625 mg. Now divide the daily dosage by four doses to determine the minimum safe dose to administer every 6 hours:

$$X = \frac{625 \text{ mg}}{4 \text{ doses}}$$

$$X = 156.25, \text{ or } 156 \text{ mg/dose}$$

The safe daily dosage range is 625 mg to 1,250 mg per day for this child. The doctor ordered 250 mg every 6 hours (or four doses per day) or a total dosage of 1,000 mg (250 mg/dose × four doses). This falls within the safe daily range.

• The child can safely receive 250 mg every 6 hours. Lastly, calculate the volume to give for each dose by setting up a proportion with the unknown volume and the amount in one dose on one side and the available dose on the other side:

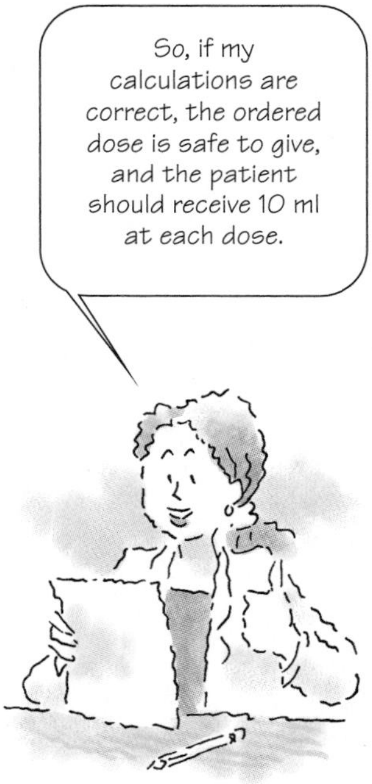

So, if my calculations are correct, the ordered dose is safe to give, and the patient should receive 10 ml at each dose.

$$\frac{X}{250 \text{ mg}} = \frac{5 \text{ ml}}{125 \text{ mg}}$$

$$X \times 125 \text{ mg} = 5 \text{ ml} \times 250 \text{ mg}$$

• Solve for X by dividing each side of the equation by 125 mg and canceling units that appear in both the numerator and denominator:

$$\frac{X \times \cancel{125 \text{ mg}}}{\cancel{125 \text{ mg}}} = \frac{5 \text{ ml} \times 250 \cancel{\text{ mg}}}{125 \cancel{\text{ mg}}}$$

$$X = \frac{5 \text{ ml} \times 250}{125}$$

$$X = \frac{1{,}250 \text{ ml}}{125}$$

$$X = 10 \text{ ml}$$

You should administer 10 ml of the drug at each dose.

I.V. guidelines

I.V. fluids and drugs are administered by continuous or intermittent infusion. Because pediatric I.V. drug administration is so complex, be sure to follow all written guidelines and protocols about dosages, fluid volumes for dilution, and administration rates when giving the drug.

Continuous infusions

A continuous infusion is used when the pediatric patient requires around-the-clock fluids, drug therapy, or both. Fluids may be infused to maintain volume or to correct an existing fluid or electrolyte imbalance.

To prepare for a continuous drug infusion, add the drug to a small-volume bag of I.V. fluid or a volume-control device. Be sure to follow the manufacturer's guidelines for mixing the solution carefully. Remember that pediatric patients can tolerate only small amounts of fluid.

Usually, a volume-control device such as the Buretrol set, which maintains flow rate by using a positive-pressure pumping mechanism, is used for continuous as well as intermittent infusion. A small-volume bag of I.V. fluid with a microdrip set is another option. (See *I.V. infusion control.*)

Infusion basics: 5 steps

Follow these steps to start a continuous infusion:

1. Calculate the dosage.
2. Draw up the drug in a syringe; then add the drug to the I.V. bag or fluid chamber through the drug additive port, using aseptic technique.
3. Mix the drug thoroughly.
4. Label the I.V. bag or fluid chamber with the drug's name, the dosage, the time and date it was mixed, and your initials.
5. Verify the patient's identity using two patient identifiers, and then hang the solution and administer the drug by infusion pump at the prescribed flow rate.

I.V. infusion control

Accurate fluid administration is extremely important for pediatric patients. So syringes, infusion pumps, and other volume-control devices are used extensively to regulate continuous and intermittent I.V. infusions. One typical device, the Buretrol set, is shown below.

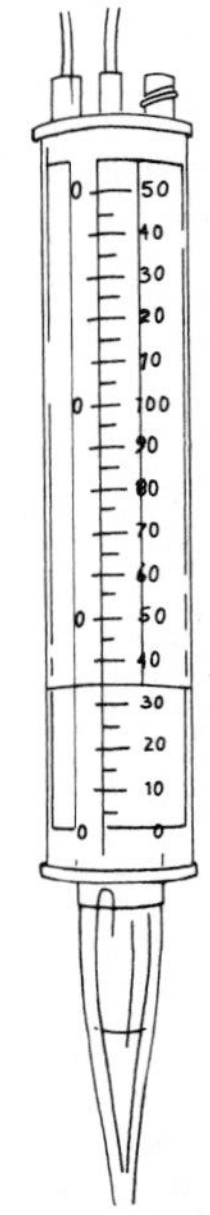

Intermittent infusions

Intermittent infusion is used commonly in acute and home care settings. If the pediatric patient is capable of normal enteral fluid intake, I.V. fluids or drug infusions may be necessary only at periodic intervals. A vascular access device can be kept in place, eliminating the need for continuous fluid infusion. The child can remain mobile, minimizing the potential for volume overload.

Adjusting the volume

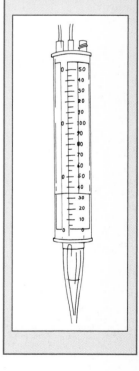

Volume-control devices have 100- to 150-ml fluid chambers, which are calibrated in 1-ml increments to allow accurate fluid administration. Medication-filled syringes with microtubing can also be used to infuse small volumes via syringe pumps. Accuracy is especially important with pediatric patients because children can't tolerate as much fluid as adults and are more prone to fluid and electrolyte imbalances. The rate of I.V. infusion must be carefully controlled to ensure proper absorption and to prevent or minimize toxicity associated with rapid infusion. Use an infusion pump whenever possible.

Starting an infusion: 10 steps

If you're using a volume-control device, follow these steps to start an intermittent infusion:

- Carefully calculate the prescribed volume of drug. Some facilities consider the drug volume as part of the diluent volume. For example, if 100 mg of a drug is contained in 5 ml of fluid and the total fluid volume should be 50 ml, add 45 ml of diluent because 45 ml of diluent plus 5 ml of fluid drug volume equals a total of 50 ml.
- After careful calculation, draw up the prescribed volume of drug into a syringe.
- Add the drug to the fluid chamber through the drug additive port, using aseptic technique.
- Mix the drug thoroughly.
- Attach the volume-control device to an electronic infusion pump to control the infusion rate. If you're using a small-volume I.V. bag instead of a volume-control device and pump, use a microdrip set, which has a drop factor of 60 gtt/ml.
- Calculate the appropriate flow rate, verify the patient's identity using two patient identifiers, and infuse the drug.
- Label the volume-control device with the name of the drug, the dosage, the time and date it was mixed, and your initials.
- When the infusion is complete, flush the line to clear the tubing of the drug. A specific flush volume may be ordered by the doctor or a standard volume protocol is followed based on the tubing volume, the patient's condition, or both. Administer the flush at the same rate as the drug. Label the volume-control device to indicate that the flush is infusing.
- With an intermittent infusion, disconnect the device when the flush is complete.
- During the infusion, check the I.V. site frequently for infiltration because children's veins are more prone to this problem.

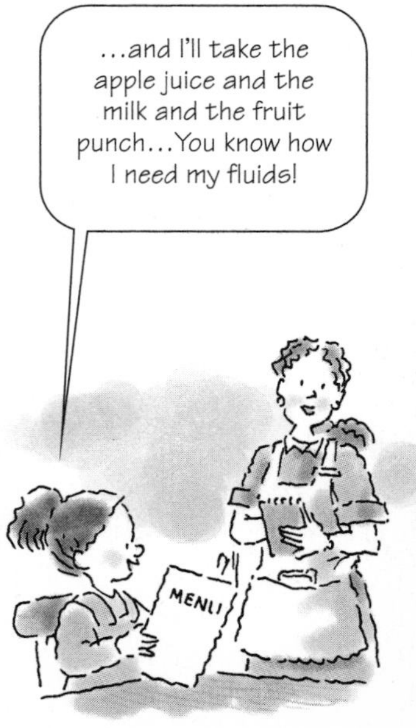

...and I'll take the apple juice and the milk and the fruit punch...You know how I need my fluids!
MENU

Calculating pediatric fluid needs

Children's fluid needs are proportionally greater than those of adults, so children are more vulnerable to changes in fluid and electrolyte balance. Because their extracellular fluid has a higher percentage of water, children's fluid exchange rates are two to three times greater than those of adults, leaving them more susceptible to dehydration.

Three ways to figure fluids

Determining and meeting the fluid needs of children are important nursing responsibilities. You can calculate the number of milliliters of fluid a child needs based on:

- weight in kilograms
- metabolism (calories required)
- BSA in square meters.

Although results may vary slightly, all three methods are appropriate. Keep in mind that fluid replacement can also be affected by clinical conditions that cause fluid retention or loss. Children with these conditions should receive fluids based on their individual needs.

Fluid needs based on weight

You may use three different formulas to calculate a child's fluid needs based on his weight.

Fluid formula for tiny tots

A child who weighs less than 10 kg requires 100 ml of fluid per kilogram of body weight. To determine this child's fluid needs, first convert his weight from pounds to kilograms. Then multiply the results by 100 ml/kg/day.

Here's the formula:

$$\text{weight in kg} \times 100\ \text{ml/kg/day} = \text{fluid needs in ml/day}$$

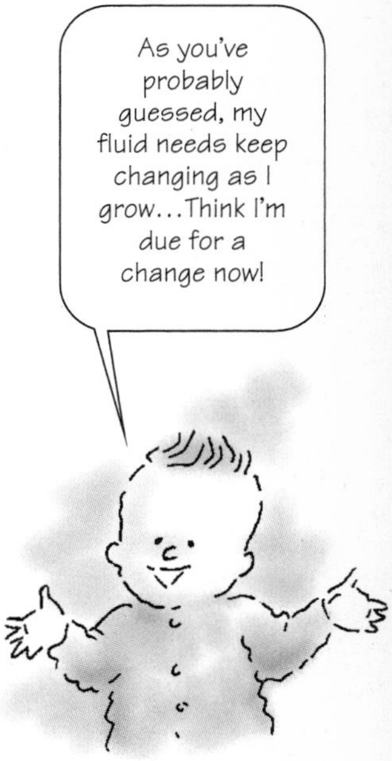

As you've probably guessed, my fluid needs keep changing as I grow...Think I'm due for a change now!

Fluid formula for middleweights

A child weighing 10 to 20 kg requires 1,000 ml of fluid per day for the first 10 kg plus 50 ml for every kilogram over 10. To determine this child's fluid needs, follow these steps:

- Convert his weight from pounds to kilograms.
- Subtract 10 kg from the child's total weight, and then multiply the result by 50 ml/kg/day to find the child's additional fluid needs.

Here's the formula:

$$(\text{total kg} - 10\ \text{kg}) \times 50\ \text{ml/kg/day} = \text{additional fluid need in ml/day}$$

- Add the additional daily fluid need to the 1,000 ml/day required for the first 10 kg. The total is the child's daily fluid requirement:

$$1{,}000\ \text{ml/day} + \text{additional fluid need} = \text{fluid needs in ml/day}$$

Fluid formula for bigger kids

A child weighing more than 20 kg requires 1,500 ml of fluid for the first 20 kg plus 20 ml for each additional kilogram. To determine this child's fluid needs, follow these steps:

- Convert the child's weight from pounds to kilograms.
- Subtract 20 kg from the child's total weight, and then multiply the result by 20 ml/kg to find the child's additional fluid need.

Here's the formula:

$$(\text{total kg} - 20\ \text{kg}) \times 20\ \text{ml/kg/day} = \text{additional fluid need in ml/day}$$

- Because the child needs 1,500 ml of fluid per day for the first 20 kg, add the additional fluid need to 1,500 ml. The total is the child's daily fluid requirement:

$$1{,}500\ \text{ml/day} + \text{additional fluid need} = \text{fluid needs in ml/day}$$

Use this information to solve the following problem.

Finding a fluid solution

How much fluid should you give a 44-lb patient over 24 hours to meet his maintenance needs?

- First, convert 44 lb to kilograms by setting up a proportion with fractions. (Remember that 1 kg equals 2.2 lb.)

$$\frac{44\ \text{lb}}{X} = \frac{2.2\ \text{lb}}{1\ \text{kg}}$$

- Cross-multiply the fractions, and then solve for X by dividing both sides of the equation by 2.2 lb and canceling units that appear in both the numerator and denominator:

$$X \times 2.2\ \text{lb} = 44\ \text{lb} \times 1\ \text{kg}$$

$$\frac{X \times \cancel{2.2\ \text{lb}}}{\cancel{2.2\ \text{lb}}} = \frac{44\ \cancel{\text{lb}} \times 1\ \text{kg}}{2.2\ \cancel{\text{lb}}}$$

$$X = \frac{44\ \text{kg}}{2.2}$$

$$X = 20\ \text{kg}$$

- The child weighs 20 kg. Now, subtract 10 kg from the child's weight, and multiply the result by 50 ml/kg/day to find the child's additional fluid need:

$$X = (20\ \text{kg} - 10\ \text{kg}) \times 50\ \text{ml/kg/day}$$

$$X = 10\ \cancel{\text{kg}} \times 50\ \text{ml/}\cancel{\text{kg}}\text{/day}$$

$$X = 500\ \text{ml/day additional fluid need}$$

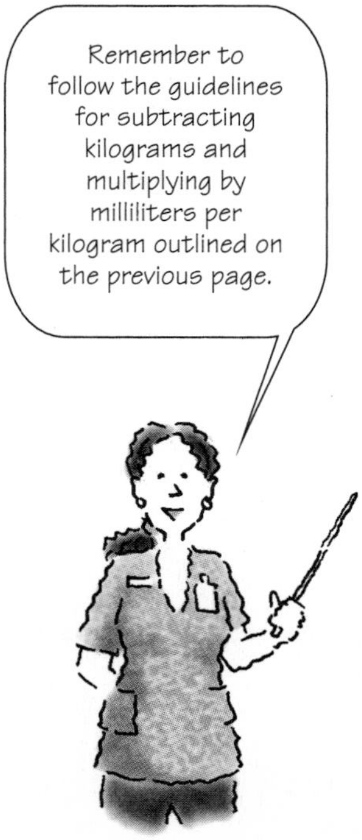

Remember to follow the guidelines for subtracting kilograms and multiplying by milliliters per kilogram outlined on the previous page.

• Next, add the additional fluid need to the 1,000 ml/day required for the first 10 kg (because the child weighs between 10 and 20 kg).

$$X = 1{,}000 \text{ ml/day} + 500 \text{ ml/day}$$

$$X = 1{,}500 \text{ ml/day}$$

The child should receive 1,500 ml of fluid in 24 hours to meet his fluid maintenance needs.

Fluid needs based on calories

You can calculate fluid needs based on calories because water is necessary for metabolism. A child should receive 120 ml of fluid for every 100 kilocalories (kcal) of metabolism, also commonly called *calories.*

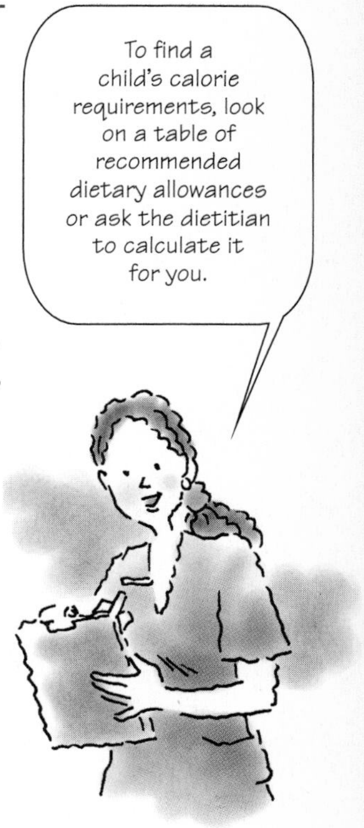
To find a child's calorie requirements, look on a table of recommended dietary allowances or ask the dietitian to calculate it for you.

Fluids help burn calories

To calculate fluid requirements based on calorie requirements, follow these steps:

• Find the child's calorie requirements. You can take this information from a table of recommended dietary allowances for children, or you can have a dietitian calculate it.

• Divide the calorie requirements by 100 kcal because fluid requirements are determined for every 100 calories.

• Multiply the results by 120 ml, the amount of fluid required for every 100 kcal. Here's the formula:

$$\text{fluid requirements in ml/day} = \frac{\text{calorie requirements}}{100 \text{ kcal}} \times 120 \text{ ml}$$

Use the information above to solve the following problem.

Calorie-conscious problem

Your pediatric patient uses 900 calories/day. What are his daily fluid requirements?

• Set up the formula, inserting the appropriate numbers and substituting X for the unknown amount of fluid:

$$X = \frac{900 \cancel{\text{kcal}}}{100 \cancel{\text{kcal}}} \times 120 \text{ ml}$$

$$X = 9 \times 120 \text{ ml}$$

$$X = 1{,}080 \text{ ml}$$

The patient needs 1,080 ml of fluid per day.

Fluid needs based on BSA

Another method for determining pediatric maintenance fluid requirements is based on the child's BSA. To calculate the daily fluid needs of a child who isn't dehydrated, multiply the BSA by 1,500, as shown in this formula:

$$\text{fluid maintenance needs in ml/day} = \text{BSA in m}^2 \times 1{,}500 \text{ ml/day/m}^2$$

Use this formula to solve the following problem.

BSA-based problem

Your patient is 36″ tall and weighs 40 lb (18.1 kg). If his BSA is 0.72 m^2, how much fluid does he need each day?

- Set up the equation, inserting the appropriate numbers and substituting *X* for the unknown amount of fluid. Then solve for *X*:

$$X = 0.72 \cancel{\text{m}^2} \times 1{,}500 \text{ ml/day/}\cancel{\text{m}^2}$$

$$X = 1{,}080 \text{ ml/day}$$

The child needs 1,080 ml of fluid per day.

Real world problem

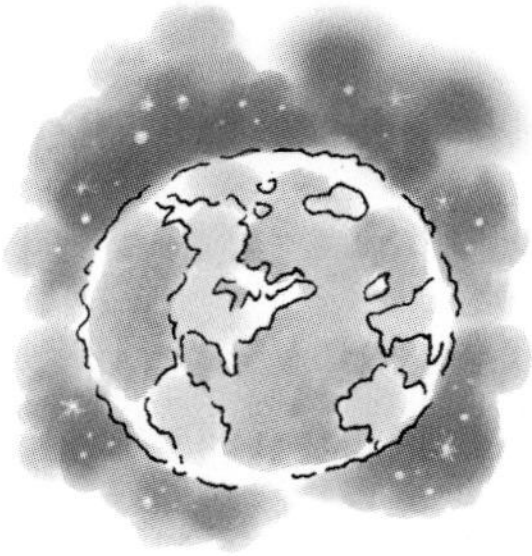

Use your calculation skills to solve the following pediatric dosage problem.

An ampicillin answer

The doctor orders a single dose of 360 mg of ampicillin for an infant who weighs 8 lb. Your pediatric drug handbook states that the usual (recommended) ampicillin dose is 100 mg/kg/dose. After reconstituting with sterile water, the ampicillin is available in a concentration of 500 mg/5 ml. Is the dose ordered correct for the patient? What volume of ampicillin should you administer to the infant?

First, you'll need to determine whether the dose ordered is correct.

- Set up the proportion to determine the child's weight in kilograms. Remember that 1 kg = 2.2 lb:

$$\frac{X}{8 \text{ lb}} = \frac{1 \text{ kg}}{2.2 \text{ lb}}$$

- Cross-multiply the fractions:

$$X \times 2.2 \text{ lb} = 8 \text{ lb} \times 1 \text{ kg}$$

- Solve for *X* by dividing both sides of the equation by 2.2 lb and canceling units that appear in both the numerator and denominator:

$$\frac{X \times \cancel{2.2 \text{ lb}}}{\cancel{2.2 \text{ lb}}} = \frac{8 \cancel{\text{lb}} \times 1 \text{ kg}}{2.2 \cancel{\text{lb}}}$$

$$X = \frac{8 \times 1 \text{ kg}}{2.2}$$

$$X = 3.63 \text{ kg}$$

The infant weighs 3.63 kg, rounded off to 3.6 kg.

- Next, set up a proportion with the recommended dosage (from the pediatric drug reference) in one fraction and the unknown dosage and the patient's weight in the other fraction:

$$\frac{100 \text{ mg}}{1 \text{ kg/dose}} = \frac{X}{3.6 \text{ kg/dose}}$$

- Cross-multiply the fractions:

$$X \times 1 \text{ kg/dose} = 100 \text{ mg} \times 3.6 \text{ kg/dose}$$

- Solve for X by dividing each side of the equation by 1 kg/dose and canceling units that appear in both the numerator and denominator:

$$\frac{X \times \cancel{1 \text{ kg/dose}}}{\cancel{1 \text{ kg/dose}}} = \frac{100 \text{ mg} \times 3.6 \cancel{\text{ kg/dose}}}{1 \cancel{\text{ kg/dose}}}$$

$$X = \frac{100 \text{ mg} \times 3.6}{1}$$

$$X = 360 \text{ mg}$$

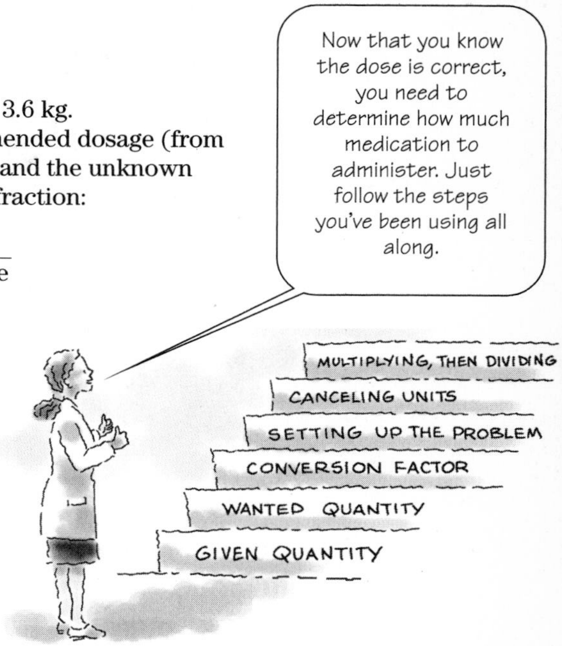

Now that you know the dose is correct, you need to determine how much medication to administer. Just follow the steps you've been using all along.
MULTIPLYING, THEN DIVIDING

SETTING UP THE PROBLEM

So, the doctor's order was correct: 100 mg/kg/dose for a child who weighs 8 lb (or 3.6 kg) is 360 mg.

Next, determine the volume of drug you should administer to the infant.

- Set up a proportion with the known concentration in one fraction and the desired dose and unknown volume in the other fraction:

$$\frac{500 \text{ mg}}{5 \text{ ml}} = \frac{360 \text{ mg}}{X}$$

- Cross-multiply the fractions:

$$500 \text{ mg} \times X = 360 \text{ mg} \times 5 \text{ ml}$$

- Solve for X by dividing both sides of the equation by 500 mg and canceling units that appear in both the numerator and denominator:

$$\frac{\cancel{500 \text{ mg}} \times X}{\cancel{500 \text{ mg}}} = \frac{360 \cancel{\text{ mg}} \times 5 \text{ ml}}{500 \cancel{\text{ mg}}}$$

$$X = \frac{360 \times 5 \text{ ml}}{500 \text{ mg}}$$

$$X = 3.6 \text{ ml}$$

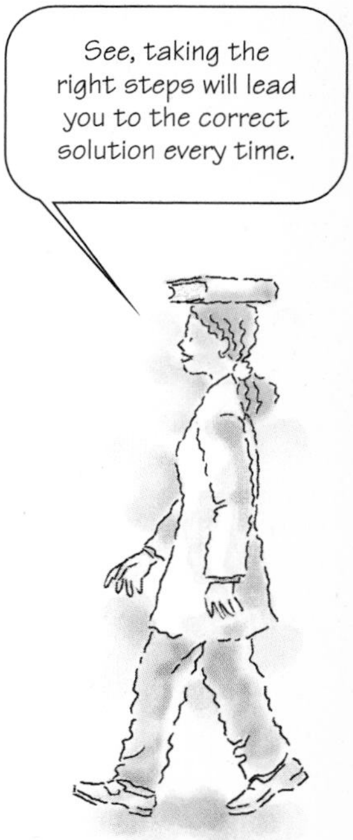

See, taking the right steps will lead you to the correct solution every time.

You should administer 3.6 ml of reconstituted ampicillin to give the patient 360 mg.

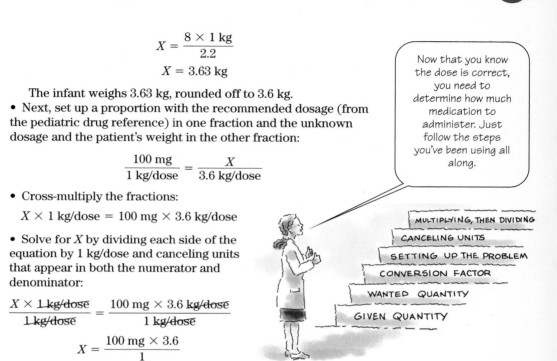

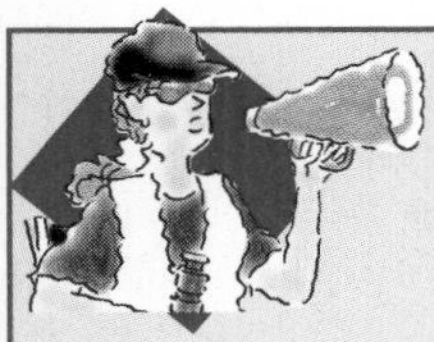

That's a wrap!

Calculating pediatric dosages review

When determining pediatric dosage calculations, be sure to keep these points in mind.

Route guidelines

- P.O. medications may be given as liquid suspensions.
  - Mix drug before measuring out dose.
  - Never crush timed-release capsules or tablets or enteric-coated drugs.
- SubQ is route commonly used for childhood immunizations and insulin injections.
  - Make sure injection contains no more than 1 ml of solution.
  - Administer in any area with sufficient subcutaneous tissue.
- I.M. is route commonly used for vaccines.
  - Never inject more than 1 ml of solution.
  - Administer in the vastus lateralis or ventrogluteal muscles.
- I.V. drugs should be diluted carefully and administered cautiously.
  - Use an infusion pump with infants and small children.
- For topical route, absorption is greater in infants and small children.
  - Wipe off any remaining drug after application.
  - Apply according to doctor's order and drug manufacturer's recommendations.

Dosage per kilogram

- Dosages are expressed as *mg/kg/day* or *mg/kg/dose.*
- Multiply the child's weight in kilograms by the required milligrams of drug per kilogram.

BSA

- Measured in m^2
- Determined through intersection of height and weight on a nomogram
- Multiplied by the prescribed dose in mg/m^2/day to calculate safe pediatric dosages

Weight-based formulas for fluid needs

- A child weighing less than 10 kg: weight in kg $\times$ 100 ml $=$ fluid needs in ml/day
- A child weighing 10 to 20 kg: (total kg $-$ 10 kg) $\times$ 50 ml $=$ additional fluid need in ml/day; 1,000 ml/day $+$ additional fluid need $=$ fluid needs in ml/day
- A child weighing more than 20 kg: (total kg $-$ 20 kg) $\times$ 20 ml $=$ additional fluid need in ml/day; 1,500 ml/day $+$ additional fluid need $=$ fluid needs in ml/day

Calorie-based formula for fluid needs

- Fluid-to-calorie ratio: 120 ml per 100 kcal
- Fluid requirements in ml/day $=$ (calorie requirements $\div$ 100 kcal) $\times$ 120 ml

BSA-based formula for fluid needs

- For a nondehydrated child: fluid maintenance needs in ml/day $=$ BSA in m^2 $\times$ 1,500 ml/day/m^2

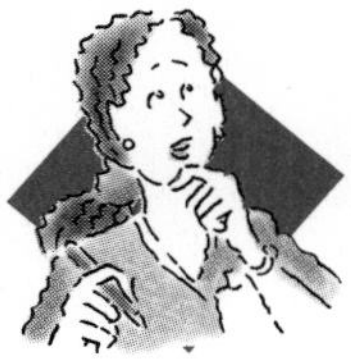

Quick quiz

1. If the suggested pediatric dosage for a drug is 35 mg/kg/day, the amount to give an infant weighing 5 kg is:

A. 250 mg.
B. 175 mg.
C. 75 mg.
D. 50 mg.

Answer: B. To solve this problem, set up a proportion with the suggested dosage in one ratio and the unknown quantity in the other. Multiply the means and extremes, and then divide each side of the equation by the value that appears on the *X* side of the equation. Cancel units that appear in the numerator and denominator.

2. A child who uses 1,000 calories per day has daily fluid requirements of:

A. 1,200 ml.
B. 1,000 ml.
C. 500 ml.
D. 200 ml.

Answer: A. Use the equation for calculating fluid needs based on kilocalories, inserting the appropriate numbers. Then solve for *X*.

3. If a patient is 40″ tall, weighs 64 lb, and has a BSA of 0.96 m^2, how much fluid does he require per day?

A. 140 ml
B. 1,040 ml
C. 1,400 ml
D. 1,440 ml

Answer: D. Use the equation for calculating fluid needs based on BSA, inserting the appropriate numbers. Then solve for *X*.

4. Your patient weighs 8 kg. What are his daily fluid needs?

A. 1,000 ml/day
B. 900 ml/day
C. 800 ml/day
D. 600 ml/day

Answer: C. Set up the equation using the formula weight in kilograms multiplied by 100 ml/kg/day. Cancel like units.

8 ~~kg~~ × 100 ml/~~kg~~/day

800 ml/day

5. The chart used to determine BSA is the:

A. monogram.
B. nomogram.
C. pediagram.
D. infogram.

Answer: B. A nomogram lets you plot the patient's height and weight to determine BSA.

Scoring

☆☆☆ If you answered all five items correctly, way to go! You're the pride and joy of precise pediatric dosages.

☆☆ If you answered four items correctly, we're impressed! There's nothing infantile about your abilities.

☆ If you answered fewer than four items correctly, review and try again! You'll be a specialist in special calculations before you know it.

15

Calculating obstetric drug dosages

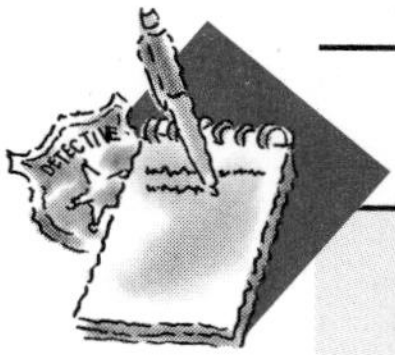

Just the facts

In this chapter, you'll learn:

- how to assess the mother and fetus during medication administration
- common obstetric drugs and their adverse effects
- how to calculate obstetric dosages.

A look at obstetric drug administration

During pregnancy, labor and delivery, and the postpartum period, drugs are commonly given to the mother for four reasons:

1. to control pregnancy-induced hypertension
2. to inhibit preterm labor
3. to induce labor
4. to prevent postpartum hemorrhage.

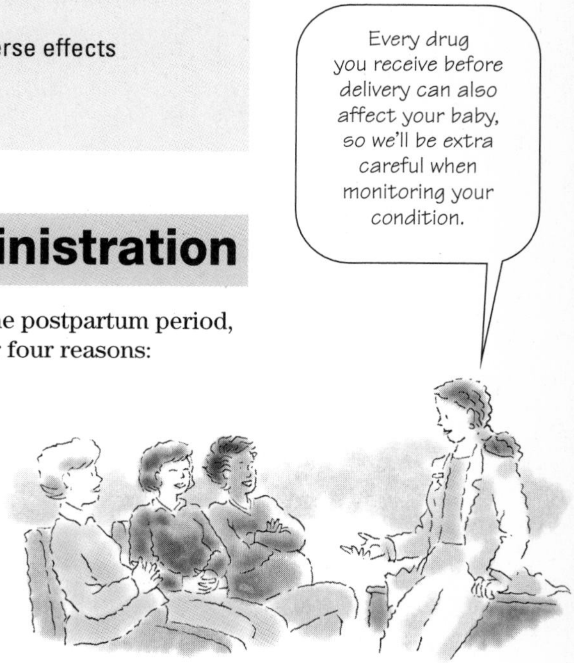
Every drug you receive before delivery can also affect your baby, so we'll be extra careful when monitoring your condition.

Because drugs administered to the mother before delivery can also affect the fetus, both mother and fetus require meticulous monitoring. *Remember:* You're caring for two patients at once, so there's a narrow margin for error.

Assessing the mother and fetus

When administering medications, frequently check the mother's vital signs, urine output, uterine contractions, and deep tendon reflexes. Carefully assess fluid intake and output along with breath

Assessing the mother's body systems

Assessment is a critical part of obstetric nursing. Here's what to assess in each of the mother's body systems.

Neurologic system
- Deep tendon reflexes when magnesium sulfate is infusing
- Pain
- Orientation (because disorientation can indicate hypoxemia or water intoxication)

Cardiovascular system
- Vital signs
- Extremities for peripheral edema with large-volume infusions
- Pulses and skin temperature in the lower extremities for evidence of deep vein thrombosis; also for Homans' sign by dorsiflexing the foot while supporting the leg (deep calf pain may indicate thrombophlebitis)
- I.V. site to check for infiltration

Respiratory system
- Breath sounds
- Oxygenation
- Lungs for pulmonary edema with large-volume infusions

GI system
- Abdomen for contractions when oxytocin is infusing
- Abdomen for bowel sounds after delivery
- Ability to pass flatus or move bowels before discharge

Genitourinary system
- Urine output
- Fluid balance to check for decreased renal function

sounds to reduce the mother's risk of fluid overload, which can lead to acute pulmonary edema. (See *Assessing the mother's body systems.*)

Fluid monitoring is especially critical in women with pregnancy-induced hypertension, which can cause decreased renal function. It's also important with drugs given to inhibit preterm labor because of their antidiuretic effect.

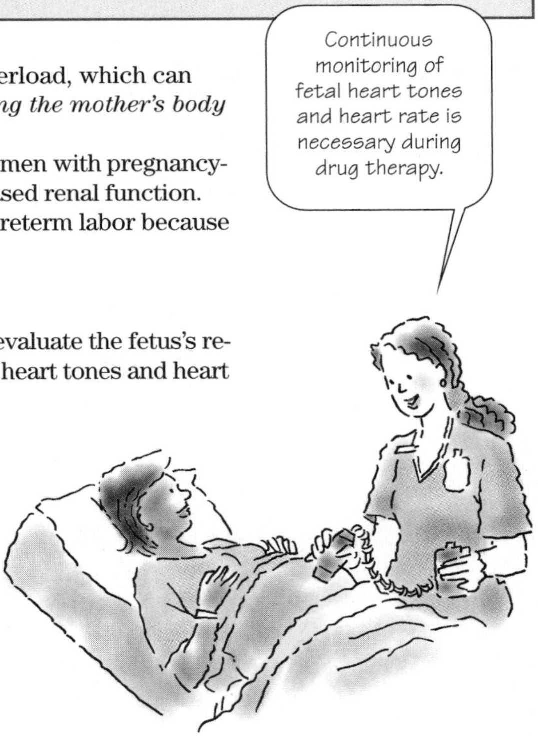

Continuous monitoring of fetal heart tones and heart rate is necessary during drug therapy.

The fetus is also the focus

While you're evaluating the mother, be sure to evaluate the fetus's response to drug therapy. Constantly assess fetal heart tones and heart rate by connecting the mother to an electronic fetal monitor. This monitor records the heart rate and also provides a tracing of it.

Be alert for a sudden increase or decrease in fetal heart rate, which may signal an adverse reaction to treatment. If either occurs, discontinue the drug immediately. (See *It's got a good beat: Contractions and fetal heart rate.*)

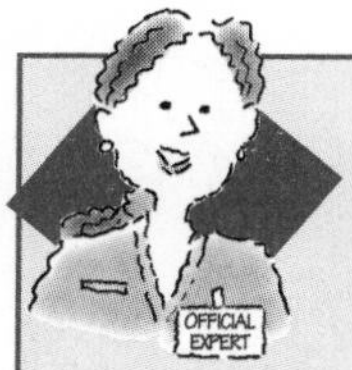

Advice from the experts

It's got a good beat: Contractions and fetal heart rate

Electronic fetal monitoring allows you to assess the mother's contractions as well as the fetal heart rate. Follow these steps.

1. Evaluate the mother's contraction pattern.

2. Note the characteristics of the contractions.
- What's the frequency?
- What's the duration?
- What's the intensity?

3. Evaluate the fetal heart rate after establishing a baseline.
- Is the rate within normal range?
- Is tachycardia present?
- Is bradycardia present?

4. Determine the fetal heart rate variability.
- What's the short-term variability (only with internal fetal monitoring)?
- What's the long-term variability?

5. Assess for changes in fetal heart rate characteristics.
- Is acceleration or increased heart rate present with contractions?
- Is deceleration or decreased heart rate present with contractions?
- Is the heart rate waveform regular and uniform in shape?
- Is the heart rate waveform irregular in shape?

Common obstetric drugs

Drugs used during pregnancy, labor and delivery, and the postpartum period include:
- terbutaline
- magnesium sulfate
- dinoprostone (Cervidil)
- oxytocin (Pitocin). (See *The lowdown on four obstetric drugs*, pages 316 and 317.)

Terbutaline

Terbutaline is used to inhibit preterm labor. It stimulates the $beta_2$-adrenergic receptors in the uterine smooth muscle and inhibits contractility.

A preterm proposition

To administer terbutaline, mix it in a compatible I.V. solution and administer it through an infusion pump. Then titrate the dose every 10 minutes until the contractions subside, the maximum dose is reached, or the patient is unable to tolerate the drug because of its adverse effects.

(Text continues on page 318.)

Before you give that drug!

The lowdown on four obstetric drugs

This table lists some common drugs used in the obstetric setting along with their actions, adverse reactions, and nursing considerations.

Drug	Action	Adverse reactions	Nursing considerations
terbutaline	Relaxes uterine muscle by acting on beta$_2$-adrenergic receptors; inhibits uterine contractions	***Maternal*** • *Blood:* increased liver enzymes • *Central nervous system (CNS):* seizures, nervousness, tremor, headache, drowsiness, flushing, sweating • *Cardiovascular (CV):* increased heart rate, changes in blood pressure, palpitations, chest discomfort • *Eye, ear, nose, and throat (EENT):* tinnitus • *GI:* nausea, vomiting, altered taste • *Respiratory:* dyspnea, wheezing	• Use cautiously in patients with diabetes, hypertension, hyperthyroidism, severe cardiac disease, seizure disorder, and arrhythmias. • Protect from light. *Don't use if discolored.* • Explain the need for the drug to the patient and family. • Give subQ injection in lateral deltoid area. • Warn the patient about the possibility of paradoxical bronchospasm. • Tell the patient she may use tablets and aerosol concomitantly. • Tell the patient how to administer a metered dose. • Although not approved by the Food and Drug Administration for treatment of preterm labor, this drug is considered very effective and is used in many hospitals. • Monitor the patient's blood glucose level with long-term use. • Monitor the neonate for hypoglycemia.
magnesium sulfate	May decrease acetylcholine released by nerve impulse; prevents seizures by blocking neuromuscular transmission	***Maternal*** • *CNS:* sweating, drowsiness, depressed reflexes, flaccid paralysis, hypothermia, flushing, blurred vision • *CV:* hypotension, circulatory collapse, depressed cardiac function, heart block • *Other:* fatal respiratory paralysis, hypocalcemia with tetany	• Use cautiously in labor and in those with impaired renal function, myocardial damage, or heart block. • This drug may be used as a tocolytic agent to inhibit premature labor; it can decrease the frequency and force of uterine contractions. • Keep calcium gluconate available to reverse magnesium sulfate intoxication. • Use cautiously in patients undergoing digitalization because arrhythmias may occur. • Watch for respiratory depression. • Monitor intake and output. • Monitor deep tendon reflexes. • Maximum infusion is 150 mg/minute. • Signs of hypermagnesemia begin to appear at blood levels of 4 mEq/L. • This drug should be stopped at least 2 hours before delivery to avoid fetal respiratory depression. • Monitor the neonate for magnesium sulfate toxicity.

The lowdown on four obstetric drugs *(continued)*

Drug	Action	Adverse reactions	Nursing considerations
dinoprostone (Cervidil)	A prostaglandin that produces strong, prompt contractions of uterine smooth muscle; facilitates cervical dilations by directly softening the cervix	***Maternal*** • *CNS:* fever, headache, dizziness, anxiety, paresthesia, weakness, syncope • *CV:* chest pain, arrhythmias, hypotension • *EENT:* blurred vision, eye pain • *GI:* nausea, vomiting, diarrhea • *Genitourinary:* vaginal pain, vaginitis, endometritis ***Fetal*** • *CNS:* hypotonia, hyperstimulation • *Respiratory:* respiratory depression • *CV:* bradycardia • *Other:* intrauterine fetal sepsis	• Use only with the patient in or near a delivery suite. Critical care facilities should be available. • After administration of the gel form of the drug, the patient should remain supine for 10 minutes. • Have the patient remain supine for 2 hours after insertion of the vaginal insert form of the drug. • Remove the vaginal insert with onset of active labor or 12 hours after insertion. • Monitor the fetus accordingly. • If hyperstimulation of the uterus occurs, gently flush the vagina with sterile saline solution. • Treat dinoprostone-induced fever (usually self-limiting and transient) with water sponging and increased fluid intake, not with aspirin.
oxytocin (Pitocin)	Causes potent and selective stimulation of uterine and mammary gland smooth muscle	***Maternal*** • *Blood:* afibrinogenemia (may be from postpartum bleeding) • *CNS:* subarachnoid hemorrhage resulting from hypertension; seizures or coma resulting from water intoxication • *CV:* hypotension, increased heart rate, systemic venous return, increased cardiac output, arrhythmias • *Other:* hypersensitivity, tetanic uterine contractions, abruptio placentae, impaired uterine blood flow, increased uterine motility, uterine rupture ***Fetal*** • *Blood:* hyperbilirubinemia, hypercapnia • *CV:* bradycardia, tachycardia, premature ventricular contractions, variable deceleration of heart rate • *Respiratory:* hypoxia, asphyxia, death • *CNS:* brain damage, seizures • *EENT:* retinal hemorrhage • *GI:* hepatic necrosis	• Oxytocin is contraindicated in cephalopelvic disproportion; where delivery requires conversion, as in transverse lie; in fetal distress; when delivery isn't imminent; and in other obstetric emergencies. • Administer by piggyback infusion so the drug can be discontinued without interrupting the I.V. line. *Don't give by I.V. bolus injection.* • Don't infuse in more than one site. • Monitor and record uterine contractions, heart rate, blood pressure, intrauterine pressure, fetal heart rate, and character of blood loss every 15 minutes. • Have magnesium sulfate (20% solution) available for relaxation of myometrium. • Monitor fluid intake and output. Antidiuretic effect may lead to fluid overload, seizures, and coma.

Magnesium sulfate

Another drug used during labor and delivery is magnesium sulfate, which prevents or controls seizures that may be caused by pregnancy-induced hypertension. The drug may decrease acetylcholine levels, but its exact anticonvulsant mechanism is unknown.

Control those seizures

To administer magnesium sulfate, first give a loading dose (a high dose given over a short time to rapidly reach a therapeutic drug level). This should be followed by an infusion at a lower dose, as prescribed.

During the infusion, closely assess knee jerk and patellar reflexes; loss of these signal drug toxicity. If toxicity is suspected, immediately stop the infusion and notify the doctor. Calcium gluconate may be ordered as an antidote.

Dinoprostone

Dinoprostone, a drug used to induce labor, is used to dilate the cervix in pregnant patients at or near term.

Scope it out

Dinoprostone is available as an endocervical gel, a vaginal insert, or a vaginal suppository. In some states in the United States, administration of this drug doesn't fall within a nurse's scope of practice, and it must be administered by a doctor.

Warm and...gel-like

For administration of dinoprostone, have the patient lie on her back; the cervix will then be examined using a speculum. Then assist with insertion of the gel, using aseptic technique. A catheter provided with the drug is used to administer the gel into the cervical canal just below the level of the internal os. Warm the gel to room temperature before using. It isn't necessary to warm the vaginal inserts before giving; however, a minimal amount of water-soluble jelly may be used to aid insertion.

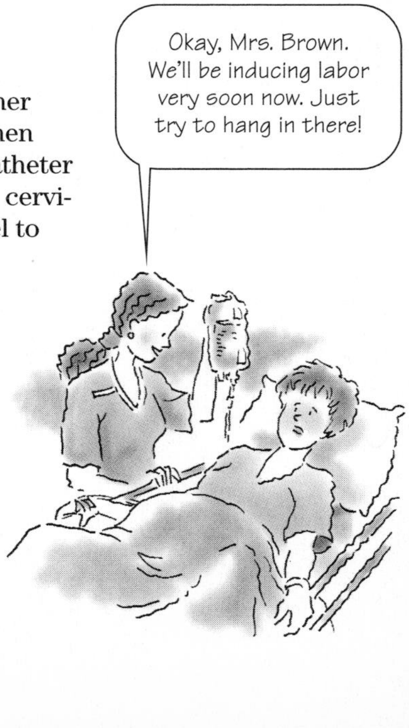

Okay, Mrs. Brown. We'll be inducing labor very soon now. Just try to hang in there!

Oxytocin

Oxytocin — the drug most commonly used to induce labor — selectively stimulates uterine smooth muscle.

Compelling contractions

After mixing oxytocin with a compatible solution, administer it by piggyback with an I.V. infusion pump and titrate until a normal contraction pattern occurs. When labor is firmly established, the doctor may prescribe a decrease in the infusion rate. Carefully monitor contraction strength because the drug can cause severe contractions that can lead to uterine rupture as well as fetal and maternal death.

Bleeding blockade

Oxytocin may also be used to control bleeding after delivery of the placenta. To control bleeding, add the drug to 1 L of I.V. fluid, and then infuse it at a rate that controls bleeding but doesn't exceed 20 milliunits per minute. Don't administer oxytocin by I.V. push.

Dosage calculations

In the labor and delivery unit, you must be especially careful to calculate and administer drugs accurately. For one thing, you may be dealing with life-threatening problems, such as hemorrhage and seizures caused by pregnancy-induced hypertension.

Administering accurate dosages to the mother helps avoid fetal complications. Be sure to examine drug labels closely. They contain valuable information for calculating dosages.

Real world problems

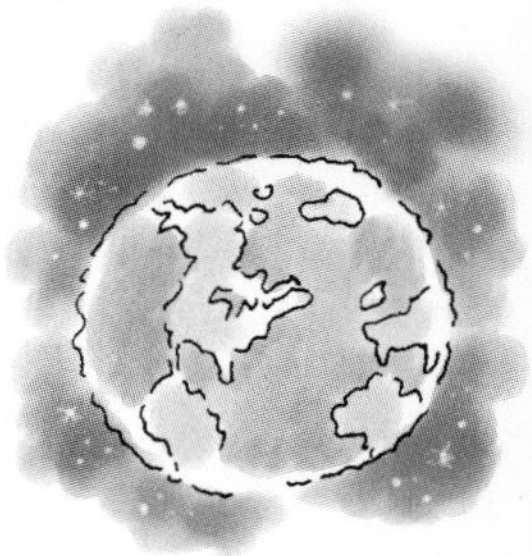

These examples show how to calculate obstetric drugs using proportions.

Overdue? Order oxytocin

Your patient is 10 days overdue, so the doctor prescribes oxytocin to stimulate labor. The order reads *1 ml (10 units) oxytocin in 1 L (1,000 ml) NSS; infuse via pump at 2 milliunits/minute for 20 minutes and then increase flow rate to 3 milliunits/minute.* What's the solution's concentration? What's the flow rate needed to deliver 2 milliunits/minute for 20 minutes? What's the flow rate needed to deliver 3 milliunits/minute thereafter?

- Determine the concentration of the solution by setting up a proportion with the ordered concentration in one fraction and the unknown concentration in the other fraction:

$$\frac{10 \text{ units}}{1{,}000 \text{ ml}} = \frac{X}{1 \text{ ml}}$$

- Cross-multiply the fractions:

$$X \times 1{,}000 \text{ ml} = 10 \text{ units} \times 1 \text{ ml}$$

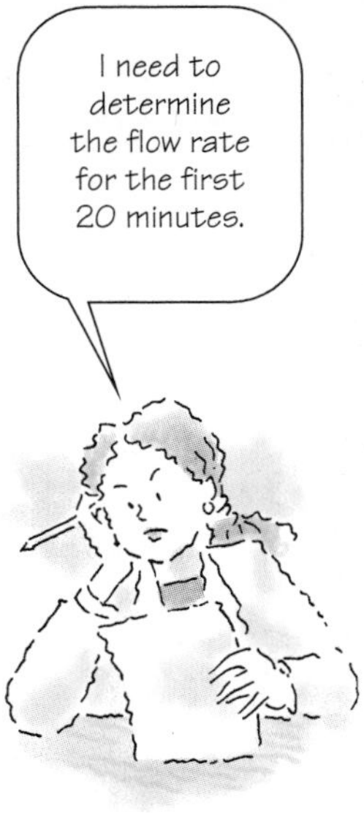

• Solve for X by dividing both sides of the equation by 1,000 ml and canceling units that appear in both the numerator and denominator:

$$\frac{X \times \cancel{1{,}000\text{ ml}}}{\cancel{1{,}000\text{ ml}}} = \frac{10\text{ units} \times 1\ \cancel{\text{ml}}}{1{,}000\ \cancel{\text{ml}}}$$

$$X = \frac{10\text{ units}}{1{,}000}$$

$$X = 0.01\text{ unit}$$

• The amount 0.01 unit can be written in milliunits: 1 milliunit is 1/1,000 of a unit; 1,000 milliunits is 1 unit. Therefore, 0.01 unit times 1,000 equals 10 milliunits. So the concentration is 10 milliunits/ml.

• Next, determine the flow rate. If the prescribed dosage of oxytocin is 2 milliunits/minute for 20 minutes, the patient receives a total of 40 milliunits. To calculate the rate needed to provide that dose, set up a proportion with the known concentration in one fraction and the total oxytocin dose and unknown flow rate in the other:

$$\frac{10\text{ milliunits}}{1\text{ ml}} = \frac{40\text{ milliunits}}{X}$$

• Cross-multiply the fractions:

$$X \times 10\text{ milliunits} = 1\text{ ml} \times 40\text{ milliunits}$$

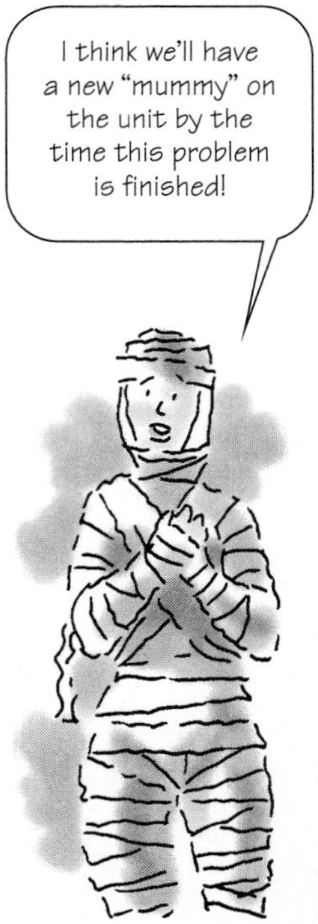

I think we'll have a new "mummy" on the unit by the time this problem is finished!

• Solve for X by dividing both sides of the equation by 10 milliunits and canceling units that appear in both the numerator and denominator:

$$\frac{X \times \cancel{10\text{ milliunits}}}{\cancel{10\text{ milliunits}}} = \frac{1\text{ ml} \times 40\ \cancel{\text{milliunits}}}{10\ \cancel{\text{milliunits}}}$$

$$X = \frac{40\text{ ml}}{10}$$

$$X = 4\text{ ml}$$

• The flow rate is 4 ml/20 minutes. Because this drug must be delivered by infusion pump, compute the hourly flow rate by multiplying the 20-minute rate by 3:

$$4\text{ ml/20 minutes} \times 3 = 12\text{ ml/hour}$$

• The hourly flow rate is 12 ml/hour. Lastly, calculate the flow rate to be used after the first 20 minutes, resulting in 3 milliunits/minute (180 milliunits/hour). Having calculated the solution's concentration as 10 milliunits/ml, set up a proportion with the known concentration in one fraction and the increased oxytocin dose and the unknown flow rate in the other fraction:

$$\frac{10 \text{ milliunits}}{1 \text{ ml}} = \frac{180 \text{ milliunits}}{X}$$

- Cross-multiply the fractions:

$$X \times 10 \text{ milliunits} = 1 \text{ ml} \times 180 \text{ milliunits}$$

- Solve for X by dividing both sides of the equation by 10 milliunits and canceling units that appear in both the numerator and denominator:

$$\frac{X \times \cancel{10 \text{ milliunits}}}{\cancel{10 \text{ milliunits}}} = \frac{1 \text{ ml} \times 180 \cancel{\text{ milliunits}}}{10 \cancel{\text{ milliunits}}}$$

$$X = \frac{180 \text{ ml}}{10}$$

$$X = 18 \text{ ml}$$

- After 20 minutes, reset the pump to deliver 18 ml/hour. That's 18 ml/60 minutes, or 0.3 ml/minute. Because there are 10 milliunits/ml, multiply 10 by 0.3 ml/minute to verify that this flow rate does provide 3 milliunits/minute.

Seizure? Stop it with magnesium sulfate.

Your patient is at risk for a seizure due to pregnancy-induced hypertension. The doctor orders *4 g (4,000 mg) magnesium sulfate in 250 ml D_5W to be infused at 2 g/hour.* What's the flow rate in milliliters per hour?

Here's one approach to solving this problem:

- Set up a proportion with the known concentration in one fraction and the flow rate in grams and the unknown flow rate in milliliters in the other fraction:

$$\frac{4 \text{ g}}{250 \text{ ml}} = \frac{2 \text{ g}}{X}$$

- Cross-multiply the fractions:

$$X \times 4 \text{ g} = 250 \text{ ml} \times 2 \text{ g}$$

- Solve for X by dividing each side of the equation by 4 g and canceling units that appear in both the numerator and denominator:

$$\frac{X \times \cancel{4 \text{ g}}}{\cancel{4 \text{ g}}} = \frac{250 \text{ ml} \times 2 \cancel{\text{ g}}}{4 \cancel{\text{ g}}}$$

$$X = \frac{250 \text{ ml} \times 2}{4}$$

$$X = \frac{500 \text{ ml}}{4}$$

$$X = 125 \text{ ml}$$

The magnesium sulfate solution should be infused at 125 ml/hour.

Let's seize that problem again

Here's another approach to solving the same problem.

- First, calculate the strength of the solution by setting up a proportion with the known strength in one fraction and the unknown strength in the other fraction:

$$\frac{4\text{ g}}{250\text{ ml}} = \frac{X}{1\text{ ml}}$$

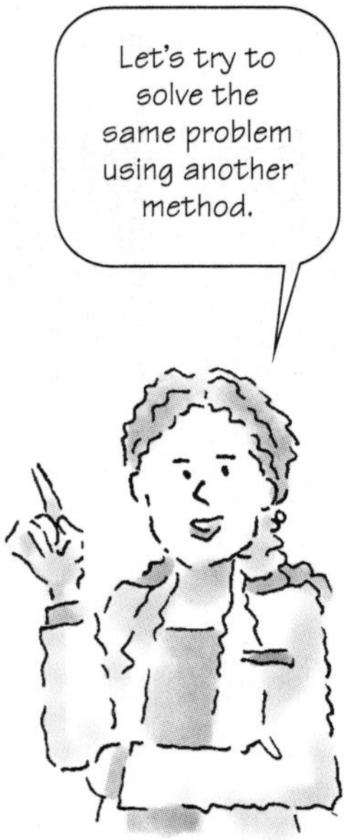

Let's try to solve the same problem using another method.

- Cross-multiply the fractions:

$$X \times 250\text{ ml} = 4\text{ g} \times 1\text{ ml}$$

- Solve for X by dividing each side of the equation by 250 ml and canceling units that appear in both the numerator and denominator:

$$\frac{X \times \cancel{250\text{ ml}}}{\cancel{250\text{ ml}}} = \frac{4\text{ g} \times 1\cancel{\text{ ml}}}{250\cancel{\text{ ml}}}$$

$$X = \frac{4\text{ g}}{250}$$

$$X = 0.016\text{ g}$$

- The solution's strength is 0.016 g/ml. Next, calculate the flow rate by setting up another proportion with the solution concentration in one fraction and the unknown flow rate in the other fraction:

$$\frac{1\text{ ml}}{0.016\text{ g}} = \frac{X}{2\text{ g}}$$

- Cross-multiply the fractions:

$$X \times 0.016\text{ g} = 1\text{ ml} \times 2\text{ g}$$

- Solve for X by dividing each side of the equation by 0.016 g and canceling units that appear in both the numerator and denominator:

$$\frac{X \times \cancel{0.016\text{ g}}}{\cancel{0.016\text{ g}}} = \frac{1\text{ ml} \times 2\cancel{\text{ g}}}{0.016\cancel{\text{ g}}}$$

$$X = \frac{2\text{ ml}}{0.016}$$

$$X = 125\text{ ml}$$

The same flow rate of 125 ml per hour is obtained using this method.

Dosage drill

Test your math skills with this drill.

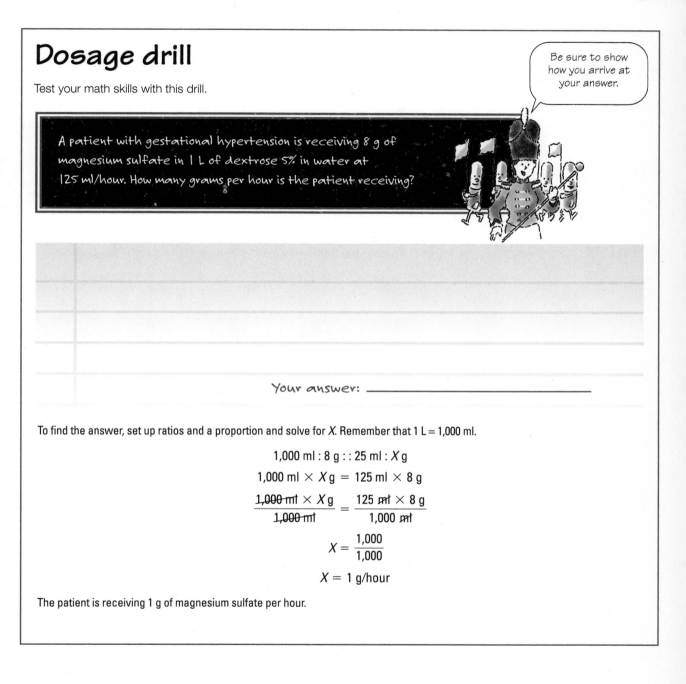

Be sure to show how you arrive at your answer.

A patient with gestational hypertension is receiving 8 g of magnesium sulfate in 1 L of dextrose 5% in water at 125 ml/hour. How many grams per hour is the patient receiving?

Your answer: ______________________

To find the answer, set up ratios and a proportion and solve for X. Remember that 1 L = 1,000 ml.

$$1{,}000 \text{ ml} : 8 \text{ g} :: 25 \text{ ml} : X \text{ g}$$

$$1{,}000 \text{ ml} \times X \text{ g} = 125 \text{ ml} \times 8 \text{ g}$$

$$\frac{\cancel{1{,}000 \text{ ml}} \times X \text{ g}}{\cancel{1{,}000 \text{ ml}}} = \frac{125 \cancel{\text{ ml}} \times 8 \text{ g}}{1{,}000 \cancel{\text{ ml}}}$$

$$X = \frac{1{,}000}{1{,}000}$$

$$X = 1 \text{ g/hour}$$

The patient is receiving 1 g of magnesium sulfate per hour.

Preterm labor? Try terbutaline

Your patient is in preterm labor. The doctor prescribes *10 mg terbutaline sulfate in 250 ml D_5W to infuse at 5 mcg/minute.* What's the flow rate for this solution?

- First, find the solution's strength. Set up a proportion with the known strength in one fraction and the unknown strength in the other fraction:

$$\frac{10 \text{ mg}}{250 \text{ ml}} = \frac{X}{1 \text{ ml}}$$

- Cross-multiply the fractions:

$$X \times 250 \text{ ml} = 10 \text{ mg} \times 1 \text{ ml}$$

- Solve for X by dividing each side of the equation by 250 ml and canceling units that appear in both the numerator and denominator:

$$\frac{X \times \cancel{250 \text{ ml}}}{\cancel{250 \text{ ml}}} = \frac{10 \text{ mg} \times 1 \cancel{\text{ml}}}{250 \cancel{\text{ml}}}$$

$$X = \frac{10 \text{ mg}}{250}$$

$$X = 0.04 \text{ mg}$$

- The strength of the solution is 0.04 mg/ml. Next, convert to micrograms (mcg) by multiplying by 1,000 (0.04 mg × 1,000 = 40 mcg/ml). Then calculate the flow rate needed to deliver the prescribed dose of 5 mcg/minute. To do this, set up a proportion with the known solution strength in one fraction and the unknown flow rate in the other:

$$\frac{1 \text{ ml}}{40 \text{ mcg}} = \frac{X}{5 \text{ mcg}}$$

- Cross-multiply the fractions:

$$X \times 40 \text{ mcg} = 1 \text{ ml} \times 5 \text{ mcg}$$

- Solve for X by dividing each side of the equation by 40 mcg and canceling units that appear in both the numerator and denominator:

$$\frac{X \times \cancel{40 \text{ mcg}}}{\cancel{40 \text{ mcg}}} = \frac{1 \text{ ml} \times 5 \cancel{\text{mcg}}}{40 \cancel{\text{mcg}}}$$

$$X = \frac{5 \text{ mcg}}{40}$$

$$X = 0.125 \text{ ml}$$

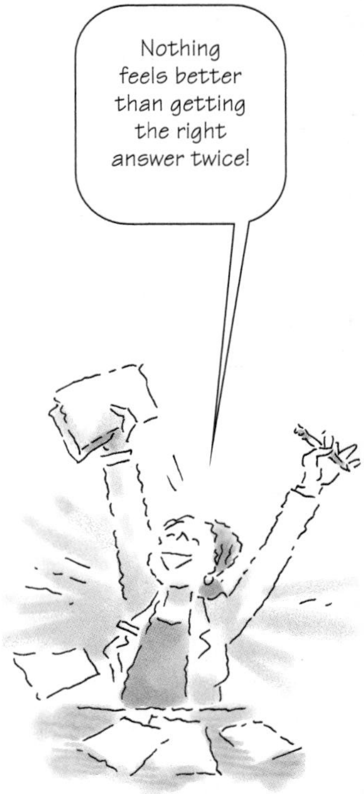

Nothing feels better than getting the right answer twice!

• The flow rate is 0.125 ml/minute. Because the infusion must be administered with a pump, compute the hourly flow rate by setting up a proportion with the known flow rate per minute in one fraction and the unknown flow rate per hour in the other fraction:

$$\frac{0.125 \text{ ml}}{1 \text{ minute}} = \frac{X}{60 \text{ minutes}}$$

• Cross-multiply the fractions:

$$X \times 1 \text{ minute} = 0.125 \text{ ml} \times 60 \text{ minutes}$$

• Solve for X by dividing each side of the equation by 1 minute and canceling units that appear in both the numerator and denominator:

$$\frac{X \times \cancel{1 \text{ minute}}}{\cancel{1 \text{ minute}}} = \frac{0.125 \text{ ml} \times 60 \cancel{\text{ minutes}}}{1 \cancel{\text{ minute}}}$$

$$X = 7.5 \text{ ml}$$

Round off the answer of 7.5 ml to the nearest milliliter, and set the infusion pump to deliver 8 ml/hour.

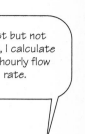

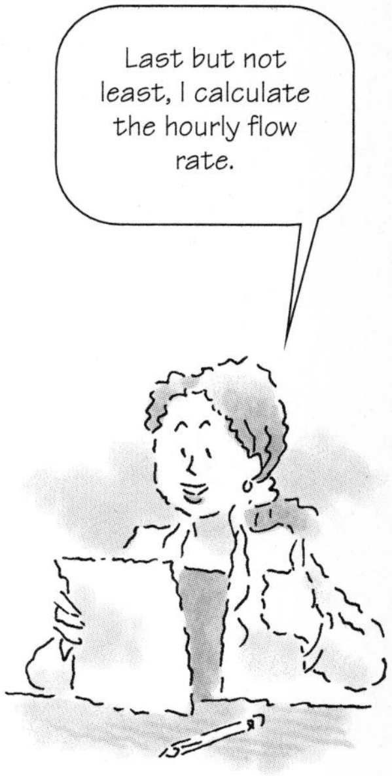
Last but not least, I calculate the hourly flow rate.

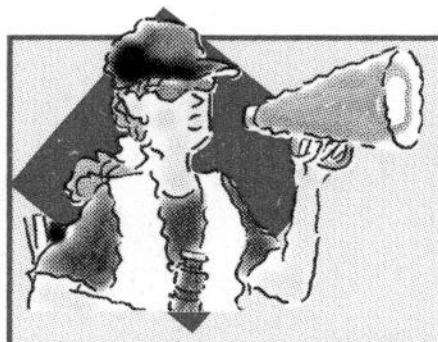

That's a wrap!

Calculating obstetric drug dosages review

Here are some important facts about obstetric drug dosages to keep in mind.

Assessing the mother during drug administration

• Frequently check vital signs, urine output, uterine contractions, and deep tendon reflexes.
• Monitor and record fluid intake and output.
• Assess breath sounds.

Evaluating fetal response to drug therapy

• Monitor fetal heart rate during mother's drug therapy.
• If sudden increase or decrease occurs, immediately discontinue the drug.

Common obstetric drugs

Terbutaline

• Inhibits preterm labor
• Administered via an infusion pump and titrated every 10 minutes as needed

Magnesium sulfate

• Prevents or controls seizures caused by pregnancy-induced hypertension
• Given as a loading dose first, then followed with infusion at a lower dose
• Suspected toxicity requires stopping infusion immediately and notifying doctor

Oxytocin

• Selectively stimulates uterine smooth muscle to induce labor
• May also be used to control bleeding after delivery of the placenta

(continued)

Calculating obstetric drug dosages review *(continued)*

- Administered I.V. piggyback with an infusion pump and titrated until normal contraction pattern occurs
- Requires careful monitoring of contraction strength because drug can cause severe contractions and even death

Dinoprostone

- Ripens the cervix (to induce labor) in pregnant patients at or near term
- Available as endocervical gel, vaginal inserts, or vaginal suppositories

Dosage calculations

- Accurate dosages of drugs given to the mother help avoid fetal complications.
- Proportions can be used to solve obstetric dosage calculations.

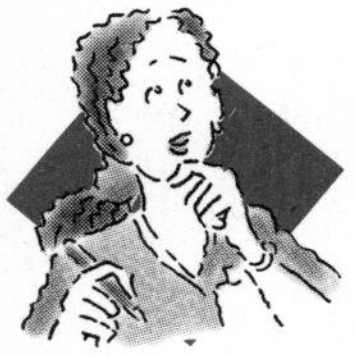

Quick quiz

1. If the order reads *20 units oxytocin (Pitocin) in 1,000 ml of lactated Ringer's solution*, the solution's concentration is:

A. 20 units/ml.
B. 2 units/ml.
C. 0.2 unit/ml.
D. 0.02 unit/ml.

Answer: D. To solve this problem, set up a proportion with the known concentration in one fraction and the unknown concentration in the other fraction. Then solve for *X*.

2. A sudden increase or decrease in the fetal heart rate after drug treatment is a:

A. sign that the infant is about to be delivered.
B. sign of an adverse reaction to the drug.
C. temporary reaction to many obstetric drugs.
D. sign indicating that the drug has reached its peak level.

Answer: B. Changes in the fetal heart rate may signal an adverse reaction to the drug; therefore, discontinue the drug immediately.

3. Which drug should be kept readily available to reverse magnesium sulfate intoxication?

A. Potassium chloride
B. Atropine
C. Calcium gluconate
D. Sodium chloride

Answer: C. During magnesium sulfate infusion, calcium gluconate should be readily available to reverse magnesium intoxication should it occur.

4. If an order says *infuse 20 mg terbutaline sulfate in 1,000 ml D_5W at 0.01 mg/minute for 20 minutes*, the flow rate should be:

A. 1 ml.
B. 10 ml.
C. 100 ml.
D. 200 ml.

Answer: B. First, calculate the concentration, which is 0.02 mg/ml. Then determine the amount of drug provided in 20 minutes by multiplying 0.01 by 20 minutes to get 0.2 mg. Lastly, set up a proportion with the concentration in one fraction and the total amount of medication and the unknown flow rate in the other fraction. Solve for *X*.

5. If 5 g of magnesium sulfate are added to 1 L of normal saline solution, the concentration of magnesium sulfate is:

A. 0.05 mg/ml.
B. 0.5 mg/ml.
C. 5 mg/ml.
D. 50 mg/ml.

Answer: C. First, convert 5 g to 5,000 mg and 1 L to 1,000 ml. Then divide the 1,000 into 5,000 to obtain the concentration: 5 mg/ml.

6. If the doctor orders *20 g magnesium sulfate in 1,000 ml D_5W to be infused at 2 g/hour*, the flow rate in milliliters per hour is:

A. 1 ml/hour.
B. 10 ml/hour.
C. 100 ml/hour.
D. 300 ml/hour.

Answer: C. To solve this problem, set up a proportion with the ordered concentration in one fraction and the flow rate in grams and the unknown flow rate in milliliters in the other. Solve for *X*.

7. The best way to administer oxytocin is by:

A. I.V. piggyback infusion.
B. I.V. bolus injection.
C. direct I.V. infusion.
D. I.M. injection.

Answer: A. Administer oxytocin by I.V. piggyback infusion using an infusion pump so that the drug can be discontinued without interrupting the I.V. line.

Scoring

☆☆☆ If you answered all seven items correctly, fantastic! Your labors have helped you become a confident calculator.

☆☆ If you answered five or six items correctly, keep at it! You'll soon be able to deftly deliver drugs in any delivery unit.

☆ If you answered fewer than five items correctly, chin up! You still have one chapter left to conquer the Quick quiz.

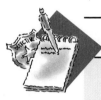

16

Calculating critical care dosages

Just the facts

In this chapter, you'll learn:

- special points to consider when giving critical care drugs
- how to calculate dosages for I.V. push drugs
- how to calculate I.V. flow rates for critical care drugs
- how to calculate drugs not ordered at a specific flow rate or dosage.

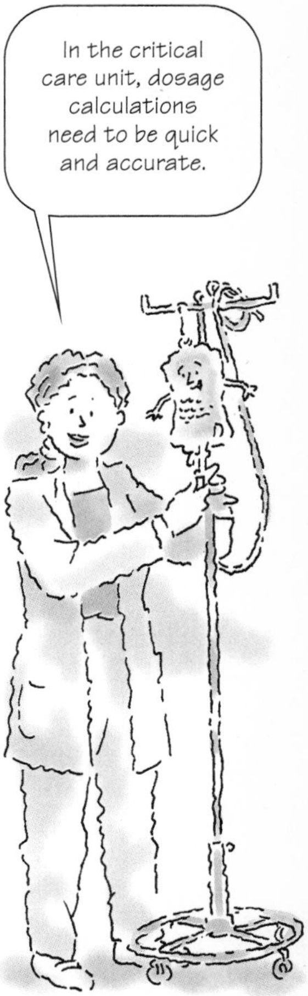
In the critical care unit, dosage calculations need to be quick and accurate.

A look at critical care dosages

If you work on a critical care unit, not only do you need to perform dosage calculations accurately, you also need to perform them quickly because of the patient's life-threatening condition. (See *Quick list of critical care meds and measurements*, page 330.)

Many I.V. drugs — such as the antiarrhythmics amiodarone, lidocaine, and procainamide, the vasodilators sodium nitroprusside and nitroglycerin, and the adrenergics norepinephrine and dopamine — are administered in life-threatening situations. The nurse's job is to prepare the drug for infusion, give it to the patient, and then observe him to evaluate the drug's effectiveness.

Administering I.V. injections

Many drugs administered on critical care units are given by direct injection, also called I.V. push. These potent, fast-acting drugs rapidly control heart rate, respirations, blood pressure, cardiac output, or kidney function. They usually have a short duration of action, so you can evaluate their effectiveness immediately and begin other treatment promptly if they aren't working.

One critical difference

Generally, the doctor orders I.V. push drugs by dosage, which can sometimes include the specific unit of measure to administer over a short time (such as mg/minute or mcg/kg/minute). Calculate dosages on the critical care unit the same as you would on other units. However, take extra care because drugs used on critical care units are extremely potent and have serious adverse effects, which can include death.

Be prepared to be under stress

You're responsible for calculating and administering the dose accurately, following any special instructions. Many drugs used on critical care units come in small vials, so double-check the label to make sure you're giving the right dose or concentration. For example, epinephrine comes in two concentrations (1:1,000 and 1:10,000). Giving the wrong concentration could be fatal.

Because calculating dosages during an emergency is stressful, and stress makes you more error-prone, do everything you can to be prepared. (See *Stress busters*.)

> **Quick list of critical care meds and measurements**
>
> The lists below show some of the common critical care drugs and associated units of measure. Memorizing these units of measure will help speed your calculations.
>
> **mg/minute**
> - lidocaine
> - procainamide
>
> **mcg/minute**
> - epinephrine
> - nitroglycerin
> - norepinephrine
> - phenylephrine
>
> **mcg/kg/minute**
> - dobutamine
> - dopamine
> - milrinone
> - nitroprusside

Calculating dosages

The following examples demonstrate how to use proportions to calculate I.V. push drugs. Note that the calculations are very similar to those for intramuscular (I.M.) drugs.

Also note how the administration times vary. If you aren't sure how slowly or quickly to push a drug, look it up or call the pharmacist. It's better to be safe than sorry with rapid-acting drugs.

Are you label able?

Your patient is admitted with frequent ventricular arrhythmias. The doctor orders procainamide 100 mg every 5 minutes by slow I.V. push (no faster than 25 to 50 mg/minute) until arrhythmias disappear. If the drug label says the dose strength is 50 mg/ml, how many milliliters of procainamide should you give to the patient every 5 minutes?

- Set up a proportion with the ordered dose and the unknown volume in one fraction and the dose strength in milligrams per milliliter in the other fraction:

$$\frac{100 \text{ mg}}{X} = \frac{50 \text{ mg}}{1 \text{ ml}}$$

- Cross-multiply the fractions:

$$X \times 50 \text{ mg} = 1 \text{ ml} \times 100 \text{ mg}$$

- Solve for X by dividing each side of the equation by 100 mg and canceling the units that appear in both the numerator and denominator:

$$\frac{X \times \cancel{50\text{ mg}}}{\cancel{50\text{ mg}}} = \frac{1\text{ ml} \times 100\ \cancel{\text{mg}}}{50\ \cancel{\text{mg}}}$$

$$X = \frac{100\text{ ml}}{50}$$

$$X = 2\text{ ml}$$

You should administer 2 ml of procainamide. According to the package insert, you should administer the drug only I.M. or I.V. Also, note that when giving procainamide I.V., the drug must be diluted.

Rapid heartbeat riddle

Your patient suddenly develops supraventricular tachycardia. The doctor orders *6 mg adenosine rapid I.V. push.* If the only vial available contains 3 mg/ml, how many milliliters should you give?

- Set up a proportion with the available solution in one ratio and the ordered dose and the unknown volume in the other ratio:

$$3\text{ mg} : 1\text{ ml} :: 6\text{ mg} : X$$

- Multiply the means and the extremes:

$$X \times 3\text{ mg} = 1\text{ ml} \times 6\text{ mg}$$

- Solve for X by dividing both sides of the equation by 3 mg and canceling units that appear in both the numerator and denominator:

$$\frac{X \times \cancel{3\text{ mg}}}{\cancel{3\text{ mg}}} = \frac{1\text{ ml} \times 6\ \cancel{\text{mg}}}{3\ \cancel{\text{mg}}}$$

$$X = \frac{6\text{ ml}}{3}$$

$$X = 2\text{ ml}$$

You should administer 2 ml of the solution. According to the package insert, this drug should be administered by rapid I.V. push because of its very short half-life. It also should be administered directly into the vein or in the most proximal port, followed by a rapid saline flush.

Advice from the experts

Stress busters

Here are four hot tips to help reduce your stress level when calculating drugs during an emergency:

- Carry a list of all the drug-calculation formulas.
- Carry a calculator for quick use.
- Convert your patients' weights into kilograms, and keep the information at their bedsides.
- Become familiar with the different critical care drugs given I.V. as well as your unit's medication protocols.

Dosage drill

Test your math skills with this drill.

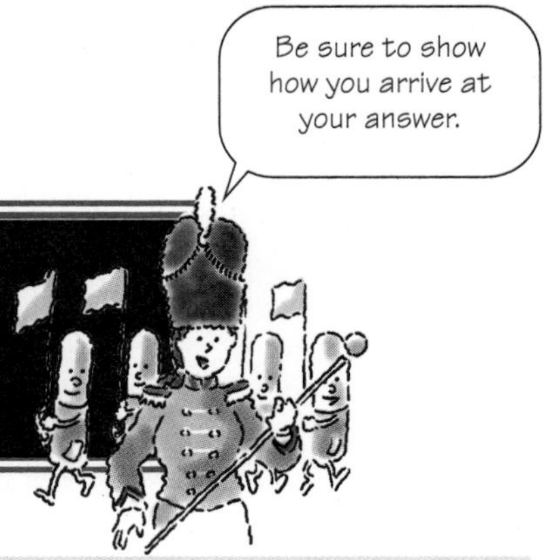
Be sure to show how you arrive at your answer.

The doctor orders amiodarone 150 mg I.V. stat for your patient with ventricular tachycardia. If the vial you have available contains 50 mg/ml, how many milliliters should you give?

Your answer: ______________________

To find the answer, first set up a proportion.

$$50 \text{ mg} : 1 \text{ ml} :: 150 \text{ mg} : X$$

Next, set up the equation, multiplying the means and extremes.

$$50 \text{ mg} \times X = 150 \text{ mg} \times 1 \text{ ml}$$

Solve for *X*.

$$\frac{\cancel{50 \text{ mg}} \times X}{\cancel{50 \text{ mg}}} = \frac{150 \cancel{\text{ mg}} \times 1 \text{ ml}}{50 \cancel{\text{ mg}}}$$

$$\frac{150 \text{ ml}}{50} = X$$

$$X = 3 \text{ ml}$$

You should give 3 ml of amiodarone.

Digoxin difficulty

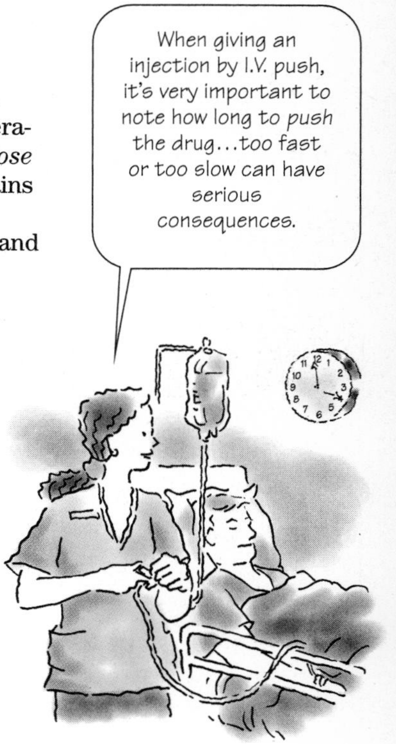

When giving an injection by I.V. push, it's very important to note how long to push the drug...too fast or too slow can have serious consequences.

Your patient has a history of rapid atrial fibrillation and takes digoxin at home. When his digoxin level is found to be subtherapeutic, the doctor orders *0.125 mg I.V. digoxin as a single dose* to control his heart rate. The only available digoxin vial contains 0.25 mg/ml. How many milliliters should you give?

- Set up a proportion with the available solution in one ratio and the ordered dose and the unknown volume in the other ratio:

$$0.25\text{ mg} : 1\text{ ml} :: 0.125\text{ mg} : X$$

- Multiply the means and the extremes:

$$X \times 0.25\text{ mg} = 1\text{ ml} \times 0.125\text{ mg}$$

- Solve for X by dividing both sides of the equation by 0.25 mg and canceling units that appear in both the numerator and denominator:

$$\frac{X \times \cancel{0.25\text{ mg}}}{\cancel{0.25\text{ mg}}} = \frac{1\text{ ml} \times 0.125\text{ }\cancel{\text{mg}}}{0.25\text{ }\cancel{\text{mg}}}$$

$$X = \frac{0.125\text{ ml}}{0.25}$$

$$X = 0.5\text{ ml}$$

You should administer 0.5 ml of digoxin. According to the package insert, the drug should be given by I.V. push over 5 minutes (not 1 minute, as with some other critical care drugs).

Calculating I.V. flow rates

Because many drugs given on the critical care unit are used to treat life-threatening problems, you can't waste any time when calculating I.V. flow rates. You must swiftly do the calculations, prepare the drug for infusion, administer it, and then observe the patient closely to evaluate the drug's effectiveness.

Three critical calculations

You may need to perform three calculations before administering critical care drugs:

- concentration of the drug in the I.V. solution
- flow rate required to deliver the desired dose
- number of micrograms needed, based on the patient's weight in kilograms. You may need to perform this calculation if the drug

is ordered in micrograms per kilogram of body weight per minute. *Remember:* If you need to convert milligrams to micrograms, multiply by 1,000.

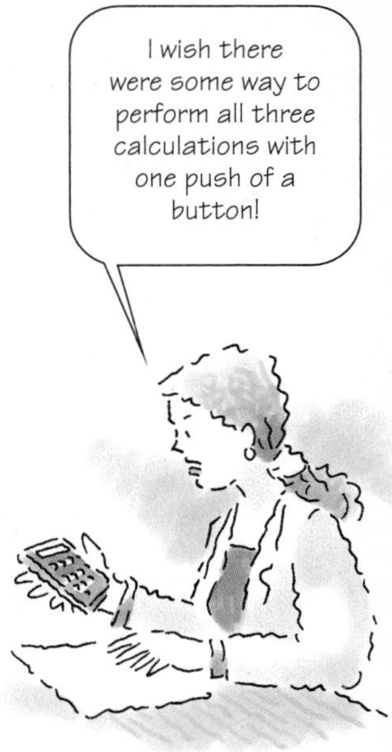

I wish there were some way to perform all three calculations with one push of a button!

Concentrate on this formula

To calculate the drug's concentration, use this formula:

$$\text{concentration in mg/ml} = \frac{\text{mg of drug}}{\text{ml of fluid}}$$

- If you need to express the concentration in mcg/ml, multiply the answer by 1,000.

Figure the flow rate

You can determine the I.V. flow rate per minute using this formula:

$$\frac{\text{dose/minute}}{X} = \frac{\text{concentration of solution}}{\text{1 ml of fluid}}$$

- To calculate the hourly flow rate, first multiply the ordered dose, given in milligrams or micrograms per minute, by 60 minutes to determine the hourly dose. Then use this proportion to compute the hourly flow rate:

$$\frac{\text{hourly dose}}{X} = \frac{\text{concentration of solution}}{\text{1 ml of fluid}}$$

Determine the dosage

To determine the dosage in milligrams per kilogram of body weight per minute, perform the following steps:

- First, determine the concentration of the solution in milligrams per milliliter. To determine the dose in milligrams per hour, multiply the hourly flow rate by the concentration using this formula:

$$\text{dose in mg/hour} = \text{hourly flow rate} \times \text{concentration}$$

- To calculate the dose in milligrams per minute, first divide the hourly dose by 60 minutes. Here's the formula:

$$\text{dose in mg/minute} = \frac{\text{dose in mg/hour}}{\text{60 minutes}}$$

- Then divide the dose per minute by the patient's weight, using this formula:

$$\text{mg/kg/minute} = \frac{\text{mg/minute}}{\text{patient's weight in kg}}$$

No time for books?

Suppose you don't have time to refer to your dosage calculation book in a critical situation. Keep these formulas on a card with your calculator for quick reference. They're foolproof!

- To find out how many micrograms per kilogram per minute your patient is receiving, use this formula:

$$\frac{\text{mg}}{\text{volume of bag}} \times 1{,}000 \div 60 \div \text{kg} \times \text{infusion rate} = \text{mcg/kg/min}$$

- To find out how many milliliters per hour you should give, use this formula:

$$\frac{\text{weight in kg} \times \text{dose in mcg/kg/min} \times 60}{\text{concentration in 1 L}} = \text{ml/hr}$$

- After you've performed these calculations, make sure that the drug is being given within a safe and therapeutic range. Compare the amount in milligrams per kilogram per minute to the safe range shown in a drug reference book. (See *No time for books?*)

Real world problems

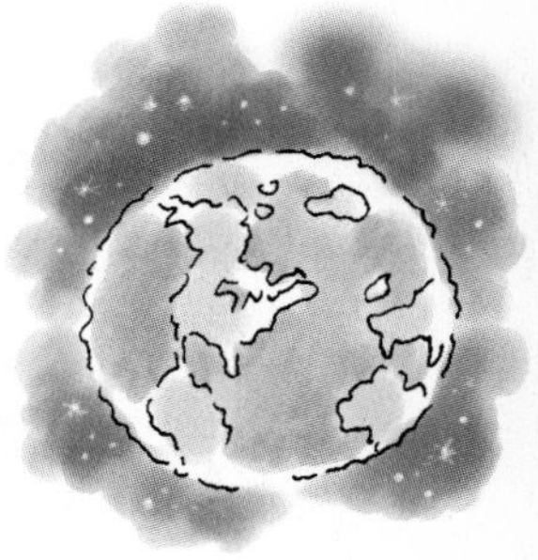

The following examples show how to calculate an I.V. flow rate using the different formulas.

A lidocaine lifeline

Your patient is having frequent runs of ventricular tachycardia that subside after 10 to 12 beats. The doctor orders *2 g (2,000 mg) lidocaine in 500 ml D_5W to infuse at 2 mg/minute.* What's the flow rate in milliliters per minute? In milliliters per hour?

- First, find the solution's concentration by setting up a proportion with the unknown concentration in one fraction and the ordered dose in the other fraction:

$$\frac{X}{1 \text{ ml}} = \frac{2{,}000 \text{ mg}}{500 \text{ ml}}$$

- Cross-multiply the fractions:

$$X \times 500 \text{ ml} = 2{,}000 \text{ mg} \times 1 \text{ ml}$$

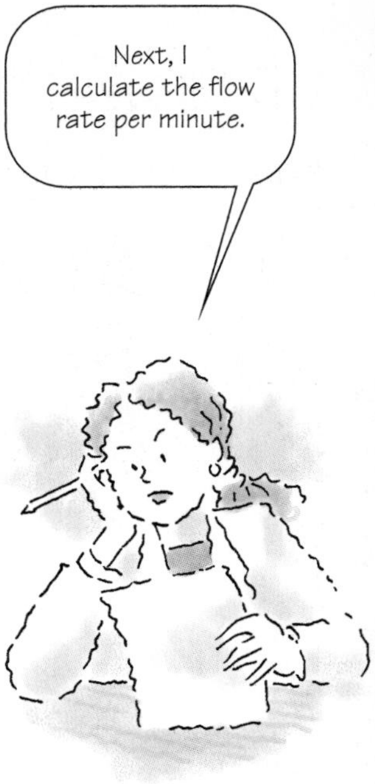
Next, I
calculate the flow
rate per minute.

- Solve for X by dividing each side of the equation by 500 ml and canceling units that appear in both the numerator and denominator:

$$\frac{X \times \cancel{500\text{ ml}}}{\cancel{500\text{ ml}}} = \frac{2{,}000\text{ mg} \times 1\ \cancel{\text{ml}}}{500\ \cancel{\text{ml}}}$$

$$X = \frac{2{,}000\text{ mg}}{500}$$

$$X = 4\text{ mg}$$

- The solution's concentration is 4 mg/ml. Next, calculate the flow rate per minute needed to deliver the ordered dose of 2 mg/minute. To do this, set up a proportion with the unknown flow rate per minute in one fraction and the solution's concentration in the other fraction:

$$\frac{2\text{ mg}}{X} = \frac{4\text{ mg}}{1\text{ ml}}$$

- Cross-multiply the fractions:

$$X \times 4\text{ mg} = 1\text{ ml} \times 2\text{ mg}$$

- Solve for X by dividing each side of the equation by 4 mg and canceling units that appear in both the numerator and denominator:

$$\frac{X \times \cancel{4\text{ mg}}}{\cancel{4\text{ mg}}} = \frac{1\text{ ml} \times 2\ \cancel{\text{mg}}}{4\ \cancel{\text{mg}}}$$

$$X = \frac{2\text{ ml}}{4}$$

$$X = 0.5\text{ ml}$$

- The patient should receive 0.5 ml/minute of lidocaine. Because lidocaine must be infused through an infusion pump, compute the hourly flow rate. Do this by setting up a proportion with the unknown flow rate per hour in one fraction and the flow rate per minute in the other fraction:

$$\frac{X}{60\text{ minutes}} = \frac{0.5\text{ ml}}{1\text{ minute}}$$

- Cross-multiply the fractions:

$$X \times 1\text{ minute} = 0.5\text{ ml} \times 60\text{ minutes}$$

Dosage drill

Test your math skills with this drill.

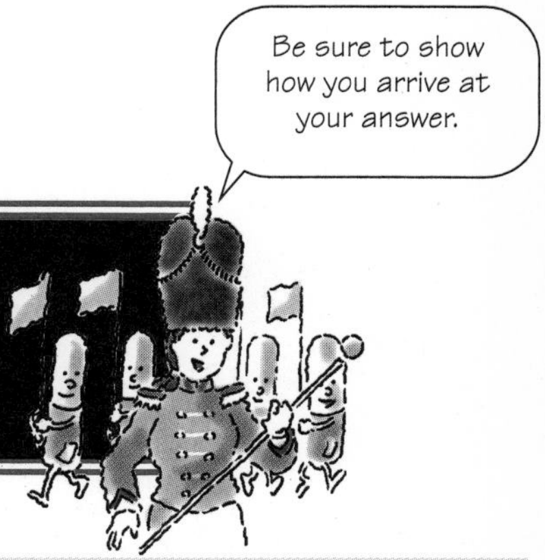
Be sure to show how you arrive at your answer.

An infusion of norepinephrine (Levophed) containing 4 mg in 250 ml of D5W is running at 30 ml/hour. How many micrograms of norepinephrine are infusing each minute?

Your answer: ________________

First set up ratios and a proportion to determine the solution's concentration.

$$4 \text{ mg} : 250 \text{ ml} :: X \text{ ml} : 1 \text{ min}$$

$$X \text{ mg} \times 250 \text{ ml} = 1 \text{ ml} \times 4 \text{ mg}$$

$$\frac{X \text{ mg} \times \cancel{250 \text{ ml}}}{\cancel{250 \text{ ml}}} = \frac{1 \cancel{\text{ ml}} \times 4 \text{ mg}}{250 \cancel{\text{ ml}}}$$

$$X = \frac{4 \text{ mg}}{250}$$

$$X = 0.016 \text{ mg/ml, or } 16 \text{ mcg/ml}$$

Next determine the flow rate in ml/minute.

$$30 \text{ ml} : 60 \text{ minutes} :: X \text{ ml} : 1 \text{ minute}$$

$$30 \text{ ml} \times 1 \text{ minute} = 60 \text{ minutes} \times X \text{ ml}$$

$$\frac{30 \text{ ml} \times 1 \cancel{\text{ minute}}}{60 \cancel{\text{ minutes}}} = \frac{\cancel{60 \text{ minutes}} \times X \text{ ml}}{\cancel{60 \text{ minutes}}}$$

$$X = \frac{30}{60}$$

$$X = 0.5 \text{ ml/minute}$$

Finally, determine how many micrograms of the drug the patient will receive per minute.

$$X = 0.5 \text{ ml/minute} \times 16 \text{ mcg/ml}$$

$$X = 8 \text{ mcg/minute}$$

There are 8 micrograms of norepinephrine infusing each minute.

• Solve for X by dividing each side of the equation by 1 minute and canceling units that appear in both the numerator and denominator:

$$\frac{X \times 1\ \cancel{\text{minute}}}{1\ \cancel{\text{minute}}} = \frac{0.5\text{ ml} \times 60\ \cancel{\text{minutes}}}{1\ \cancel{\text{minute}}}$$

$$X = 30\text{ ml}$$

Set the infusion pump to deliver 30 ml/hour.

Don't doubt dobutamine

A 200-lb patient is to receive an I.V. infusion of dobutamine at 10 mcg/kg/minute. The label instructs to check the package insert. There it states to dilute 250 mg of the drug in 50 ml of D_5W.

Because the drug vial contains 20 ml of solution, the total to be infused is 70 ml (50 ml of D_5W + 20 ml of solution). How many milliliters of the drug should the patient receive each minute? Each hour?

• First, compute the patient's weight in kilograms. To do this, set up a proportion with the weight in pounds and the unknown weight in kilograms in one fraction and the number of pounds per kilogram in the other fraction:

$$\frac{200\text{ lb}}{X} = \frac{2.2\text{ lb}}{1\text{ kg}}$$

• Cross-multiply the fractions:

$$X \times 2.2\text{ lb} = 1\text{ kg} \times 200\text{ lb}$$

• Solve for X by dividing each side of the equation by 2.2 lb and canceling units that appear in both the numerator and denominator:

$$\frac{X \times \cancel{2.2\text{ lb}}}{\cancel{2.2\text{ lb}}} = \frac{1\text{ kg} \times 200\ \cancel{\text{lb}}}{2.2\ \cancel{\text{lb}}}$$

$$X = \frac{200\text{ kg}}{2.2}$$

$$X = 90.9\text{ kg}$$

• The patient weighs 90.9 kg. Next, determine the dose in milliliters per minute by setting up a proportion with the patient's weight in kilograms and the unknown dose in micrograms per minute in one fraction and the known dose in micrograms per kilogram per minute in the other fraction:

$$\frac{90.9\text{ kg}}{X} = \frac{1\text{ kg}}{10\text{ mcg/minute}}$$

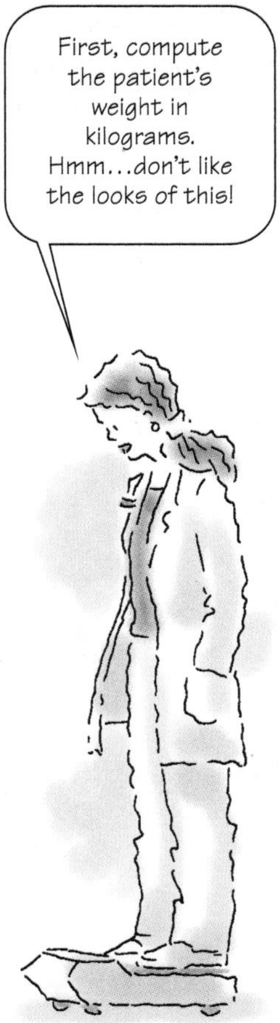
First, compute the patient's weight in kilograms. Hmm...don't like the looks of this!

• Cross-multiply the fractions:

$$X \times 1\ \text{kg} = 10\ \text{mcg/minute} \times 90.9\ \text{kg}$$

• Solve for X by dividing each side of the equation by 1 kg and canceling units that appear in both the numerator and denominator:

$$\frac{X \times \cancel{1\ \text{kg}}}{\cancel{1\ \text{kg}}} = \frac{10\ \text{mcg/minute} \times 90.9\ \cancel{\text{kg}}}{1\ \cancel{\text{kg}}}$$

$$X = 909\ \text{mcg/minute}$$

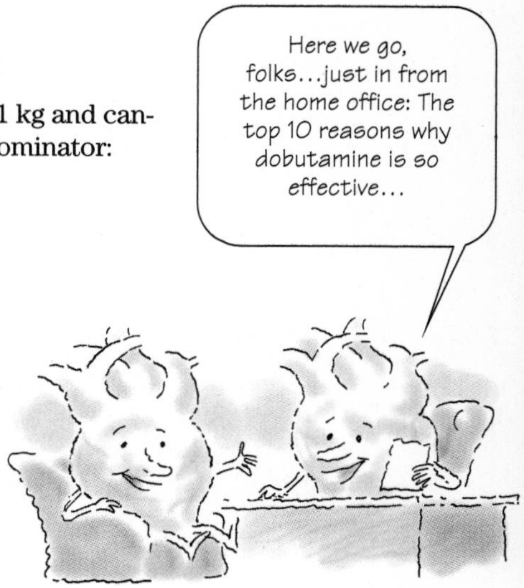

Here we go, folks...just in from the home office: The top 10 reasons why dobutamine is so effective...

• The patient should receive 909 mcg of dobutamine every minute, or 0.909 mg every minute. To determine the flow rate in milliliters per minute, set up a proportion using the solution's concentration and solve for X:

$$\frac{0.909\ \text{mg}}{X} = \frac{250\ \text{mg}}{70\ \text{ml}}$$

$$\frac{\cancel{250\ \text{mg}} \times X}{\cancel{250\ \text{mg}}} = \frac{0.909\ \cancel{\text{kg}} \times 70\ \text{ml}}{250\ \cancel{\text{mg}}}$$

$$X = \frac{63.63\ \text{ml}}{250}$$

$$X = 0.25\ \text{ml/minute}$$

• To find the flow rate in milliliters per hour, multiply by 60.

$$0.25\ \text{ml/minute} \times 60\ \text{minutes/hour} = 15\ \text{ml/hour}$$

The patient should receive dobutamine at a rate of 15 ml/hr.

Special cases

Critical care drugs aren't always ordered at a specific flow rate or dosage. Sometimes, they're prescribed according to the patient's heart rate, blood pressure, or other parameters.

In some cases, the doctor may order a starting dose and a maximum dose to which the drug can be titrated. To deliver the correct amount of drug, you must calculate the starting dose and the maximum dose.

Here are some examples of drug calculations that you may use in special cases.

Dosage drill

Test your math skills with this drill.

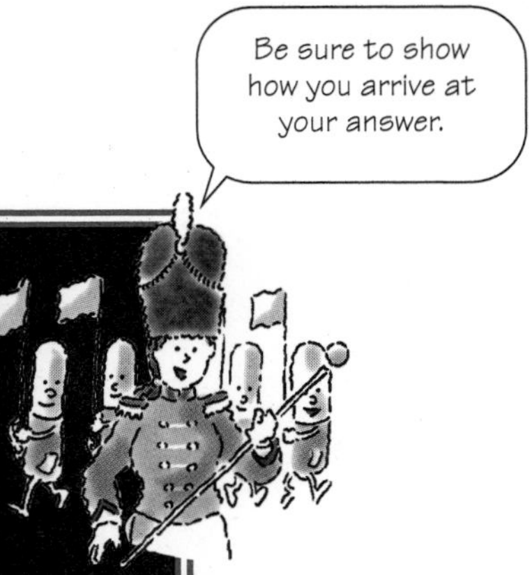
Be sure to show how you arrive at your answer.

A patient with supraventricular tachycardia is ordered esmolol hydrochloride (Brevibloc) at 50 mcg/kg/minute. The solution contains 2.5 g esmolol in 250 ml of D_5W. The patient weighs 73 kg. How should the nurse set the pump to deliver the correct milliliters per hour so the patient receives the ordered dose?

Your answer: ______________________

First determine the dose in micrograms per minute.

$$73 \text{ kg} : X \text{ mcg/minute} :: 1 \text{ kg} : 50 \text{ mcg/minute}$$

$$73 \text{ kg} \times 50 \text{ mcg/minute} = 1 \text{ kg} \times X \text{ mcg/minute}$$

$$\frac{73 \cancel{\text{kg}} \times 50 \text{ mcg/minute}}{1 \cancel{\text{kg}}} = \frac{\cancel{1 \text{ kg}} \times X \text{ mcg/minute}}{\cancel{1 \text{ kg}}}$$

$$X = 3{,}650 \text{ mcg/minute}$$

Next set up an equation to determine the volume infused per minute.

$$3.65 \text{ mg} : X \text{ ml} :: 2{,}500 \text{ mg} : 250 \text{ ml}$$

$$3.650 \text{ mg} \times 250 \text{ ml} = X \text{ ml} \times 2{,}500 \text{ mg}$$

$$\frac{3.650 \cancel{\text{mg}} \times 250 \text{ ml}}{2{,}500 \cancel{\text{mg}}} = \frac{X \text{ ml} \times \cancel{2{,}500 \text{ mg}}}{\cancel{2{,}500 \text{ mg}}}$$

$$X = \frac{912.5}{2{,}500}$$

$$X = 0.365 \text{ ml/minute}$$

Finally, multiply by 60 minutes/hour to determine the correct flow rate in ml/hour.

$$0.365 \text{ ml/minute} \times 60 \text{ minutes/hour} = 21.9 \text{ ml/hour}$$

Rounding off, the nurse should set the pump to deliver 22 ml/hour.

Nitroprusside number cruncher

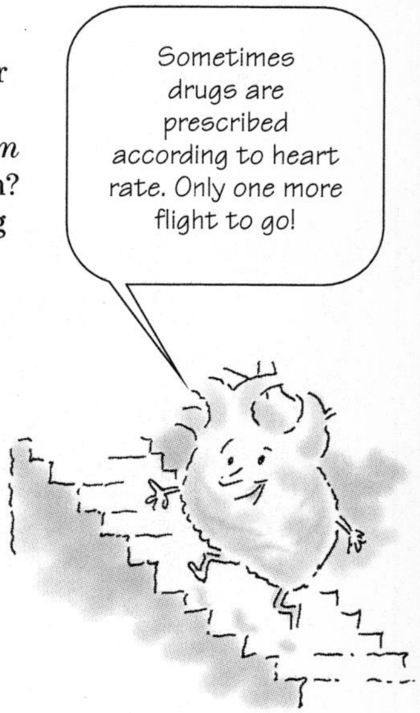

Sometimes drugs are prescribed according to heart rate. Only one more flight to go!

A patient with severe hypertension weighs 85 kg. The doctor's order reads *nitroprusside 50 mg in 250 ml D_5W. Start at 0.5 mcg/kg/minute. Titrate to keep systolic BP less than 170 mm Hg. Maximum dose is 10 mcg/kg/minute.* At what rate should you start the infusion?

- First, find the concentration of the infusion. Start by converting 50 mg to 50,000 mcg.

$$\frac{50{,}000 \text{ mcg}}{250 \text{ ml}} = 200 \text{ mcg/ml}$$

- Then set up the following equation:

$$X = \frac{85 \text{ kg} \times 0.5 \text{ mcg/kg/min} \times 60}{200 \text{ mcg/ml}}$$

$$X = 12.75 \text{ ml/hr}$$

The starting dose is 13 ml/hour.

Keep the phenylephrine flowing

A patient with terminal Hodgkin's disease who weighs 90 lb (41 kg) has been hypotensive for several hours despite receiving I.V. fluid boluses. The doctor orders *100 mg phenylephrine in 250 ml of normal saline solution.* The drug is to start at 30 mcg/minute and then be titrated to keep the systolic blood pressure at 90 mm Hg. What's the flow rate in milliliters per minute?

- First, determine the solution's concentration by dividing the ordered dose of phenylephrine by the amount of normal saline solution:

$$X = \frac{100 \text{ mg}}{250 \text{ ml}}$$

$$X = 0.4 \text{ mg/ml}$$

- The concentration is 0.4 mg/ml. Next, convert milligrams to micrograms by multiplying by 1,000:

$$0.4 \text{ mg/ml} \times 1{,}000 = 400 \text{ mcg/ml}$$

- The concentration is 400 mcg/ml. Now calculate the flow rate by setting up a proportion with the starting flow rate and the unknown flow rate in one fraction and the concentration in the other fraction:

$$\frac{30 \text{ mcg/minute}}{X \text{ ml/minute}} = \frac{400 \text{ mcg}}{1 \text{ ml}}$$

- Cross-multiply the fractions:

$$X \text{ ml/minute} \times 400 \text{ mcg} = 30 \text{ mcg/minute} \times 1 \text{ ml}$$

Dosage drill

Test your math skills with this drill.

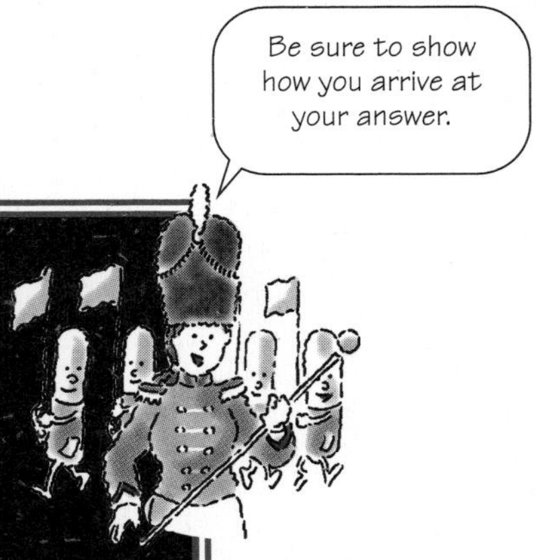
Be sure to show how you arrive at your answer.

An 80-kg patient is admitted with urosepsis. The doctor's order reads Dopamine 800 mg in 500 ml dextrose 5% in water, start at 5 mcg/kg/minute. Titrate to keep systolic blood pressure greater than 90 mm Hg. Maximum dose is 15 mcg/kg/minute. At what rate should you start the infusion?

Your answer: ______________________

First, find the concentration of the solution. Start by converting 800 mg to 800,000 mcg.

$$\frac{800{,}000 \text{ mcg}}{500 \text{ ml}} = 1{,}600 \text{ mcg/ml}$$

Then set up the following equation:

$$X = \frac{80 \text{ kg} \times 5 \text{ mcg/kg/min} \times 60 \text{ min}}{1{,}600 \text{ mcg/ml}}$$

$$X = 15 \text{ ml/hr}$$

You should start the infusion at 15 ml/hour.

- Solve for X by dividing each side of the equation by 400 mcg and canceling units that appear in both the numerator and denominator:

$$\frac{X \text{ ml/minute} \times \cancel{400 \text{ mcg}}}{\cancel{400 \text{ mcg}}} = \frac{30 \cancel{\text{mcg}}\text{/minute} \times 1 \text{ ml}}{400 \cancel{\text{mcg}}}$$

$$X = \frac{30 \text{ ml/minute}}{400}$$

$$X = 0.075 \text{ ml/minute}$$

- The flow rate is 0.075 ml/minute. To calculate the hourly flow rate, multiply 0.075 ml by 60:

$$0.075 \text{ ml} \times 60 = 4.5 \text{ ml}$$

The hourly flow rate is 4.5 ml, which can be rounded off to 5 ml/hour.

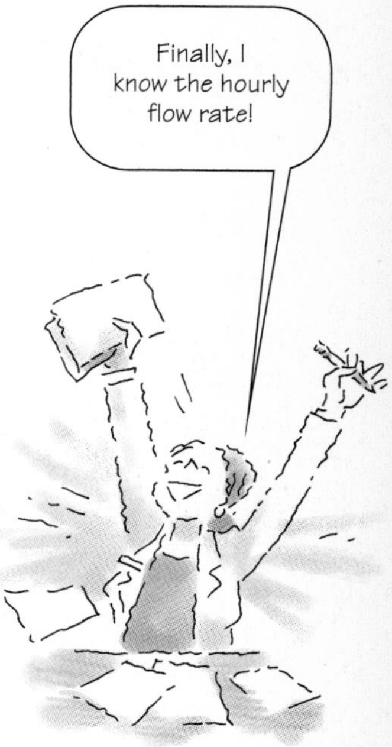
Finally, I know the hourly flow rate!

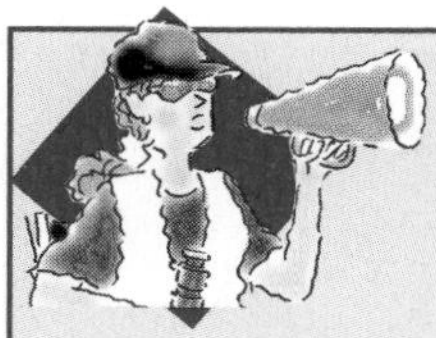

That's a wrap!

Calculating critical care dosages review

When working with critical care dosages, keep in mind these important facts.

Calculating I.V. push dosages

- Use proportions to calculate dosages.
- Determine administration time.

Calculating a drug's concentration

$$\text{Concentration in mg/ml} = \frac{\text{mg of drug}}{\text{ml of fluid}}$$

- Remember to multiply the answer by 1,000 if you need to express concentration in mcg/ml.

Calculating the flow rate

- Per minute:

$$\frac{\text{dose/minute}}{X} = \frac{\text{concentration of solution}}{1 \text{ ml of fluid}}$$

- Per hour:

$$\frac{\text{hourly dose}}{X} = \frac{\text{concentration of solution}}{1 \text{ ml of fluid}}$$

Calculating a dosage in mg/kg of body weight/minute

- Determine the dose in milligrams per hour: hourly flow rate × concentration
- Calculate the dose in milligrams per minute: dose in mg/hour ÷ 60 minutes
- Solve for mg/kg/minute: mg/minute ÷ patient's weight in kg

More formulas!

- To determine how many micrograms per kilogram per minute a patient is receiving:

$$\frac{\text{mg}}{\text{volume of bag}} \times 1{,}000 \div 60 \div \text{kg} \times \text{infusion rate} = \text{mcg/kg/minute}$$

- To determine how many milliliters per hour to give:

$$\frac{\text{weight in kg} \times \text{dose in mcg/kg/min} \times 60}{\text{concentration in 1 L}} = \text{ml/hr}$$

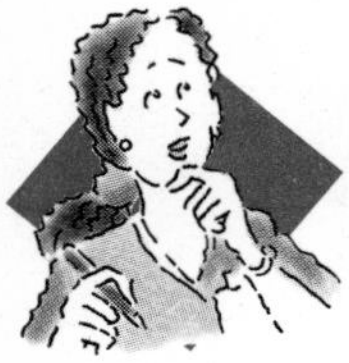

Quick quiz

1. If a patient has a dopamine drip of 800 mg in 500 ml D_5W, the concentration is:

A. 0.16 mg/ml.
B. 1.6 mg/ml.
C. 16 mg/ml.
D. 160 mg/ml.

Answer: B. Concentration is determined by dividing the total in milligrams (800 mg) by the volume (500 ml).

2. Procainamide is measured in:

A. mg/minute.
B. mcg/kg/minute.
C. mg/hour.
D. mcg/minute.

Answer: A. This information is necessary before you can calculate dosages of procainamide.

3. To convert milligrams to micrograms, multiply by:

A. 10.
B. 60.
C. 100.
D. 1,000.

Answer: D. When converting a number from milligrams to micrograms, move the decimal three spaces to the right.

4. How many kilograms does a 250-lb man weigh?

A. 11.4 kg
B. 114 kg
C. 550 kg
D. 125 kg

Answer: B. To convert pounds to kilograms, divide by 2.2 and round off the number.

5. The doctor's order reads *Lasix 80 mg I.V. as a single dose.* The available vial contains 100 mg in 10 ml of normal saline solution. What volume should you give to administer this dose?

A. 0.08 ml
B. 0.8 ml
C. 1.8 ml
D. 8 ml

Answer: D. Set up a proportion with the available solution in one ratio and the ordered dose and the unknown volume in the other ratio. Solve for *X*.

6. If a patient weighs 50 kg, his weight in pounds is:
- A. 28 lb.
- B. 100 lb.
- C. 110 lb.
- D. 200 lb.

Answer: C. To convert kilograms to pounds, multiply by 2.2.

7. A patient requires nitroprusside to lower his blood pressure. This dose should be ordered in:
- A. mcg/hour.
- B. mcg/minute.
- C. mg/minute.
- D. mcg/kg/minute.

Answer: D. Nitroprusside should be ordered in doses of mcg/kg/minute.

Scoring

☆☆☆ If you answered all seven items correctly, fantastic! You can calculate confidently in critical cases.

☆☆ If you answered five or six items correctly, that isn't bad! You're a cool, calm, and collected calculator.

☆ If you answered fewer than five items correctly, keep at it! You have the best dosage calc book ever. Keep it with you always and refer to it frequently.

Appendices and index

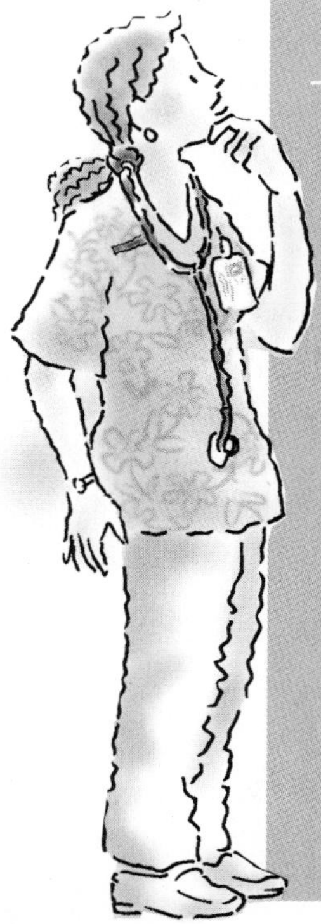

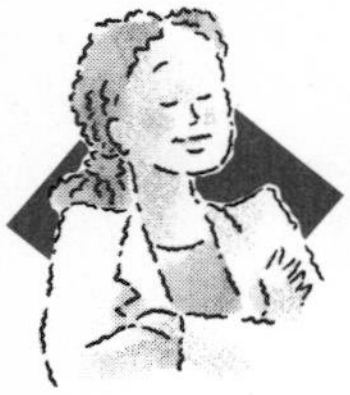

Practice makes perfect

1. The improper fraction $\frac{11}{2}$ converted into a mixed number is:

A. $\frac{2}{11}$.
B. $5\frac{1}{11}$.
C. $5\frac{1}{2}$.
D. $\frac{22}{11}$.

2. The sum of $\frac{1}{2} + \frac{3}{4} + \frac{6}{10}$ is:

A. $1\frac{8}{10}$.
B. $1\frac{17}{20}$.
C. $2\frac{1}{4}$.
D. $\frac{10}{16}$.

3. The complex fraction $\frac{1}{75}$ divided by the complex fraction $\frac{1}{25}$ equals:

A. $\frac{1}{3}$.
B. 3.
C. $\frac{1}{100}$.
D. $\frac{2}{3}$.

4. The decimal fraction 4.3 divided by 8.6 yields:

A. 0.5.
B. 2.
C. 20.
D. 50.

5. When 21.3478 is rounded off to the nearest hundredth, it becomes:

A. 21.34.
B. 21.3.
C. 21.348.
D. 21.35.

6. 31% of 105 is:

A. 3.15.
B. 31.5.
C. 32.55.
D. 33.3.

7. When 20% is converted to a decimal fraction, it becomes:

A. 0.02.
B. 2.0.
C. 0.2.
D. 2.2.

8. In fraction form, the proportion 1 : 4 :: 4 : 16 is:

A. $4/1 = 4/16$.
B. $1/4 = 4/16$.
C. $4/4 = 1/16$.
D. $4/1 = 16/4$.

9. If a vial has 20 mg of drug in 50 ml of solution, the amount of drug in 10 ml of solution is:

A. 15 mg.
B. 10 mg.
C. 5 mg.
D. 4 mg.

10. In the proportion 3 : 9 :: 9 : *X*, *X* equals:

A. 81.
B. 3.
C. 27.
D. 18.

11. How much chlorine bleach should you add to 500 ml of water to make a solution that contains 10 ml of chlorine bleach for every 100 ml of water?

A. 5 ml
B. 50 ml
C. 10 ml
D. 100 ml

12. A patient weighs 70 kg. How many pounds is this?

A. 140 lb
B. 154 lb
C. 70 lb
D. 32 lb

13. A patient has been ordered ampicillin 250 mg. The medication is supplied as an oral suspension, 125 mg per 5 ml. How many milliliters should the patient receive?

A. 10 ml
B. 5 ml
C. 25 ml
D. 1 ml

14. The doctor prescribes meperidine 75 mg. The pharmacy stocks a multidose vial containing 100 mg/ml. How many milliliters should you administer?

A. 7.5 ml
B. 5 ml
C. 1.5 ml
D. 0.75 ml

15. Convert 0.025 kl to liters.
- A. 250 L
- B. 2.5 L
- C. 0.25 L
- D. 25 L

16. During a 24-hour period, a patient received 600 ml, 1.25 L, and 2.5 L of I.V. fluid. How many milliliters did he receive altogether?
- A. 43,500 ml
- B. 43.5 ml
- C. 4,350 ml
- D. 435 ml

17. The weight in kilograms of an infant who weighs 8,300 g is:
- A. 8,300 kg
- B. 8.3 kg
- C. 83.0 kg
- D. 830 kg

18. A patient receives 0.25 mg of digoxin (Lanoxin). How many grams did he receive?
- A. 25 g
- B. 2.5 g
- C. 0.25 g
- D. 0.00025 g

19. According to the medication order, a patient is to receive 2 gr of a drug. The bottle is labeled 120 mg/ml. How many milliliters will you give?
- A. 1 ml
- B. 2 ml
- C. 10 ml
- D. 30 ml

20. A patient's fingerstick glucose level was 365 mg/dl. The doctor has ordered 10 units of regular insulin for the patient. The bottle is labeled 100 units/ml. The volume of insulin you'll administer is:
- A. 0.01 ml.
- B. 0.1 ml.
- C. 1 ml.
- D. 10 ml.

21. A patient needs 20 mEq of potassium chloride oral solution. The solution contains 60 mEq in every 15 ml. How many milliliters of solution should you give the patient?
- A. 5 ml
- B. 2.5 ml
- C. 7.5 ml
- D. 3 ml

22. The Arabic numeral 148 in Roman numerals is:
A. CXLVIII.
B. CXXXIIIIIIII.
C. DLXVIII.
D. DXXXVIII.

23. A doctor prescribes *digoxin 0.125 mg P.O. 0900 daily* for a patient with heart failure. How should you interpret this order?
A. Give 125 grams of digoxin orally at 9 a.m. every other day.
B. Give 0.125 milligrams of digoxin orally every day at 9 p.m.
C. Give 0.125 milligrams of digoxin orally every day at 9 a.m.
D. Give 0.125 micrograms of digoxin orally at 9 a.m. every other day.

24. Which doctor's order is incomplete?
A. *Tylenol elixir 1 tsp P.O. STAT*
B. *Aspirin 325 P.O. q a.m.*
C. *Seconal 100 mg P.O. at bedtime. p.r.n.*
D. *Rocephin 1 g I.V. daily*

25. The doctor prescribes *metoprolol 5 mg I.V. q 6 hours* for a patient with an acute myocardial infarction. You should understand that this drug is to be given:
A. four times per day.
B. in a suspension.
C. as needed.
D. intravenously.

26. You're administering medication to a 58-year-old patient who was admitted with heart failure. In giving a regularly scheduled drug, you must:
A. give the drug one-half hour before or after the ordered time.
B. give the drug 1 hour before or after the ordered time.
C. give the drug 15 minutes before or after the ordered time.
D. give the drug exactly at the ordered time.

27. You need to administer morphine to a patient who just returned from the postanesthesia care unit after undergoing a laminectomy. The information recorded on the perpetual inventory record when you remove a controlled substance from a locked storage site should include:
A. date and time of removal, patient's name, drug dose, and your initials.
B. date and time of removal, patient's name, drug dose, and your signature.
C. date and time of removal, patient's name, doctor's name, drug dose, and your signature.
D. date and time of removal, patient's initials, doctor's name, and your initials.

28. You're caring for a 49-year-old patient with metastatic breast cancer. You need to administer her 9 a.m. medications. When administering regularly scheduled drugs, you should:

A. document the time of administration before giving the drug to the patient.
B. document the time of administration after giving the drug to the patient.
C. document the time of administration for all regularly scheduled drugs on your shift at the beginning of the shift.
D. document the time of administration at the end of your shift.

29. A patient tells you that she typically takes two ibuprofen tablets for menstrual cramps. If one tablet of ibuprofen contains 200 mg, how many milligrams does she usually take?

A. 500 mg
B. 600 mg
C. 400 mg
D. 300 mg

30. Before administering a patient's medication, you should compare the drug ordered with the drug's label. The nonproprietary name on a drug label is the drug's:

A. trade name.
B. generic name.
C. manufacturer name.
D. chemical name.

31. The doctor orders *minoxidil 5 mg P.O. daily* for treatment of hypertension in a 52-year-old patient. The medication is supplied as 2.5 mg per tablet. How many tablets should be administered?

A. ½ tablet
B. 1 tablet
C. 1½ tablets
D. 2 tablets

32. An 83-year-old patient complains that she hasn't had a bowel movement for 4 days and she's very uncomfortable. The doctor orders *Milk of Magnesia 1½ tbs P.O. at bedtime.* How many milliliters is this?

A. 17.5 ml
B. 15.5 ml
C. 22.5 ml
D. 7.5 ml

33. A patient is ordered *Tylenol 240 mg supp per rectum* to treat a fever. You have Tylenol 120 mg supp available. What should be prepared?

A. 1½ supp
B. 1 supp
C. 2 supp
D. ½ supp

34. A doctor orders a 2.5-mg suppository for a child, but only 5-mg suppositories are on hand. How much should be given?

A. 2 supp
B. 1½ supp
C. 1 supp
D. ½ supp

35. A patient is ordered bacitracin for treatment of a wound he received in a motor vehicle accident. Before giving the patient a topical preparation, it's important to read the label first because:

A. you want to know the manufacturer's name.
B. the patient may be allergic to the ingredients.
C. you like to read small print.
D. there's probably no package insert.

36. A 52-year-old patient requires transdermal nitroglycerin to control his angina. You know that transdermal nitroglycerin should be removed 12 to 14 hours after application to:

A. prevent it from falling off while the patient sleeps.
B. prevent it from irritating the patient's skin.
C. prevent the patient from developing a tolerance to the drug.
D. prevent toxicity.

37. A patient returns from the postanesthesia care unit after undergoing an exploratory laparotomy and a lysis of adhesions. The doctor orders *meperidine 75 mg I.M. q4h p.r.n.* for pain. The medication is available in a prefilled syringe containing 100 mg of meperidine per 1 ml. How many milliliters of meperidine should you administer?

A. 1 ml
B. 0.75 ml
C. 0.5 ml
D. 0.25 ml

38. The doctor orders *Dilaudid 3 mg I.M. q6h p.r.n.* for a patient with postoperative pain. The medication is available in a prefilled syringe containing 4 mg per ml. How many milliliters of Dilaudid should you waste?

A. 0.25 ml
B. 0.75 ml
C. 0.5 ml
D. 1 ml

39. The doctor orders *heparin 8,000 units subcutaneously q8h* for a patient with deep vein thrombosis. The heparin available is 20,000 units per 1 ml. How many milliliters of heparin should you give?

A. 0.2 ml
B. 0.3 ml
C. 0.4 ml
D. 0.5 ml

40. A patient with type 1 diabetes mellitus is ordered 45 units of NPH insulin subcutaneously in the morning daily. You have NPH insulin 100 units per ml available. Using a U-100 syringe, how many milliliters will be in the syringe?

A. 0.045 ml
B. 0.45 ml
C. 4.5 ml
D. 5 ml

41. A patient needs an infusion of D_5W at 100 ml/hour. If the tubing set is calibrated at 15 gtt/ml, what's the drip rate?

A. 31 gtt/minute
B. 33 gtt/minute
C. 25 gtt/minute
D. 30 gtt/minute

42. A patient diagnosed with pneumonia needs 2,000 ml of fluid over 24 hours. What's the flow rate?

A. 150 ml/hour
B. 125 ml/hour
C. 110 ml/hour
D. 83 ml/hour

43. You're about to administer a continuous infusion of 25,000 units of heparin in 500 ml of half-normal saline solution. If the patient is to receive 750 units/hour, what's the flow rate?

A. 25 ml/hour
B. 15 ml/hour
C. 10 ml/hour
D. 5 ml/hour

44. A 4-year-old patient weighs 46 lb. How many kilograms is this?

A. 21 kg
B. 20 kg
C. 23 kg
D. 12 kg

45. The doctor orders a single dose of acetaminophen 10 mg/kg/dose oral suspension for a child with a fever who weighs 6 kg. What's the dose in milligrams?

A. 1.6 mg
B. 16 mg
C. 60 mg
D. 80 mg

46. A child weighing 66 lb is admitted with appendicitis. How much maintenance I.V. fluid should the child receive in 24 hours?

A. 1,500 ml/day
B. 1,700 ml/day
C. 1,800 ml/day
D. 1,900 ml/day

47. A 25-year-old primagravida has been in labor for 20 hours with little progress. The doctor prescribes oxytocin for her. The order reads *10 units oxytocin in 1,000 ml NSS to infuse via pump at 1 milliunit/minute for 15 minutes; then increase flow rate to 2 milliunits/minute.* What's the flow rate needed to deliver 1 milliunit/minute for 15 minutes?

A. 4 ml/hour
B. 6 ml/hour
C. 8 ml/hour
D. 12 ml/hour

48. Use the calculations in the previous problem. After 15 minutes, the pump needs to be reset to deliver 2 milliunits/minute. What's the flow rate?

A. 10 ml/hour
B. 20 ml/hour
C. 12 ml/hour
D. 15 ml/hour

49. The doctor orders *4 g magnesium sulfate in 250 ml D_5W infused at 1 g/hour* for a patient with preeclampsia. What's the flow rate?

A. 125 ml/hour
B. 250 ml/hour
C. 25 ml/hour
D. 63 ml/hour

50. The doctor orders *150 mg of ritodrine in 500 ml D_5W to infuse at 0.15 mg/minute* for a patient admitted in preterm labor. What's the flow rate?

A. 30 ml/hour
B. 15 ml/hour
C. 10 ml/hour
D. 5 ml/hour

51. A 170-lb patient with minimal urine output has an order to receive dopamine at 5 mcg/kg/minute. The premixed bag of dopamine contains 800 mg in 500 ml D_5W. How many milliliters of solution containing dopamine will the patient receive each hour?

A. 17 ml
B. 16 ml
C. 15 ml
D. 14 ml

52. A patient experiencing an acute myocardial infarction is to receive nitroglycerin 10 mcg/minute I.V. The I.V. solution contains 250 ml D_5W with 25 mg nitroglycerin. How many milliliters should the patient receive each hour?

A. 16 ml
B. 10 ml
C. 6 ml
D. 4 ml

53. A patient experienced a sustained ventricular tachycardia that required cardioversion. The doctor orders *1 g lidocaine in 250 ml D_5W to infuse at 3 mg/minute* to help maintain a normal sinus rhythm. What's the flow rate?

A. 30 ml/hour
B. 45 ml/hour
C. 60 ml/hour
D. 70 ml/hour

54. The doctor writes an order for 2 L of lactated Ringer's solution to be infused over 16 hours. The drop factor of the administration set is 20 gtt/ml. What should the drip rate be?

A. 25 gtt/minute
B. 33 gtt/minute
C. 20 gtt/minute
D. 42 gtt/minute

55. The nurse is to administer Rocephin 2 g in 500 ml over 10 hours. What hourly flow rate should the nurse set the infusion pump to deliver?

A. 50 ml/hour
B. 65 ml/hour
C. 35 ml/hour
D. 15 ml/hour

56. The nurse receives a doctor's order to administer 4,000 ml of normal saline solution I.V. over 12 hours. What should the drip rate be if the drop factor of the tubing is 15 gtt/ml?

A. 46 gtt/ml
B. 91 gtt/ml
C. 166 gtt/ml
D. 83 gtt/ml

57. The doctor writes a single-dose order for ketorolac tromethamine 15 mg I.V. for pain. Ketorolac tromethamine is available in a vial containing 60 mg/2 ml. How many milliliters should the nurse administer?

A. 0.5 ml
B. 5 ml
C. 0.2 ml
D. 2 ml

58. A 150-lb patient is to receive gentamicin 3 mg/kg daily in 3 divided doses. Gentamicin is available to the nurse in 80 mg/2 ml. How many milliliters should the nurse administer every 8 hours?

A. 1.7 ml
B. 4 ml
C. 2.7 ml
D. 1.3 ml

59. The doctor orders digoxin 250 mcg P.O. every day. The pharmacy stocks digoxin 0.5-mg scored tablets. How many tablets should the nurse administer?

A. ¼ tab
B. 1 tab
C. ½ tab
D. 2 tabs

60. The doctor orders Dilantin suspension 300 mg P.O. every day. Dilantin is available to the nurse in a suspension of 125 mg/5 ml. How many milliliters should the nurse administer per dose?

A. 18 ml
B. 12 ml
C. 6 ml
D. 2.1 ml

61. The doctor orders Imuran 75 mg P.O. every day. Imuran is available to the nurse in 50-mg unscored tablets. How should the nurse administer the dose?

A. Administer 2 tablets.
B. Administer 1½ tablets.
C. Administer 1 tablet.
D. Withhold the dose until the pharmacy sends a 75-mg tablet.

62. An infant weighing 2.3 kg is ordered to receive gentamicin 2.5 mg/kg/dose I.V. q 12 hours. The pharmacy stocks gentamicin in a solution of 2 mg/ml. How many milliliters of the solution should the nurse administer for each dose?

A. 3.2 ml
B. 2.6 ml
C. 1.9 ml
D. 2.9 ml

63. An infant weighing 8 lb is about to receive a blood transfusion of 15 ml/kg of packed red blood cells over 4 hours. What hourly flow rate should the nurse set the infusion pump to deliver?

A. 8 ml/hour
B. 10.6 ml/hour
C. 13.5 ml/hour
D. 15.2 ml/hour

64. The doctor orders *ferrous sulfate 5 gr.* Ferrous sulfate is available to the nurse in 150-mg tablets. How many tablets should the nurse administer? _____

65. The doctor orders *Rocephin 1 g in 10 ml of D_5W, give 250 mg I.V. q12h.* How many milliliters should the nurse administer for each dose? _____

66. The doctor orders *meperidine 60 mg I.M. stat.* The drug is available in a prefilled, 1-ml syringe containing 100 mg/ml. How many milliliters should the nurse waste before administering the ordered dose?

_____

67. Which conversion factors are correct? Select all that apply.

A. 2.2 kilograms = 1 pound
B. 1,000 milligrams = 1 gram
C. 1 teaspoon = 5 milliliters
D. 1 kilogram = 2.2 pounds
E. 1 milliliter = 30 ounces
F. 1 liter = 1,000 milliliters

Answers

1. C. Divide the numerator (11) by the denominator (2). The calculation looks like this:

$$\frac{11}{2} = 11 \div 2 = 5\frac{1}{2}$$

You get 5 with 1 left over. The 1 becomes the new numerator and the denominator stays the same.

2. B. Determine the lowest common denominator (20). Then convert each to the lowest common denominator: $1/2 = 10/20$, $3/4 = 15/20$, $6/10 = 12/20$. Add all the numerators and place over the denominators: $10/20 + 15/20 + 12/20 = 37/20$. Reduce to lowest terms: $1\,17/20$.

3. A. Divide the dividend $1/75$ by the divisor $1/25$. Invert the divisor ($1/25$) and multiply $1/75 \times 25/1 = 25/75$. Reduce to lowest terms: $1/3$.

4. A. Move the decimal points of both the divisor and the dividend one place to the right before dividing. Place the quotient's decimal point over the new decimal point in the dividend.

5. D. The number 4 is in the hundredth place. Look at the number to the right of it, which is 7. Seven is greater than 5 so add 1 to 4 to round off the number.

6. C. To solve this, restate the question as a decimal fraction by removing the percent sign and moving the decimal point two places to the left. (The decimal fraction is 0.31.) Then multiply 0.31 by 105.

7. C. Remove the percent sign and move the decimal point two places to the left.

8. B. Make the ratio on both sides into fractions by substituting slashes for colons; replace the double colon in the center with an equal sign.

9. D. Substitute X for the amount of drug in 10 ml of solution; then set up a proportion with ratios or fractions and solve for X:

$$X : 10 \text{ ml} :: 20 \text{ mg} : 50 \text{ ml} \quad or \quad \frac{X}{10 \text{ ml}} = \frac{20 \text{ mg}}{50 \text{ ml}}$$

10. C. Multiply the means and the extremes. Put the products of the means and extremes into an equation. Solve for X by dividing both sides by 3. The calculation looks like this:

$$9 \times 9 = 3 \times X$$

$$81 = 3X$$

$$X = 27$$

11. B. Substitute X for the amount of chlorine bleach in 500 ml of water. Then set up a proportion with ratios or fractions and solve for X. The setup looks like this:

$$X \text{ ml bleach/500 ml of water} = 10 \text{ ml bleach/100 ml water}$$

or

$$X \text{ ml bleach} : 500 \text{ ml water} :: 10 \text{ ml bleach} : 100 \text{ ml water}$$

12. B. Use the conversion factor 1 kg equals 2.2 lb to find that 70 kg equals 154 lb.

13. A. Use the conversion factor 125 mg equals 5 ml to find that the patient should receive 10 ml.

14. D. Set up the following equation and solve for X (X represents the milliliters needed to administer 75 mg.):

$$\frac{100 \text{ mg}}{1 \text{ ml}} = \frac{75 \text{ mg}}{X}$$

15. D. Using the *Amazing metric decimal place finder*, page 90, count the number of places to the right or left of kiloliters to reach liters. In this case, it's three places to the right, so move the decimal three places to the right.

16. C. Knowing that there are 1,000 ml in 1 L, convert all the measurements to milliliters and add all the numbers together.

17. B. Knowing that 1 kg equals 1,000 g, set up an equation with X as the unknown quantity:

$$\frac{1 \text{ kg}}{1{,}000 \text{ g}} = \frac{X}{8{,}300 \text{ g}}$$

Cross-multiply and then divide both sides of the equation by 1,000 g to isolate X, canceling like units. Finish solving for X.

18. D. Using the *Insta-metric conversion table*, page 89, you'll see that 1 g is equal to 1,000 mg. Set up the equation with X as the unknown quantity:

$$\frac{X}{0.25 \text{ mg}} = \frac{1 \text{ g}}{1{,}000 \text{ mg}}$$

Cross-multiply and then divide both sides of the equation by 1,000 mg to isolate *X*, canceling like units. Finish the math.

19. A. The known equivalent is 60 mg equals 1 gr. Set up an equation to determine how many milligrams there are in 2 grains by solving for *X* as the unknown quantity:

$$\frac{X}{2\ \text{gr}} = \frac{60\ \text{mg}}{1\ \text{gr}}$$

Cross-multiply the equation, divide both sides by 1 gr, and then cancel like units to isolate *X*. There are 120 mg in 2 gr. The bottle is labeled 120 mg/ml; therefore, you should administer 1 ml.

20. B. Set up the equation with *X* as the unknown quantity:

$$\frac{X}{10\ \text{units}} = \frac{1\ \text{ml}}{100\ \text{units}}$$

Cross-multiply both sides of the equation. To isolate *X*, divide both sides by 100 units. Finish the math.

21. A. Set up the equation using *X* as the unknown quantity:

$$\frac{X}{20\ \text{mEq}} = \frac{15\ \text{ml}}{60\ \text{mEq}}$$

Cross-multiply the fractions. Then find *X* by dividing both sides by 60 mEq to isolate *X* and cancel like units. Finish the math.

22. A. To convert 148, break it into its component parts (100, 40, and 8); then translate into Roman numerals.

23. C. In the correct answer, *daily* is interpreted as "every day" and *0900* is the military time for 9 a.m. Also, *mg* stands for milligrams not grams or micrograms and *P.O.* means "by mouth" or "orally."

24. B. This answer is incomplete because the unit of measure for the dose is missing.

25. D. I.V. is the abbreviation for intravenous, which means the drug should be injected through an intravenous catheter.

26. A. Scheduled drugs are considered on time if they're given one-half hour before or after the ordered time.

27. C. When a controlled substance is removed from the locked storage site, the date and time the dose is removed, the patient's full name, the doctor's name, the drug dose, and your signature must be recorded on the perpetual inventory record. You may also be required to note the amount of the controlled substance remaining in the locked storage site.

28. B. Document the time of administration of a drug immediately after giving the drug to the patient to keep from mistakenly giving the drug again.

29. C. Set up the equation with 200 mg per 1 tablet as the known amount and X as the unknown factor:

$$\frac{200\text{ mg}}{1\text{ tablet}} = \frac{X}{2\text{ tablets}}$$

Solve for X.

30. B. The generic name is the accepted nonproprietary name, which is a simplified form of the drug's chemical name.

31. D. Set up the equation with 2.5 mg equals 1 tablet as the known factor and X as the unknown factor:

$$\frac{2.5\text{ mg}}{1\text{ tablet}} = \frac{5\text{ mg}}{X}$$

Solve for X.

32. C. Set up the equation with 1 tbs equals 15 ml as the known factor and X as the unknown factor:

$$\frac{1\text{ tbs}}{15\text{ ml}} = \frac{1.5\text{ tbs}}{X}$$

Solve for X.

33. C. Set up the equation with 120 mg per 1 supp as the known factor and X as the unknown factor:

$$120\text{ mg} : 1\text{ supp} :: 240\text{ mg} : X$$

Solve for X.

34. D. Set up the equation with 5 mg equals 1 supp as the known factor and X as the unknown factor:

$$5\text{ mg} : 1\text{ supp} :: 2.5\text{ mg} : X$$

Solve for X.

35. B. Topical preparations may contain one or more ingredients and you need to make sure the patient isn't allergic to any of them.

36. C. A new patch is applied daily (usually in the morning) and removed after 12 to 14 hours to prevent the patient from developing a tolerance to the drug.

37. B. Set up the equation with the known factor 100 mg/1 ml and X as the unknown factor:

$$\frac{100\text{ mg}}{1\text{ ml}} = \frac{75\text{ mg}}{X}$$

Solve for X.

38. A. Set up the equation with the known factor 4 mg/1 ml and X as the unknown factor:

$$\frac{4 \text{ mg}}{1 \text{ ml}} = \frac{3 \text{ mg}}{X}$$

Solve for X. Then subtract the answer (0.75 ml) from 1 ml to determine the amount to waste.

39. C. Set up the equation with 20,000 units/1 ml as the known factor and X as the unknown factor:

$$\frac{20{,}000 \text{ units}}{1 \text{ ml}} = \frac{8{,}000 \text{ units}}{X}$$

Solve for X.

40. B. Set up the equation with 100 units/1 ml as the known factor and X as the unknown factor:

$$\frac{100 \text{ units}}{1 \text{ ml}} = \frac{45 \text{ units}}{X}$$

Solve for X. Cross-multiply the fractions. Then find X by dividing both sides by 100 units to isolate X and cancel like units. Finish the math.

41. C. Convert hours to minutes. Then set up the equation using this formula to find drops/minute: Total ml/total minutes × drop factor in drops/ml.

$$X = \frac{100 \text{ ml}}{60 \text{ min}} \times \frac{15 \text{ gtt}}{1 \text{ ml}}$$

Multiply the fraction by the drop factor and cancel like units. Solve for X by dividing the numerator by the demoninator.

42. D. Set up the equation using the formula total volume ordered ÷ number of hours.

43. B. Set up the equation using 25,000 units/500 ml as the known factor and X ml as the unknown factor:

$$\frac{25{,}000 \text{ units}}{500 \text{ ml}} = \frac{750 \text{ units}}{X}$$

Solve for X.

44. A. Divide the weight in pounds by 2.2 kg (1 kg = 2.2 lb), and round off the answer (20.9) to 21.

45. C. Set up the proportion with the ordered dosage in one fraction and the unknown dosage and the patient's weight in the other fraction:

$$\frac{10 \text{ mg}}{1 \text{ kg}} = \frac{X}{6 \text{ kg}}$$

Cross-multiply, cancel like units, and solve for *X*.

46. B. First, convert the child's weight to kilograms by dividing by 2.2. Then calculate the dosage, remembering that the first 20 kg of a child's weight requires 1,500 ml and each additional kilogram of weight requires 20 ml/kg. Because the child weighs 30 kg, he needs 1,500 ml for the first 20 kg and 200 ml for the additional 10 kg of weight.

47. B. First determine the concentration of the solution by setting up the equation with 10 units/1,000 ml as the known factor and *X* as the unknown factor:

$$\frac{10 \text{ units}}{1{,}000 \text{ ml}} = \frac{X}{1 \text{ ml}}$$

Cross-multiply and solve for *X*. Then convert to milliunits by multiplying by 1,000. Next, determine the flow rate by setting up the equation with 10 milliunits/1 ml as the known factor and 15 milliunits/*X* as the unknown factor:

$$\frac{10 \text{ milliunits}}{1 \text{ ml}} = \frac{15 \text{ milliunits}}{X}$$

Cross-multiply and solve for *X*. Convert to an hourly rate by multiplying by 4 (60 minutes/15 minutes = 4).

48. C. Using the calculation for the solution above, 10 milliunits/1 ml, determine that the patient needs 120 milliunits in 1 hour (2 milliunits/minute × 60 minutes). Set up the equation with 10 milliunits/1 ml as the known factor and 120 milliunits/*X* as the unknown factor:

$$\frac{10 \text{ milliunits}}{1 \text{ ml}} = \frac{120 \text{ milliunits}}{X}$$

Cross-multiply and solve for *X*.

49. D. Set up the equation with 4 g/250 ml as the known factor and 1 g/*X* as the unknown factor:

$$\frac{4 \text{ g}}{250 \text{ ml}} = \frac{1 \text{ g}}{X}$$

Cross-multiply and solve for *X*. Round off the answer.

50. A. First find the fluid's strength by setting up the equation 150 mg/500 ml as the known factor and *X*/1 ml as the unknown factor:

$$\frac{150 \text{ mg}}{500 \text{ ml}} = \frac{X}{1 \text{ ml}}$$

Cross-multiply and solve for *X* to determine 0.3 mg/ml of ritodrine. Next, set up the equation with 1 ml/0.3 mg as the known factor and *X*/0.15 mg as the unknown factor:

$$\frac{1 \text{ ml}}{0.3 \text{ mg}} = \frac{X}{0.15 \text{ mg}}$$

Cross-multiply and solve for *X*. Convert to hourly flow rate by multiplying by 60.

51. D. First determine the patient's weight in kilograms by dividing his weight in pounds by 2.2 kg (170 ÷ 2.2 = 77 kg).

Next, determine the concentration of medication in micrograms by multiplying milligrams by 1,000. Then divide by 500 ml to determine the concentration in 1 ml.

$$\frac{800 \text{ \sout{mg}}}{500 \text{ ml}} \times \frac{1{,}000 \text{ mcg}}{1 \text{ \sout{mg}}} = \frac{800{,}000 \text{ mcg}}{500 \text{ ml}} = \frac{1{,}600 \text{ mcg}}{1 \text{ ml}}$$

To find out how many milliliters per hour you should give, use the formula: weight in kg × dose in mcg/kg/min × 60 (minutes in 1 hour) ÷ concentration in 1 ml of solution:

$$\frac{77 \text{ \sout{kg}}}{1} \times \frac{5 \text{ mcg}}{\text{\sout{kg}/min}} = \frac{385 \text{ mcg}}{1 \text{ min}}$$

$$\frac{385 \text{ mcg}}{\text{\sout{min}}} \times \frac{60 \text{ \sout{min}}}{1 \text{ hr}} = \frac{23{,}100 \text{ mcg}}{1 \text{ hr}}$$

$$\frac{23{,}100 \text{ \sout{mcg}/hr}}{1{,}600 \text{ \sout{mcg}/ml}} = 14.43 \text{ ml/hr}$$

Then round off the answer.

52. C. First, determine the concentration. It's easier to do this if you first convert the 25 mg of nitroglycerin to micrograms by multiplying by 1,000. Then divide this by the number of milliliters to determine the concentration of the solution. Then determine ml/hour by multiplying the ordered dose by 60 minutes and dividing by the concentration.

53. B. Multiply 1 g by 1,000 to convert to milligrams. Then set up the equation with 1,000 mg/250 ml as the known factor and *X* as the unknown factor to determine the concentration in 1 ml:

$$\frac{1{,}000 \text{ mg}}{250 \text{ ml}} = \frac{X}{1 \text{ ml}}$$

Cross-multiply and solve for *X*. Using this information, set up an equation with the concentration per milliliter as the known factor and 3 mg/*X* as the unknown factor:

$$\frac{4 \text{ mg}}{1 \text{ ml}} = \frac{3 \text{ mg}}{X}$$

Cross-multiply and solve for *X*. You find 0.75 ml for 3 mg of lidocaine. Now set up the final equation to determine hourly flow rate with 0.75 ml/1 minute and *X*/60 minutes. Cross-multiply and solve for *X*.

54. D. First, convert 2 L to milliliters by setting up an equation with the conversion of 1,000 ml/1 L:

$$\frac{1 \text{ L}}{1{,}000 \text{ ml}} = \frac{2 \text{ L}}{X}$$

The total to be infused is 2,000 ml.

Next, convert 16 hours to minutes by multiplying by 60 to determine that the solution needs to be infused over 960 minutes. Then determine the drip rate using the formula: total ml/total minutes × drop factor in drops/ml.

$$\text{Drip rate} = \frac{2{,}000 \text{ ml}}{960 \text{ min}} \times \frac{20 \text{ gtt}}{\text{ml}}$$

Multiply the fraction by the drip rate and cancel like units. Then divide the numerator by the denominator, and round off the answer.

55. A. Use the formula: total volume ordered ÷ number of hours. In this case, it would be 500 ml ÷ 10 hours.

56. D. First, convert 12 hours to minutes by multiplying by 60 to determine that the fluid must be infused over 720 minutes. Then determine the drip rate using the formula: total ml/total minutes × drop factor in drops/ml.

$$\text{Drip rate} = \frac{4{,}000 \text{ ml}}{720 \text{ min}} \times \frac{15 \text{ gtt}}{\text{ml}}$$

Multiply the fraction by the drip rate and cancel like units. Then divide the numerator by the denominator, and round off the answer.

57. A. Set up an equation using 60 mg/2 ml as the known factor and 15 mg/X as the unknown factor:

$$\frac{60 \text{ mg}}{2 \text{ ml}} = \frac{15 \text{ mg}}{X}$$

Cross-multiply and solve for X by dividing both sides of the equation by 60 mg and canceling units that appear in both the numerator and denominator.

58. A. First, convert the patient's weight in pounds to kilograms by dividing by 2.2. Then determine the number of milligrams the patient is to receive per day by multiplying the desired dose per day (3 mg) by the weight in kilograms (68 kg).

Then determine the number of milligrams to administer every 8 hours by dividing the total number of milligrams per day (204 mg) by 3.

Lastly, determine the number of milliliters to administer every 8 hours by cross-multiplying the drug's available concentration (80 mg/2 ml) and the unknown factor (68 mg/X) and solving for X.

59. C. Convert the dose in micrograms to milligrams by dividing by 1,000 (1 mg = 1,000 mcg). Then set up an equation using 0.5 mg/tablet as the known factor, and 0.25 mg/X as the unknown factor:

$$\frac{0.5 \text{ mg}}{1 \text{ tab}} = \frac{0.25 \text{ mg}}{X}$$

Solve for X by cross-multiplying, dividing both sides by 0.5 mg, and canceling units that appear in both the numerator and denominator. Because the tablet is scored, the nurse may administer ½ of a tablet.

60. B. Set up an equation using the drug's available concentration as the known factor, and the desired dose as the unknown factor:

$$\frac{125 \text{ mg}}{5 \text{ ml}} = \frac{300 \text{ mg}}{X}$$

Cross-multiply and solve for X, canceling units that appear in both the numerator and denominator.

61. D. Determine the number of tablets to administer by setting up an equation using 50 mg/tablet as the known factor and 75 mg/X as the unknown factor, and solve for X.

Because the tablet is unscored, the nurse shouldn't break it in half to administer the necessary 1½ tablet dose. The nurse must call the pharmacy to have the dose sent as a single tablet or, if this is unavailable, the pharmacist should crush and measure out the tablet so that the nurse may administer the most accurate dosage.

62. D. First, determine the number of milligrams per dose by multiplying the infant's weight in kg (2.3 kg) by the ordered dose

(2.5 mg/kg). Then cross-multiply the known drug concentration (2 mg/1 ml) by the unknown factor (5.75 mg/X) and solve for X to calculate the number of milliliters to administer for each dose.

63. C. Convert the infant's weight to kilograms by dividing the weight in pounds by 2.2. Then multiply the child's weight in kilograms (3.6 kg) by 15 ml/kg to determine the total volume of the blood transfusion. Calculate the hourly flow rate by dividing the total volume of the transfusion (54 ml) by the number of hours (4).

64. 2. Convert the dose in grains to milligrams using the conversion factor 1 gr = 60 mg, to get a dosage of 300 mg. Then calculate the number of tablets needed by setting up an equation using 150 mg/1 tablet as the known factor, and 300 mg/X as the unknown factor.

$$\frac{150 \text{ mg}}{1 \text{ tab}} = \frac{300 \text{ mg}}{X}$$

Cross-multiply, and solve for X by dividing both sides of the equation by 150 mg, canceling units that appear in the numerator and denominator.

65. 2.5. Determine the concentration of the solution in milligrams using the conversion factor 1 g = 1,000 mg. Calculate the final concentration of the solution by cross-multiplying the known factor of 1,000 mg/10 ml and the unknown factor of X/1 ml, to get the final concentration of 100 mg/1 ml.

Then calculate the dose in milliliters:

$$\frac{100 \text{ mg}}{1 \text{ ml}} = \frac{250 \text{ mg}}{X}$$

Cross-multiply, and solve for X by dividing both sides of the equation by 100 mg and canceling units that appear in the numerator and denominator.

66. 0.4. First, determine the required dose in milliliters using 100 mg/1 ml as the known factor and 60 mg/X as the unknown factor. The patient should receive 0.6 ml of meperidine. Subtract the volume of the dose (0.6 ml) from the total volume of the syringe (1 ml) to determine the volume to be wasted.

67. B, C, D, F. Commit frequently used conversion factors to memory to administer dosages quickly and accurately.

Drug therapy conversions

Metric weight

1 kilogram (kg)	= 1,000 grams (g)
1 g	= 1,000 milligrams (mg)
1 mg	= 1,000 micrograms (mcg)
0.6 g	= 600 mg
0.3 g	= 300 mg
0.1 g	= 100 mg
0.06 g	= 60 mg
0.03 g	= 30 mg
0.015 g	= 15 mg
0.001 g	= 1 mg

Metric volume

1 liter (L)	= 1,000 milliliters (ml)
1 ml	= 1,000 microliters (μl)
Household	***Metric***
1 teaspoon (tsp)	= 5 ml
1 tablespoon (T or tbs)	= 15 ml
2 tbs	= 30 ml
8 ounces	= 240 ml
1 pint (pt)	= 473 ml
1 quart (qt)	= 946 ml
1 gallon (gal)	= 3,785 ml

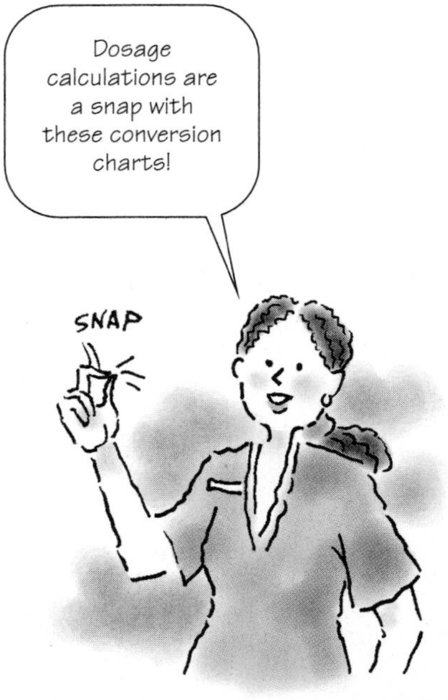

Dosage calculations are a snap with these conversion charts!
SNAP

Weight conversion

To convert a patient's weight in pounds to kilograms, divide the number of pounds by 2.2 kg; to convert a patient's weight in kilograms to pounds, multiply the number of kilograms by 2.2 lb.

Pounds	Kilograms
10	4.5
20	9.1
30	13.6
40	18.2
50	22.7
60	27.3
70	31.8
80	36.4
90	40.9
100	45.5
110	50
120	54.5
130	59.1
140	63.6
150	68.2
160	72.7
170	77.3
180	81.8
190	86.4
200	90.9

Temperature conversion

To convert Fahrenheit to Celsius, subtract 32 from the temperature in Fahrenheit and then divide by 1.8; to convert Celsius to Fahrenheit, multiply the temperature in Celsius by 1.8 and then add 32.

$$(F - 32) \div 1.8 = \text{degrees Celsius}$$
$$(C \times 1.8) + 32 = \text{degrees Fahrenheit}$$

Degrees Fahrenheit (°F)	Degrees Celsius (°C)
89.6	32
91.4	33
93.2	34
94.3	34.6
95	35
95.4	35.2
96.2	35.7
96.8	36
97.2	36.2
97.6	36.4
98	36.7
98.6	37
99	37.2
99.3	37.4
99.7	37.6
100	37.8
100.4	38
100.8	38.2

Degrees Fahrenheit (°F)	Degrees Celsius (°C)
101	38.3
101.2	38.4
101.4	38.6
101.8	38.8
102	38.9
102.2	39
102.6	39.2
102.8	39.3
103	39.4
103.2	39.6
103.4	39.7
103.6	39.8
104	40
104.4	40.2
104.6	40.3
104.8	40.4
105	40.6

Dosage calculation formulas

Calculating drip rates

When calculating the flow rate of I.V. solutions, remember that the number of drops required to deliver 1 ml varies with the type of administration set you're using. To calculate the drip rate, you must know the calibration of the tubing's drip rate for each specific manufacturer's product. As a quick guide, refer to the chart below. Use this formula to calculate specific drip rates:

$$\frac{\text{volume of infusion (in ml)}}{\text{time of infusion (in minutes)}} \times \text{drip factor (in drops/ml)} = \text{drops/minute}$$

	Ordered volume					
	500 ml/24 hour or 21 ml/hour	***1,000 ml/24 hour or 42 ml/hour***	***1,000 ml/20 hour or 50 ml/hour***	***1,000 ml/10 hour or 100 ml/hour***	***1,000 ml/8 hour or 125 ml/hour***	***1,000 ml/6 hour or 166 ml/hour***
Drops/ml	**Drops/minute to infuse**					
Macrodrip						
10	4	7	8	17	21	28
15	5	11	13	25	31	42
20	7	14	17	33	42	55
Microdrip						
60	21	42	50	100	125	166

Common calculation formulas

$$\text{Body surface area in m}^2 = \sqrt{\frac{\text{height in cm} \times \text{weight in kg}}{3{,}600}}$$

$$\text{mcg/ml} = \text{mg/ml} \times 1{,}000$$

$$\text{ml/minute} = \frac{\text{ml/hour}}{60}$$

$$\text{gtt/minute} = \frac{\text{volume in ml to be infused}}{\text{time in minutes}} \times \text{drip factor in gtt/ml}$$

$$\text{mg/minute} = \frac{\text{mg in bag}}{\text{ml in bag}} \times \text{flow rate} \div 60$$

$$\text{mcg/minute} = \frac{\text{mg in bag}}{\text{ml in bag}} \div 0.06 \times \text{flow rate}$$

$$\text{mcg/kg/minute} = \frac{\text{mcg/ml} \times \text{ml/minute}}{\text{weight in kilograms}}$$

Glossary

apothecaries' system: system used to measure liquid volumes and solid weights based on the units *drop, minim,* and *grain,* with amounts expressed in Roman numerals; used before the metric system was established

avoirdupois system: measurement system used to order certain pharmaceutical products and to weigh patients; based on the units *grain, ounce,* and *pound*

body surface area (BSA): the area covered by a person's external skin calculated in square meters (m^2) according to height and weight; used to calculate safe pediatric dosages for all drugs and safe dosages for adult patients receiving extremely potent drugs or drugs requiring great precision, such as antineoplastic and chemotherapeutic agents

common factor: a number that's a factor of two different numbers (For example, 2 is a common factor of 4 and 6.)

common fraction: fraction with a whole number in both the numerator and denominator (such as $\frac{2}{3}$)

complex fraction: fraction in which the numerator and the denominator are fractions such as:

$$\frac{2/7}{5/16}$$

concentration: ratio that expresses the amount of a drug in a solution; sometimes called *drug strength*

denominator: the bottom number in a fraction, which represents the total number of equal parts of a whole (For example, in the fraction $\frac{7}{10}$, the denominator is 10.)

dividend: in division, the number to be divided (For example, in the problem 33 ÷ 7, 33 is the dividend.)

divisor: in division, the number by which the dividend is divided (For example, in the problem 33 ÷ 7, 7 is the divisor.)

dosage: the amount, frequency, and number of doses of a drug

dose: the amount of a drug to be given at one time

drip rate: the number of drops of I.V. solution to be infused per minute; based on the drop factor (number of drops delivered per millimeter) and calibrated for the selected I.V. tubing

drop factor: the number of drops to be delivered per milliliter of solution in an I.V. administration set; measured in gtt/ml (drops per milliliter); listed on the package containing the I.V. tubing administration set

enteral: within or by way of the small intestine

equianalgesic dose: amount of an opioid analgesic that provides the same pain relief as 10 mg of I.M. morphine; used to recalculate the necessary dose when substituting one analgesic for another

flow rate: the number of milliliters of I.V. fluid to administer over 1 hour; based on the total volume to be infused in milliliters and the amount of time for the infusion

fraction: representation of the division of one number by another number; mathematical expression for parts of a whole, with the bottom number (denominator) describing the total number of parts and the top number (numerator) describing the parts of the whole being considered (for example, $\frac{1}{2}$, $\frac{1}{3}$, $\frac{7}{18}$)

generic name: accepted nonproprietary name, which is a simplified form of the drug's chemical name

glucometer: device used to calculate blood glucose levels — and, thereby, insulin levels — from one drop of blood

grain: the basic unit for measuring solid weight in the Apothecaries' system

gram (g): basic unit of weight in the metric system; represents the weight of one cubic centimeter of water at 4° C

household system: system that uses familiar household items, such as teaspoons, to measure drugs

improper fraction: fraction in which the numerator is larger than or equal to the denominator, such as $\frac{3}{2}$, $\frac{10}{7}$, and $\frac{5}{5}$

International System of Units: system adopted in 1960 by the International Bureau of Weights and Measures to promote the use of standard metric abbreviations to prevent drug transcription errors

intradermal route: drug administration into the dermis of the skin

intramuscular (I.M.) route: drug administration into a muscle

intravenous (I.V.) route: drug administration into a vein

largest common divisor: in a fraction, the largest whole number that can be divided into both the numerator and denominator of a fraction (For example, in the fraction $\frac{8}{10}$, the largest common divisor is 2.)

liter (L): basic unit of fluid volume in the metric system; equivalent to $\frac{1}{10}$ of a cubic meter

lowest common denominator: smallest number that's a multiple of all denominators in a set of fractions; also called *least common multiple* (For example, for the fractions, $\frac{1}{100}$ and $\frac{3}{150}$, the lowest common denominator is 300.)

lowest terms: in a fraction, the smallest numbers possible in the numerator and denominator (Reduce a fraction to its lowest terms by dividing the numerator and denominator by the largest common divisor.

For example, in the fraction $\frac{3}{15}$, divide both the numerator and denominator by 3, the largest common divisor, to find $\frac{1}{5}$, the lowest terms of this fraction.)

meter (m): basic unit of length in the metric system; equivalent to 39.37 inches

metric system: decimal-based measurement system that uses the units *meter* (for length), *liter* (for volume), and *gram* (for weight); most widely used system for measuring amounts of drugs

milliequivalent (mEq): number of grams of a solute in 1 ml of normal solution; used to measure electrolytes

minim: basic unit for measuring liquid volume in the Apothecaries' system

mixed number: number that consists of a whole number and a fraction (such as $1\frac{1}{2}$)

multiplied common denominator: for a set of fractions, the product of all the denominators, which is found by multiplying all the denominators together (For example, for the fractions, $\frac{1}{2}$, $\frac{2}{3}$, and $\frac{3}{5}$, multiply the denominators together to find the multiplied common denominator, which is 30 [$2 \times 3 \times 5 = 30$].)

nonparenteral drugs: drugs administered by the oral, topical, or rectal route, as opposed to drugs administered by the parenteral route

nomogram: chart used to determine body surface area in square meters, based on the patient's height and weight

numerator: the top number in a fraction, which represents the number of parts being considered (For example, in the fraction $\frac{7}{10}$, the numerator is 7.)

oral route (P.O.): drug administration through the mouth

parenteral route: drug administration through a route other than the digestive tract, such as I.V., I.M., and subQ

percentage: a quantity stated as a part per hundred; written with a percent sign (%), which means "for every hundred" (For example, 50% represents 50 parts out of 100 total parts.)

prime factor: prime numbers that can be divided into some part of a mathematical expression such as the denominators in a set of fractions; used to find the lowest common denominator for a set of fractions (For example, the prime factors for the denominators in the fractions $\frac{1}{10}$ and $\frac{2}{3}$ are 5, 2, and 3.)

prime number: whole number that's evenly divisible only by 1 and itself, such as 2, 3, 5, and 7

product: the answer of a multiplication problem (For example, in the equation, $4 \times 5 = 20$, the product is 20.)

proper fraction: fraction with a numerator that's smaller than the denominator (such as $\frac{1}{2}$)

proportion: set of equivalent ratios or fractions (An example of a proportion expressed by ratios is 2 : 3 :: 8 : 12, which is read as "2 is to 3 as 8 is to 12." The same proportion expressed with fractions is $\frac{2}{3} = \frac{8}{12}$.)

quotient: the answer of a division problem (For example, in the equation $20 \div 5 = 4$, the quotient is 4.)

ratio: numerical way to compare items or show a relationship between numbers, with numbers separated by a colon, which represents the words, "is to" (For example, the ratio 4 : 5 is read as "4 is to 5." Ratios are commonly used to describe the relative proportions of ingredients such as the amount of drug relative to its solution.)

reciprocal: inverted fraction; used when dividing fractions (For example, to divide $\frac{1}{2}$ by $\frac{2}{3}$, multiply $\frac{1}{2}$ by the reciprocal of $\frac{2}{3}$, which is $\frac{3}{2}$; in other words, $\frac{1}{2} \div \frac{2}{3} = \frac{1}{2} \times \frac{3}{2} = \frac{3}{4}$. When a fraction is multiplied by its reciprocal, the product is 1; for example, the reciprocal of the fraction $\frac{2}{3}$ is $\frac{3}{2}$, and $\frac{2}{3} \times \frac{3}{2} = \frac{6}{6}$ or 1.)

rectal route (P.R.): drug administration (usually by suppository) through the rectum

reduce: to simplify a numerical expression by using the lowest possible numbers — or lowest terms — to describe it (For example, the fraction $\frac{15}{45}$ may be reduced to $\frac{1}{3}$.)

rounding off: reducing the number of decimal places used to express a number (For example, a decimal fraction that's expressed in thousandths may be rounded off to the nearest hundredths or tenths; the number 12.827 rounded off to the nearest hundredths is 12.83. The same number rounded off to the nearest tenths is 12.8.)

subcutaneous (subQ) route: drug administration into the subcutaneous tissue

topical route: drug administration through the skin (after absorption through the skin layers, the drug enters circulation), usually in cream, ointment, or transdermal patch form

trade name: the drug's name given by the manufacturer; also called the *brand* or *proprietary name*

transcribe: to write or type a copy of something; to record information by hand, tape-recorder, or computer

transdermal route: drug administration in which the drug is absorbed continuously through the skin and enters the systemic system

unit system: measurement system that expresses the amount of a drug in units, United States Pharmacopeia (USP) units, or International Units (Drugs measured in units include insulin, heparin, the topical antibiotic bacitracin, and penicillins G and V. Some forms of vitamins A and D are measured in USP units. The hormone calcitonin and the fat-soluble vitamins A, D, and E are measured in International Units.)

Selected references

Abrams, A.C., and Kirkpatrick, M.J. *Clinical Drug Therapy: Rationales for Nursing Practice*, 9th ed. Philadelphia: Lippincott Williams & Wilkins, 2008.

Aschenbrenner, D.S., et al. *Drug Therapy in Nursing*, 3rd ed. Philadelphia: Lippincott Williams & Wilkins, 2008.

Boyer, M.J. *Math for Nurses: A Pocket Guide to Dosage Calculation and Drug Preparation*, 7th ed. Philadelpia: Lippincott Williams & Wilkins, 2008.

Brown, M., and Mulholland, J.L. *Drug Calculations: Process and Problems for Clinical Practice*, 8th ed. St. Louis: Mosby, 2008.

Cochran, G.L., et al. "Errors Prevented by and Associated with Bar-Code Medication Administration Systems" *The Joint Commission Journal on Quality and Patient Safety* 33(5): 293-301, May 2007.

Dosage Calculations: An Incredibly Easy Workout. Philadelphia: Lippincott Williams & Wilkins, 2009.

Hodgson, B.B., and Kizior, R.J. *Saunders Nursing Drug Handbook 2009*. Philadelphia: Saunders, 2009.

Institute for Safe Medication Practices Guidance on the Interdisciplinary Safe Use of Automated Dispensing Cabinets. Horsham, Pa.: Institute for Safe Medication Practices, 2008.

The Joint Commission. "Sentinel Event Alert: Preventing Pediatric Medication Errors," *Sentinel Event Alert* #39, April 11, 2008.

Karch, A.M. *2009 Lippincott's Nursing Drug Guide*. Philadelphia: Lippincott Williams & Wilkins, 2008.

Karch, A.M. *Focus on Nursing Pharmacology*. Philadelphia: Lippincott Williams & Wilkins, 2008.

2009 National Patient Safety Goals. Oakbrook Terrace, Ill.: The Joint Commission, 2009.

Nursing2009 Drug Handbook, 29th ed. Philadelphia: Lippincott Williams & Wilkins, 2009.

Nursing2009 Student Drug Handbook, 10th ed. Philadelphia: Lippincott Williams & Wilkins, 2009.

"Oral Dosage Forms That Should Not Be Crushed or Chewed," *Hospital Pharmacy* 42(6) Supp., 2007.

Skidmore-Roth, L. *Mosby's 2009 Nursing Drug Reference*, 22nd ed. St. Louis: Mosby, 2009.

Index

t refers to a table; i refers to an illustration.

t refers to a table; i refers to an illustration.

t refers to a table; i refers to an illustration.

t refers to a table; i refers to an illustration.

t refers to a table; i refers to an illustration.